Chiropractic: History and Evolution of a New Profession

CHIROPRACTIC: HISTORY AND EVOLUTION OF A NEW PROFESSION

Walter I. Wardwell, Ph.D.
Professor Emeritus
Department of Sociology
University of Connecticut
Storrs, Connecticut

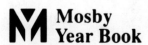 **Mosby**
Year Book

St. Louis   Baltimore   Boston   Chicago   London   Philadelphia   Sydney   Toronto

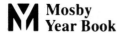
**Mosby
Year Book**

Dedicated to Publishing Excellence

Sponsoring Editor: James F. Shanahan
Assistant Editor: Joyce-Rachel John
Assistant Managing Editor, Manuscript Services: George Mary Gardner
Senior Production Assistant: Maria Nevinger
Proofroom Manager: Barbara Kelly

1 2 3 4 5 6 7 8 9 0   CL MV   96 95 94 93 92

Library of Congress Cataloging-in-Publication Data
Wardwell, Walter I.
    Chiropractic : history and evolution of a profession / Walter
I. Wardwell.
        p.   cm.
    Includes bibliographical references and index.
    ISBN 0-8016-6883-2
    1. Chiropractic—United States—History. I. Title.
    [DNLM: 1. Chiropractic—history—United States. 2. Chiropractic—
trends—United States.   WB 905.6 W266c]
    RZ225.U6W37   1992   92-8436
    615.5′34′0973—dc20   CIP
    DNLM/DLC
    for Library of Congress

Foreword

Professor Wardwell's book without doubt constitutes the definitive history to date of chiropractic since its beginnings in 1895. It will be of immense interest to all who are associated, directly or otherwise, with the chiropractic profession.

As an unbiased observer of much of chiropractic's history, Professor Wardwell has been present at some of the most significant events occurring during my 30 years of involvement in professional matters. I have known him over many years and have watched his sense of professionalism prevail when he might have been tempted to leave his obligation to objectivity. Wherever Professor Wardwell offers his opinion, he makes it clear that his conclusions are based on thorough documentation and analysis. His scholarly research, in my opinion, will stand as a historic milestone in chiropractic's development as a profession.

Our profession has not unfailingly been a picture of beauty and innocence. Initially, and for perhaps too long, chiropractic resisted advancing its educational standards, adhered too often (even to this day) to cultist concepts, displayed a siege mentality, frequently failed to insist on its rights as a legislatively authorized profession, and sometimes tended to self-isolation. All this and more is brought to our attention by Professor Wardwell. But as my brother, George McAndrews, attorney for the plaintiffs in the Wilk vs. AMA antitrust suit, has told chiropractors: "You may have some 'dirt under your fingernails' but it is clear that your profession has cared deeply and well for its patients."

There have been lofty moments in which the profession could take pride: achieving licensure in all the states of the United States and elsewhere, resisting illegal anticompetitive forces initiated and maintained over decades, and, finally, consummating a successful legal action against what a federal court called a "lengthy, systematic, successful, and illegal boycott by the American Medical Association."

Chiropractic has struggled to gain inclusion in Medicare (1972), attracted a clientele in excess of 30 million Americans, obtained approval from the U.S. Office of Education for its Council on Chiropractic Education (CCE) as the chiropractic college accrediting agency (1974), exercised its influence to obtain the first Workshop on the Research Status of Spinal Manipulative Therapy by an institute of the National Institutes of Health (1975), and, against Goliath-like odds, finally moved into the arena of significant scientific research. These research efforts can be credited to the Foundation for Chiropractic Education and Research (FCER), the chiropractic colleges, the American Chiropractic Association, the National Chiropractic Mutual Insurance Company (NCMIC), and others.

v

Ours has certainly been a century of struggle, but we are now on a rising curve of development. We should be proud of the odds we have overcome, for it is now well established that, whereas medicine is not as good as its image, chiropractic is better than its image. This book will help bring that message to its readership.

JEROME F. MCANDREWS, D.C.
Vice President for Professional Affairs
American Chiropractic Association
Former Executive Vice President of the
   International Chiropractors Association
Former President of Palmer College of Chiropractic
Arlington, Virginia

Preface

Around 1920, when I was small enough to ride on my father's shoulders, an incident occurred that convinced him that chiropractic is effective, and for which I was inadvertently responsible. His job as a draftsman had caused him eye strain and severe headaches that neither medical treatment nor glasses helped. Someone—I don't know who—persuaded him to try a chiropractor. He went to Dr. Ernest Carreiro in Boston. When I later interviewed Carreiro for my doctoral research, he told me that he had been on the faculty of J. Shelby Riley's New England College of Chiropractic in Boston, which closed in 1915. My role in the incident was to accidentally knock my father's glasses from his face onto the floor, causing them to shatter. My father then discovered that he no longer needed glasses since he no longer had headaches. He was led to understand that constant bending over his drafting board had created muscle strain, causing what chiropractors call a "subluxation" in his neck. After that he never wore glasses until he was much older and needed them for reading.

I don't know how many adjustments my father received for his eye problem, but he became thoroughly convinced of the benefits of chiropractic. Henceforth our family of five would be taken to a chiropractor whenever any one of us had symptoms of illness. In addition to the ailing person, the rest of us would be given "checkups." My father was one of what I later learned was a large class of dedicated chiropractic patients. I estimate that he alone persuaded at least 50 skeptics to "try chiropractic." As an adolescent I can remember hearing Dr. Paul Bemis of Everett, Massachusetts, who became our family chiropractor when we moved from Boston to the suburbs, saying to my father: "Fred, if you never offered to pay me, I wouldn't ask you for money; you have sent me so many patients." Sometimes after he had treated all of us and my father asked him "How much?" he would say: "Oh, give me $2, Fred." That was during the depression of the 1930s when $2 was the standard fee for one treatment. Payments usually were made in cash, because chiropractors were not licensed in Massachusetts and were always at risk of being arrested and prosecuted for practicing medicine without a license.

I wrote my first paper on chiropractic when I was a Harvard undergraduate, not for a course requirement but for a student magazine that chose not to publish it, which probably was wise. However, I did arrange a small chiropractic exhibit, mainly of illustrations from college catalogues, which was displayed in an undergraduate library. I once asked to talk with the Director of the Student Health Service about chiropractic, which was a frustrating experience for me but seemed rather to amuse him as I tried to convince him of the benefits of chiropractic. What I remember most is that he argued that any substance, even water, can be a poison to the body if taken in excessive amounts.

As a doctoral candidate in sociology at Harvard after World War II and after some casting around for an appropriate dissertation topic, I determined that an analysis of chiropractors focussed on the Massachusetts situation could be "a contribution to knowledge," the criterion for an acceptable doctoral thesis. My advisor, Talcott Parsons, the distinguished theorist who first expounded the sociologic concept of the sick role, approved my proposal. The topic permitted me to utilize my background knowledge of chiropractic and to work on a topic that had fascinated me. I was not particularly surprised that the distinguished Harvard orthopedist Joel Goldthwaite, who had written the pioneering *Body Mechanisms in Health and Disease* (1941), refused even to talk to me. My dissertation was titled *Social Strain and Social Adjustment in the Marginal Role of the Chiropractor* (1951), from which I published two papers in sociologic journals (1952, 1955) and a brief historical paper (1954). Both chiropractors and organized medicine ignored my work for nearly 15 years. Neither "side" would publish any papers I submitted. (See, for example, B.J. Palmer's criticisms of my doctoral dissertation in Chapter 4, Section 2.) The only exception was the *Journal of the National Medical Association*. I have always wondered if it accepted my paper "Public Regulation of Chiropractic" (1961) because black physicians shared with chiropractors some hostility and resentment toward the American Medical Association.

In 1968 I served on the Expert Review Committee set up by the U.S. Public Health Service for a study that Congress mandated the Surgeon General conduct in order to recommend whether the federal government should reimburse chiropractors and naturopaths under the Medicare program (Cohen WJ, 1968). As I had anticipated, the medically dominated Committee recommended against including both groups. At almost the same time, I was invited to lecture at the annual convention of the American Chiropractic Association in New York City, which was the first acknowledgment by chiropractors of my work (1968).

Over the years I have written other papers (1975, 1976b, 1978, 1980a, 1982a, 1987, 1989, 1991) and chapters in books (1963, 1976a, 1980b, 1982b, 1988) on chiropractors. Naturally I have incorporated ideas from my earlier writings into the present work. However, the reader is advised that while there are many constants in my interpretation of the development of the chiropractic profession, neither the profession nor my conception of it is the same now as it was more than 40 years ago when I wrote my doctoral dissertation. Neither I nor chiropractic should be held to what I said so long ago. Indeed, it is precisely the *evolution* of the profession and its success in changing from very dubious status to the position it holds today that constitutes the central drama of the chiropractic story and demands description and analysis.

The principal questions that have intrigued me are these: What caused chiropractic to appear? Why, unlike other dissenting groups, did it survive? How has it changed? What has been its relationship to organized medicine? What impact has it had on our health care system? In what possible future directions could it conceivably go? And which of these alternatives is it most likely to take? These questions have nurtured my curiosity throughout my professional career. This book is the culmination of my long personal and professional involvement with chiropractors, their profession, and their fate.

I should address the question of my professional objectivity, always a problem when one conducts research as a "participant observer" (to use the current phrase). As early as my 1951 dissertation I was well aware of the professional obligations of an objective social scientist. Although I always tended to sympathize with the underdog chiropractors, much as I always sympathize with oppressed ethnic groups, I was trained as a sociologist to examine evidence impartially and to look at all sides of controversial issues. For my dissertation, in addition to searching the literature I conducted interviews (today called "oral histories") with many chiropractors and medical doctors, covering not only the chiropractors' early experiences going back to 1912 but also the then current controversies between the two professions. I was also a participant observer at formal and informal gatherings of chiropractors and at legislative hearings and sessions (see especially chapter 7, Section 3).

Later when I was invited to serve on the committee for the Surgeon General's study of chiropractic in 1968 I considered my role to be both a participant observer and an informed and helpful committee member, but not partisan. My contribution may have seemed biased to orthodox physicians, but that cannot be avoided when one tries to be objective about a controversial area. Similarly, I expect that this book may disturb some of those who have been exposed only to organized medicine's antichiropractic propaganda dating from the early 1920s, when it began its campaign "to contain and then eliminate chiropractic" from the American scene. That is one reason why I have documented my argument so extensively and used many verbatim quotes from a wide variety of observers.

I have never accepted payment from chiropractors for my writing, nor been an advisor to them. I have functioned only in peripheral capacities, such as very ocasionally lecturing at meetings, reviewing articles submitted for publication in professional journals, contributing to the technical quality of the 1979 federally sponsored national survey of chiropractors (Von Kuster, 1980), and more recently serving on the board of the Association for the History of Chiropractic.

I have continued to study the literature, to observe assemblies of chiropractors, to visit schools, and to interview chiropractors and students, especially since 1974 when I devoted the first of two sabbatic leaves to this research. This book is as fair and objective as I can make it.

After an introductory chapter, in Chapter 2 I briefly survey 19th century dissenters from orthodox medicine: Thomsonists, homeopaths, Christian Scientists, osteopaths, naturopaths, and the bonesetters who first used spinal manipulation therapy. Chapter 3 presents a concise discussion of some of the basic concepts I use in the analysis. Chapters 4 and 5 cover the origins of chiropractic, in particular the roles played by D.D. and B.J. Palmer and the other leaders and founders of schools, the national associations, and the numbers of chiropractors.

Chapters 6 and 7 relate chiropractors' successful struggle, despite intense medical opposition, to obtain state licensure and to raise educational standards. Chapter 8 analyzes the conflicting relations between chiropractic and organized medicine from the earliest period to the present. Chapters 9 and 10 discuss why chiropractic "works"—its philosophic and scientific bases and the role of psychologic factors in chiropractic treatment.

Chapter 11 documents chiropractic's acceptance by patients, the public, and more recently by MDs and hospitals. Chapter 12 attempts an explanation of why it survived its many trials and tribulations. In Chapter 13 I summarize the remaining problems and dilemmas facing chiropractors, and in Chapter 14 I outline the possible future directions chiropractic could take, including the one I think is most likely.

WALTER I. WARDWELL, PH.D.

Acknowledgments

I have collected so much material over the past 50 years and the story of chiropractic is so very rich that it has been difficult to decide what to dispense with. I have sought to achieve a balance between including valuable reference material such as names, dates, schools, organizations, and books published that will benefit future scholars, on the one hand, and analytical treatment of broader issues and controversial topics that will interest the general reader, on the other.

Since I am not a historian, I must rely on secondary sources for information about the early years of chiropractic. I draw heavily from *Who's Who in Chiropractic International,* edited by Fern Dzaman et al. (1980), which contains biographies prepared by William S. Rehm, first president of the Association for the History of Chiropractic, and Russell W. Gibbons of "who's who" and "who was who" (called "the pioneers") in chiropractic; from the many insightful essays by Russell Gibbons; and from the many excellent articles published in *Chiropractic History: The Archives and Journal of the Association for the History of Chiropractic.*

Neither of the two published early histories of chiropractic is a scholarly work, but I have found them helpful for specific facts and dates: Chittenden Turner's *Rise of Chiropractic* (1931) and A. Augustus Dye's *The Evolution of Chiropractic* (1939). Dye was clearly an apologist for B.J. Palmer, and originally was employed to make stenographic records of his lectures, and subsequently served as Business Manager of the Palmer School from 1913 to 1925. Turner was a professional writer who presented the more liberal, "mixer" side of the story. Samuel Homola's *Bonesetting, Chiropractic, and Cultism* (1963), the most sophisticated analysis by a chiropractor, is finally winning due respect after many years in eclipse because it offended so many of them. I interpret its belated recognition as evidence of the growing maturity of the profession and willingness to look at its history more objectively.

I have found especially helpful Pierre-Louis Gaucher-Peslherbe's insightful *La Chiropractique: Contribution a l'Histoire d'Une Discipline Marginalisee* (1985), translated into English under the title *Chiropractic Early Concepts in Their Historical Setting,* which was his doctoral thesis in the history of medicine at the Ecole des Hautes Etudes en Sciences Sociales in Paris. It is an in-depth investigation of the historical antecedents of modern spinal manipulation and of the sources used by D.D. Palmer, usually called the "discoverer" of chiropractic. Gaucher convincingly documents that Palmer, although self-educated, was well versed in the medical and scientific literature of the time.

For the early history of the Palmers I also have used a lovingly researched small volume titled *Old Dad Chiro* by Vern Gielow (1981), for many years an administrator at the Palmer School; an unpublished *History of Chiropractic* by Willard Carver (1936), Palmer's long-time friend and sometime legal advisor; and Cyrus Lerner's *Report on the History of Chiropractic* (1954), an unpublished manuscript of 780 pages. Lerner, an attorney and journalist, had been retained by the mixer Foundation for Health Research in New York City "to re-write the history of Chiropractic and tell it truthfully for the first time," but it became available to very few persons.

I am deeply grateful to the many chiropractors I have known over many years, for their friendship, openness, and assistance in preparing this book, and particularly to the following for reviewing sections of the manuscript, research assistance, and/or counsel: medical historian Robert U. Massey, former dean of the University of Connecticut Medical School and editor of the *Journal of the History of Medicine;* John McM. Mennell, M.D.; Nicholas J. Palermo, D.O.; John H. Furlong, N.D., chiropractic historian Russell W. Gibbons; chiropractors Scott Haldeman, D.C., Ph.D., M.D., William S. Rehm, Robert A. Leach, James G. Steele, Karl Kranz, Joseph Donahue, and Paul Szwez; attorneys George P. McAndrews and Robert Hirtle; psychologists Joseph Keating and David Lindorff; Palmer College archivist Glenda Wiese; and especially to chiropractors Alan H. Adams, Pierre-Louis Gaucher-Peslherbe, Malcolm E. Macdonald, Jerome F. McAndrews, and Stephen E. Owens, for critically reviewing the entire manuscript. Of course, none of these helpful persons should be held responsible for what I have written.

WALTER I. WARDWELL, PH.D.

Contents

Chapter 1

INTRODUCTION

The rise of Chiropractic has been one of the most remarkable social phenomena in American history.

Brian Inglis (1964)

Chiropractic is a unique phenomenon. The year 1995 marks its 100th anniversary. Of all the dissenting schools of healing that have appeared in America, no other has lasted so long or been so successful. It continues to be the leading challenger of medical domination of health care in the United States. Whether in the future it will remain as it is or merge into the medical mainstream remains an unanswered and perhaps unanswerable question at this time.

My purpose is to examine a broad range of questions related to the appearance, persistence, and success of chiropractors as contenders for public and professional recognition. Since they challenge highly sophisticated medical science, questions of chiropractic's validity and worth should long ago have been resolved in academic seminars, professional journals, and research investigations, experimental or clinical. Why has that not happened? In view of the fact that chiropractic students now are taught the basic medical sciences from the same textbooks used by medical students and by university-trained teachers with advanced degrees, how can chiropractors maintain a different "philosophy" or paradigm of health from that of orthodox medicine? Why haven't the differences between the two professions been resolved? What *are* the differences between them, and why do they continue to generate so much heat?

A fundamental criticism of the practice of orthodox medicine is often voiced by chiropractors as well as by those within medicine itself: that modern medicine has tended to treat localized diseases and dysfunction rather than the person who has a disease or a dysfunction; that its therapy focuses on symptoms rather than on causes and on ways to strengthen the body's innate recuperative powers (vix medicatrix naturae); that it concentrates too much on finding drugs ("magic bullets") to counter invading bacteria or to relieve symptoms rather than on improving the resistance of

1

the whole person in his or her environment; and that its excessive use of surgery and toxic drugs causes too much iatrogenic disability.

By contrast, chiropractors advocate an alternative "natural" philosophy of illness and cure that assigns primacy to balancing the neurologic functioning of the body, viewed as highly dependent on the integrity, protection, and support of the musculo-skeletal system, especially that of the spine. Its original formulation was that mis-aligned vertebrae (subluxations) create pressure on or irritate nerves as they exit the spinal canal through the intervertebral foramina. Daniel David Palmer (1845–1913; hereinafter D.D.; Figure 1) the originator of chiropractic, stated that such impinge-ments cause disease or disability by creating either an excess or deficiency of func-tioning or of "tone" (1910, p 19). Chiropractic "adjustments" are manipulative tech-niques that replace or "balance" misaligned vertebrae and, it is argued, restore health by permitting the body to cure itself.

Although most chiropractors today do not subscribe completely to this original doctrine, and recognize the importance of other factors in disease causation, they still mainly manipulate spines to correct musculoskeletal problems and to restore neuro-logic integrity. In addition they emphasize the importance of diet, life-style, preven-tion, and psychologic factors in maintaining health. Despite disagreement among them concerning the validity of the subluxation theory of disease, their distinctive mode of therapy remains spinal adjustments. All chiropractors oppose the excessive use of surgery and medicines and favor a drugless, holistic approach to healing.

Chiropractic originally was perceived to be a close cousin of osteopathy, which preceded it by several years. However, it is well documented that there always were

FIGURE 1.
Daniel David ("D.D.") Palmer. (Courtesy of Palmer College of Chiropractic Archives.)

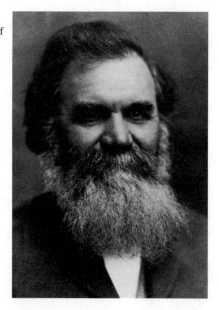

fundamental differences in their theories as well as in their manipulative techniques (see Chapter 2, Section 4). In any case, the majority of U.S. osteopaths (DOs) differ little today from medical doctors (MDs). Currently they are formally accorded the same legal privileges, are treated as equals in governmental programs, statistics, and in most reports, and have become in fact medical physicians, although they retain their own schools, degree (Doctor of Osteopathy, D.O.), national association (American Osteopathic Association), hospitals, and specialty boards. DOs now can compete for medical residencies and hospital staff appointments on a formally equal basis with MDs. Hence today they differ from doctors of chiropractic (DCs) almost as much as MDs do.

Nor is chiropractic, as a dissenting sect, similar to homeopathy, which merely advocated a different medication strategy than that used by other MDs. Homeopaths became numerous by the middle of the 19th century, reached their zenith around 1880 (Rothstein, 1972, p 246), but were losing numbers and importance by the end of the century. Although homeopathy has undergone a small revival in recent years, very few MDs now practice it. It is currently mainly of interest to naturopaths, who earn Doctor of Naturopathy (N.D.) degrees, and to a few chiropractors. Naturopaths closely resemble chiropractors in that they use spinal manipulative therapy (henceforth SMT) and because many so-called mixer chiropractors also use such naturopathic methods as heat, cold, hydrotherapy, physiotherapy, dietary supplements, and even some herbal and homeopathic remedies. That is why the traditional, or "straight," chiropractors disparagingly call the mixers "medipractors." Until the middle of the 20th century a few mixer schools offered both D.C. and N.D. degrees, either as alternatives or both together after an additional semester of study. As chiropractors achieved greater acceptance and became licensed in more states, naturopaths lost out in competition; they are now licensed in only a handful of states and support only two small schools.

At a time when much medical education was grossly inadequate, documented by Abraham Flexner in his famous Carnegie Foundation–supported report *Medical Education in the United States and Canada* (1910), and the education of osteopaths was even worse (Flexner, 1914), chiropractic schools were also of poor quality. Like most osteopathic and medical schools of the period they were privately owned, subsisted mainly on tuition, lacked good laboratories, attracted many ill-prepared students, and when successful provided a profit for their owners. Early chiropractic students often had failed or succeeded in some other profession, sometimes in one of the other healing arts. Some were attracted to the profession that had cured them of an acute or chronic disability. It is not widely known that among the first 15 students whom D.D. began teaching in 1898 in his school in Davenport, Iowa, were five MDs and that there always were MDs on the faculty of the Palmer School (Gibbons, 1981a). Hence, although the formal education of early chiropractors was spotty, the profession attracted some well-educated students. Some of them proceeded to set up their own schools. Solon Massey Langworthy was the first to do so, in Cedar Rapids, Iowa, in 1903. Willard Carver founded a school in Oklahoma City in 1906 and other schools in Denver, New York, and Washington, D.C. He rivaled the Palmers in influence on the developing profession.

D.D.'s son Bartlett Joshua Palmer (B.J.) assumed total management of the Palmer School of Chiropractic (PSC) after D.D. relinquished it to him in 1906. PSC and the profession grew rapidly in the years before the first World War, and even more rapidly immediately afterward when veterans returned. In 1921 PSC graduated a class of 1,000 students from its 12-month course, which was soon extended to 18 months (called "3 years of 6 months each"). Some of the other chiropractic schools lengthened their courses to 3 and even 4 academic years and taught a more complete program of basic medical subjects. By 1931, 37 states had licensed chiropractors.

It is documented by Pierre-Louis Gaucher-Peslherbe, a French chiropractor whose doctoral thesis in the history of medicine has been translated under the English title *Chiropractic Early Concepts in Their Historical Setting* (1992), that D.D, though not formally educated, actually had an excellent grasp of the scientific writings of his day and was meticulous in citing authors of the best scientific and medical treatises in his many debates with other chiropractors, osteopaths, and MDs. According to Gaucher-Peslherbe (1992): "The birth of the chiropractic movement was not a historical anachronism, but a logical development within the clinical sciences, and particularly the neurological sciences, of the time." Manipulation of the spine to reduce subluxations and restore health had been known and practiced for millennia in nearly every country on Earth (see Chapter 2, Section 2). In late nineteenth-century England bonesetting attracted considerable attention from the public and the medical profession, while in the United States Bonesetter Reese and the Sweet family were its best known practitioners (Joy, 1954).

The heat and emotion that D.D. generated in disputes often surpassed reason and logic. Organized medicine took little notice of chiropractic during the first 15 years of its existence (Ratledge, 1971, p 66). The first medical paper dealing with chiropractic education was published soon after Flexner's 1910 report in the *Denver Medical Times* (Schaller, 1911) and was quite favorable. But in 1912 the *Illinois Medical Journal* described B.J. as "the most dangerous man in Iowa out of a prison cell . . . insane, a paranoiac, a man whose irresponsibility is criminal" (cited by Gibbons 1987, p 9). Over the next dozen years a flurry of critical comment appeared in the medical press. Flexner (1910, p 158) already had published his impression:

> The chiropractics [sic], the mechanotherapists, and several others are not medical sectarians, though exceedingly desirous of masquerading as such; they are unconscionable quacks, whose printed advertisements are tissues of exaggeration, pretense, and misrepresentation of the most unqualifiedly mercenary character. The public prosecutor and the grand jury are the proper agencies for dealing with them.

Instruction by correspondence courses was especially condemned, and osteopathy was similarly attacked. In 1918, alongside an article belittling chiropractic, *Canada Lancet* published a disparaging obituary for A.T. Still that ended with the statement: "The whole system of osteopathy is a disgrace to this century" (Brennan, 1983a, p 27)

The most famous condemnation of chiropractic was penned by Morris Fishbein, editor of the *Journal of the American Medical Association* and Secretary of the American Medical Association (AMA), in *The Medical Follies* (1925, p 98):

> Chiropractic is the malignant tumor on the body of osteopathy. . . . Osteopathy is essentially a method of entering the practice of medicine by the back door. Chiropractic, by contrast, is an attempt to arrive through the cellar. The man who applies at the back-door at least makes himself presentable. The one who comes through the cellar is besmirched with dust and grime; he carries a crowbar and he may wear a mask.

Medical propaganda later characterized chiropractors as "mad dogs" and "killers." These are not the words of dispassionate scientific investigators. Their emotional and vindictive tone possibly hurt more than helped the AMA in its goal of arousing the public against chiropractors, although its message came through clearly. It was picked up by such writers as H.L. Mencken (1924), who referred to chiropractic as "this preposterous quackery."

Chiropractors fought back using the ancient technique of testimonials from patients cured by chiropractic after medical failure. Medicine was just beginning to use the experimental research method urged by Claude Bernard (1865), and controlled clinical trials were hardly known. Chiropractic's successes were enough to convince its practitioners of its validity. The statement "It works" was their primary weapon in debate, and it satisfied the intellectual curiosity of all but a few scientifically oriented chiropractors.

Chiropractors were no less vigorous and vindictive in their attacks on the AMA and on its spokesman, Dr. Fishbein, whom they called the *Medical Mussolini* (Bealle, 1939). The contention between them reached a level that Scotton (1974, p 23) called "a holy war between the forces of good and evil." With such heightened emotions, clearly no rational discourse or impartial evaluation of chiropractic claims could occur. Despite frequent professional interaction at the community level, at national and state levels MDs and chiropractors were not even on speaking terms. Students at the Palmer School studied from specially written chiropractic texts, although they, and especially students at the "mixer" schools, also used standard medical texts. On the medical side it appears unlikely that chiropractic claims or texts ever were seriously evaluated. However, a few individual MDs (e.g., Alfred Walton [1915]) investigated chiropractic and found it to their liking (see Chapter 2, Section 4). No joint scientific investigation of the merits of chiropractic was ever undertaken. An MD is quoted by the British chiropractor J. Henry Jones (1926, p 78) as writing to him:

> I should like to congratulate you on the results you have obtained with my friend. Had it been nineteen hundred years ago they'd have called it a miracle; in the Middle Ages they'd have said it was sorcery. Nowadays I suppose the profession to which I have the

honor to belong are the only people left who would have the impertinence to call it quackery.

During the Great Depression of the 1930s and World War II chiropractic lost ground. Its imminent demise was regularly forecast. Rushmore (1932) predicted: "Chiropractic is going the way of all sects. . . . No medical sect has ever staged a comeback. . . . The hand of death is already visible." A misinformed British barrister (Minty, 1932, p 117) erroneously wrote: "In most of the states of the Union chiropractic has already died a natural death." Many weaker schools closed (certainly a good thing) as student applications declined. (The poor quality of early chiropractic schools is discussed in Chapter 7, Section 1). After World War II, when veterans' education was financed by the GI Bill, the schools again prospered. Instruction was lengthened to a standard course of 4 years of 8 or 9 months each, improved in quality, and the 2-year preprofessional requirement, which had been instituted in some schools, was made mandatory by 1974. The schools had lost ground in the 1960s and again were predicted to disappear (Stanford Research Institute, 1960; "Inevitable Decline of Chiropractic," 1973; Pascoe 1961).

How was it possible for chiropractic to survive and prosper through the early years of this century? Two reasons were the already existing variety of health practitioners contending with each other and the public's widespread lack of confidence in MDs. In the 19th century "heroic" medical practices had been decried by herbalists, Thomsonians, eclectics, and homeopaths for their excessive reliance on bloodletting and on such harmful drugs as calomel (mercurous chloride). Medicine was later criticized by magnetists, mental healers, Christian Scientists, and osteopaths. Furthermore, there were not enough well-trained regular MDs to serve the needs of the burgeoning population, especially in the West, where frontier conditions prevailed. In the East the millions of immigrants who flooded the cities between the Civil War and World War I brought with them folk practices from Europe, including Swedish massage, bonesetting, and "Bohemian Medicine," also known as "napravit" (Zarbuck, 1986).

Quality of medical education in the 19th century varied greatly. While the best colleges (after 1893 Johns Hopkins in Baltimore was preeminent) began to imitate the great European universities, notorious "diploma mills" persisted in Chicago, Cleveland, Kansas City, and elsewhere. Many offered only didactic instruction, with little laboratory or clinical training, and competed for students with the homeopathic and eclectic schools by keeping tuition and admission requirements low. In this connection the account by Walter Cannon (1934) of the "notoriously lax" examination system at Harvard Medical School as late as the 1870s is classic:

> Nine professors representing nine different important subjects sat each at a table in the examination room. Nine students were admitted to the room in a group, and each sat down with a professor. At the end of ten minutes a bell rang and each student moved along to the next table. This process continued until at the end of ninety minutes all had been examined, whereupon they filed out. Each professor had a card, white on one side

and marked with a black spot on the other. In order to secure the individual professional judgments, uninfluenced by conference, the Dean immediately called out separately the names of the students in the group; and after each name the professors simultaneously held up their cards, the white side meaning approval, the black spot disapproval. If five professors displayed the white side of the card, that is, if the student was recognized as having passed five of the nine subjects on which he had been examined, he was granted the degree of Doctor of Medicine. Thus, at that time a young man could go forth from this School quite ignorant of four of the nine branches of medicine which he was supposed to use in his practice. I have heard from the lips of William James, who received his medical degree here in 1869, an account of his examination under this system. When he sat at the table with Oliver Wendell Holmes, he was asked to describe the circle of Willis. James briefly mentioned its position and relations, whereupon Holmes remarked, "If you know that you know everything. Now, tell me all about the folks."

Continuous bickering between schools over opposing philosophies of treatment was raised to a fine art, and continued well into the 20th century. Into this confusing mélange of claims and counterclaims, osteopathic and chiropractic schools fitted rather easily, for there was little official concern over standards. No accrediting agency separated the good from the bad, the better from the mediocre. For example, in 1921 Mecca College of Chiropractic in Newark, New Jersey, was headed by Fred Collins, "an MD who also conducted schools of medicine, osteopathy, and naturopathy with separate charters under the same roof" (Gibbons 1980a, p 346; see also "Fred Collins and His New Jersey 'Mecca,' " 1989). In the early 1920s the Illinois College of Physicians and Surgeons (which I am told graduated only one class) occupied space in the National School of Chiropractic building at 20 North Ashland Boulevard in Chicago.

No wonder the public and student candidates were confused over what was orthodox medicine or a competing school. A new form of therapy such as chiropractic could find an opening, gain a foothold, and claim the right to equal freedom in the health care market. No third-party payers (insurance companies or the government) would evaluate the care provided for the money paid. It was therefore a pure case of "client control" not "colleague control" of practice, in the terminology suggested by Eliot Freidson (1970b), inasmuch as almost all were solo practitioners. It was also an example of *caveat emptor* ("Let the buyer beware"), since the purchasers of care, the patients, are far less able to judge the quality of the service they are getting than when buying a horse or a used car, the best known American examples of where buyers were warned to be wary. Peer review had yet to be invented.

Since many diseases are self-limiting, puzzling as to cause or prognosis, unpredictable, and intractable, the value of any therapeutic intervention is problematic. Hence the therapist often receives unearned credit or blame for the outcome. Although in the early years of this century orthodox medicine was becoming more scientific and empirically grounded, it was still limited in effectiveness. Hence it was easier then than later for chiropractors to gain credit for cures and therefore public acceptance. Their training and resources were closer to those of medicine than became true later. Furthermore, as medicine successively conquered most of the conta-gious diseases, those remaining were the degenerative and chronic conditions that are less responsive to regular medical treatment. This increased the *relative* effectiveness of chiropractic care.

That was not the entire explanation for chiropractic's growth and acceptance. Also required, of course, were students able and zealous to learn the techniques of spinal manipulation in order to treat sick people, and sick people willing to try an unknown therapy. Usually they were persuaded by their failure to obtain relief or cure via the medical route. These requirements—motivated practitioners and willing patients—provided themes for the folklore on both sides that accompanied the ex-pansion of chiropractic. Organized medicine portrayed chiropractors either as out-and-out quacks motivated by greed (i.e., charlatans) or as well-meaning but ignorant and bumbling dupes of a false theory whose occasional successes convinced them of its validity and of their own healing skill. MDs explained chiropractors' successes mainly as based on illnesses that were misdiagnosed, self-limiting, imaginary, or re-sponsive to suggestion. Such stereotypes were also applied to faith healers and to any other unorthodox practitioners that the AMA disapproved of.

Contrasting stereotypes were also part of chiropractic folklore, which maintained that most chiropractors became involved in the profession because of personal benefit they had received, usually a dramatic cure following medical failure, or because a relative or friend had been impressively benefited; I have heard many such tales. Or a parent or relative was a chiropractor role model, for there is a tradition of three and even four generations of chiropractors in the same family. Chiropractic folklore says that many patients had been treated by MDs for many years without success and at long last discovered chiropractic, received remarkable results, and became dedicated supporters. The downside of this pattern is revealed in the complaint of a chiropractor whom I interviewed in Massachusetts who told me that patients come to chiropractic "when they have exhausted medical science and their money."

Certainly there have been a lot of dedicated chiropractic patients. My father was one. Such patients often were asked to help chiropractors in their struggles for licens-ing legislation or when defending against court prosecutions. Sometimes they were organized into formal pressure groups such as the Chiropractic Layman's League. The slogan "Go to jail for chiropractic" originated in 1917 in Alameda County, Cal-ifornia, after a particularly strong campaign by authorities to arrest chiropractors. Chiropractors set up their portable adjusting tables in jail and gave free treatments to patients who came to show support. The result was a large increase in public support. In 1923 Governor Friend W. Richardson pardoned all chiropractors then in jail, and a state law licensing chiropractors soon passed by initiative referendum. The record of 66 arrests was held by Charles C. Lemly of Texarkana, Texas (Dzaman 1980, p 294).

Stereotypes and folklore always contain at least a grain of truth, often more. But that is not the main reason for their importance. To the extent they are believed they govern behavior, because symbols and stereotypes determine the way the world is viewed. If the leaders of the AMA believe their own portrayals of chiropractors as charlatans or dupes, they act on that basis. Reality is distorted if they ignore other considerations. This partially accounts for the failure of their efforts designed to eliminate chiropractors and the threat they were believed to pose.

Correspondingly, to the extent chiropractors believe that their patients have not been or cannot be helped by medical treatment (usually understood to mean drugs) and that only chiropractic adjustments will cure them, their view of reality likewise is distorted. Since another part of their belief system is that medical opposition is based more on greed and jealousy over losing patients than on concern for patient welfare, they often have misperceived the purposes of public policies intended to regulate them.

Ideally reason, science, and logic should govern health behavior, but they do not. False stereotypes and folklore are only part of the problem. Economic competition and political influence are other major considerations. Practitioners must be compensated in order to survive. A consulting profession (i.e., one that serves clients), unlike pure scientists (Freidson, 1970b, p 5), depends on them for survival, because clients collectively provide the economic resources and the political strength essential to achieve a secure place in society. Larson (1977, pp 19–25) documents how the ascendance of orthodox physicians over their competitors in the 19th century in both Britain and the United States resulted more from their social advantages in education and the higher social status of their clients than from any superiority of their technology of practice.

Until third parties began paying for health care, chiropractors competed on a level playing field, economically speaking. After World War II, as more and more health care was paid for by Workers Compensation, Medicare, and Medicaid and as employee group health insurance became the predominant mode of reimbursement, chiropractors faced a crisis. Only if patients were wealthy, dedicated, or desperate would they forgo their insurance coverage and pay chiropractors out-of-pocket. Concerted action was needed to include chiropractors in health plans legislated at federal and state levels and to persuade insurance companies to reimburse chiropractors as good business practice. If insurance companies could not be persuaded, then political action was needed to pass "insurance equality laws" to coerce them. Basically the strategy worked. Despite the strongest opposition the AMA could mount and the earlier negative recommendation from the Secretary of the Department of Health, Education, and Welfare (Cohen, 1968), Congress voted in 1972 to include chiropractors under Medicare. More than half of all federal, state, and private health plans currently reimburse chiropractors.

Thus chiropractors have coped successfully with changing methods of payment for health care in the United States. Under the socialized health care plans of Canada, Australia, and New Zealand chiropractors are reimbursed on a basis comparable with MDs. If chiropractors had not gained inclusion in third-party payment plans, they might not have survived anywhere. Being a publicly supported profession also provides symbolically important official recognition.

Chiropractors' main political battles historically were for licensing laws (for details see Chapter 6). In some states, largely in the Midwest and Far West, gaining licensure was relatively easy. In the holdout states of New York and Massachusetts chiropractors did not obtain legal standing until the mid-1960s. The most troublesome controversy has been over what their legally defined scope of practice should be, caused as much by disagreement within the profession over how restrictive (straight) or broad (mixer) the definition should be as by the medical opposition. Consequently the types of law and licensing boards varied from state to state, and still do, depending on whether straights or mixers predominated, and from an all-chiropractic board to a medically dominated board, depending on the strength of the medical opposition. Beginning in 1925, 23 states established Basic Science Boards (now abandoned) to examine all health practitioner candidates, followed by separate examinations by the board responsible for each profession (Gevitz, 1988a). Chiropractors still disagree as to what their proper scope of practice should be, and hence what their licensing laws should permit or proscribe. Straights want a narrow definition limited mainly to adjustment of spinal segments by hand only, whereas mixers favor a broader definition including nearly all therapies and modalities except pharmacology and major surgery.

In 1974 Congress mandated that the United States Public Health Service (USPHS) conduct an " 'independent, unbiased' study of the fundamentals of the chiropractic profession," and suggested that up to $2 million be used for it. Consequently, in 1975 the USPHS organized a conference of international experts in the basic sciences of neurology, orthopedics, and spinal biomechanics and the leading clinicians in medicine, osteopathy, and chiropractic at the National Institutes of Health in Bethesda, Maryland. Publication of its results by the USPHS (Goldstein, 1975) symbolized for the first time convergence of the scientific and clinical interests of these professions, and more important, was recognition that chiropractors have a service to offer and a part to play in delivering health care to the American people. Soon afterward came a series of interdisciplinary conferences on the spine, and their publication (Buerger and Tobis, 1977; Korr, 1978a; Haldeman, 1980; Mazzarelli, 1982; Greenman, 1984; Buerger and Greenman, 1985). (See Chapter 9 for evaluations of chiropractic's effectiveness.)

Strictly speaking, federal funds have been available for research on chiropractic, but little money has actually been awarded. For years the only recipient was Professor Chung-Ha Suh (1974, 1975, 1980), an engineer at the University of Colorado, who did research on spinal biomechanics and neurophysiology with Seth K. Sharpless (1975) and Marvin W. Luttges and Richard A. Gerren (1980). The second grant was not awarded until 1985. Among the reasons why federal grants were slow in coming was that chiropractors and their colleges lacked experience and commitment to doing research, and until recently it was nearly impossible to undertake interdisciplinary research with MDs.

Efforts to upgrade chiropractic education were federally recognized in 1974 when United States Office of Education designated the Council on Chiropractic Education the official accrediting agency for chiropractic colleges. Two years of preprofessional college credits emphasizing the basic medical sciences plus 4 years in a chiropractic college became the minimum requirements. The better colleges now exceed this, and the quality of student applicants has risen as a result of competition for admission. No longer can the AMA claim that chiropractors are ignorant of the basic medical sciences, except for pharmacology and surgery, which chiropractors choose not to cover. While chiropractic academic programs clearly do not equal those in medical and osteopathic colleges, they are taught by university-trained instructors with advanced degrees in the basic medical sciences. Instruction in the clinical courses remains relatively weak, not primarily because the teachers are chiropractors but because the college clinics do not attract a wide variety of the seriously sick and because the facilities of medical clinics and hospitals are only beginning to become available to chiropractic students. Instruction is particularly strong in anatomy, neurology, spinal biomechanics, and related pathology, the subjects on which chiropractic is centrally focused.

Full recognition of chiropractic's improved legal and professional status by the medical and scientific communities has not yet been achieved. De facto recognition at the community level could hardly be denied, and was from the very beginning far ahead of acceptance at state and national levels. Historically, mutual referrals of patients and exchange of professional services were frequent. The taboo in the AMA code of medical ethics prohibiting association with "irregulars" became the chief weapon used by the AMA to discourage professional relationships with chiropractors. Only after five chiropractors, with organizational support, launched a massive antitrust suit against the AMA, eleven affiliated organizations, and four AMA officers (Wilk et al., 1976) was the code of ethics belatedly modified in 1980 to permit association with chiropractors provided the individual MD believed it to be in the best interests of the patient.

The Wilk antitrust suit was lost in federal court in 1981, reversed on appeal in 1983, and won in 1987. Of the four defendants found guilty only the AMA appealed the decision, which was finally denied by the United States Supreme Court in 1990. The other defendants had settled out of court, agreeing to permit all kinds of professional association with chiropractors and each paying between $25,000 and $200,000 toward the chiropractors' legal expenses. The AMA appeal to the Supreme Court produced a counterappeal by the chiropractors arguing that the Joint Commission on Accreditation of Hospitals (JCAH) also should have been found guilty, but the Court in 1990 declined to hear either appeal.

One of the most important of the court-approved settlements was that with the American Hospital Association (AHA). The AHA had abided by the mandate of the JCAH requiring exclusion of chiropractors from hospital staffs as a condition of accreditation. The settlement with AHA required that hospitals no longer arbitrarily deny chiropractors admission to their staffs, although they retain the right to screen individual applicants of any profession. Even before the settlement a few hospitals (most of them small and seeking more patients) had begun accepting chiropractors.

The symbolism of this victory for chiropractors can hardly be exaggerated, even if few chiropractors ever seek or gain hospital appointment. Chiropractors now have come full circle, in that from the earliest days some chiropractors, including D.D. himself, maintained "infirmaries" or hospitals in conjunction with their practices. And for at least the first 40 years of their existence chiropractors often treated patients in small hospitals owned or managed by MDs. Indeed, several chiropractic hospitals, a mental sanitarium, and birthing homes associated with chiropractic colleges lasted into the second half of the 20th century.

Chiropractors have come a long way since 1895. They are currently recognized licensed professionals fairly well integrated into the health care system as independent practitioners legally qualified to diagnose the conditions they can or cannot help, that is, as "portals of entry" into the system. They are no longer pariahs, but have gained widespread acceptance. Most third-party payers now reimburse them, although not at so high a level as MDs. But they know they must continue to remain alert and active politically, ready to repel legislative assaults on their hard-won legal rights, on the breadth of their scope of practice, and on their reimbursements. They continue to be especially attentive to public relations and advertising, because they sincerely believe that the public needs to become better informed as to what they do. Other political goals include acceptance in the military as commissioned officers and by the Veterans Administration (VA) as providers of care. Congressionally mandated demonstration projects involving chiropractic treatment by the VA and the Civilian Health and Medical Program of the Uniformed Services (CHAMPUS) have been carried out, but no clear-cut recognition of chiropractic has yet come from either of these medically dominated departments of the federal government.

Numerous public opinion surveys reveal how much more favorably the public now regards chiropractic and chiropractors. There is increased awareness of who they are and what they do. The public reports nearly as much satisfaction with chiropractic treatment as with medical treatment. Many who have never been to a chiropractor respond that they have a favorable impression of them and that they would consult a chiropractor if they had "a condition a chiropractor treats" (Gallup Organization, 1982; Wardwell, 1989). The surveys also reveal that the public actually has limited understanding of the range of conditions that chiropractors treat. Most respondents associate chiropractic with neck and back problems but often are unaware that other bones and joints of the body (e.g., shoulders, feet, elbows) can be manipulated with benefit and that conditions such as headaches, sciatica, and gastrointestinal problems often are helped by spinal manipulation. Many do not know that young children and pregnant women also can benefit and that patients with cancer, stroke, or heart disease, especially hypertension, often obtain relief from some of their symptoms through chiropractic adjustments, although chiropractors do not claim they can treat such conditions directly. There are also outright misconceptions regarding chiropractic. The Gallup (1982) survey of New York residents found that 20% of a representative sample of New York residents thought that chiropractors prescribe drugs, and another 17% did not know. Twenty percent of the respondents to a Pennsylvania

State University survey (Hearne and Smalley, 1985) thought that chiropractors are members of the AMA. (For documentation on the acceptance of chiropractors see Chapter 11.)

Lay persons often are confused over the differences between different professions and specialists, which is why they should have a family physician qualified to refer them to the one they need. All portal-of-entry health providers—general practitioners, dentists, podiatrists, optometrists, psychotherapists, and chiropractors—should have at least minimum skills to identify which conditions fall within their range of competence and which do not, and to know which other providers are appropriate for referral. Chiropractors have been subject to repeated allegations of failure in this regard, for which there is documentation in the medical literature (see Chapter 9, Section 2). But chiropractors provide a *conservative* therapy with much less likelihood of iatrogenic harm than can be caused by potent drugs or major surgery. If they had not been able to make what has sometimes been called a "chiropractic diagnosis" they would not have survived and prospered as well as they have. Their relatively low malpractice insurance rates (Holoweiko, 1987; Harrison JD, 1990; Campbell et al., 1990) are evidence for this conclusion. It is ironic, now that chiropractors have become more competent to diagnose and hence to avoid cases unsuitable for their treatment, that their malpractice insurance rates have risen somewhat, probably for the same reasons that the insurance rates of all health practitioners have escalated.

We cannot escape history. We are creatures of it. We cannot understand where we are or where we are likely to go in the future unless we know where we have been. Simple chronology is the unavoidable basis of history, but it is not enough. We need to understand relationships between events, especially causes and consequences. In addition to knowing these, we usually also want to influence the future. Although each event is unique and history never exactly repeats itself, there are enough common elements to permit historians and sociologists to generalize from repeated sequences. Chiropractic's history over the past century is part of the history of the U.S. health care system and is relevant to the question of how organized medicine continues to cope with its challengers. Chiropractic differs from other dissenting groups by being the only one that did not disappear, either through abandonment or absorption into the medical mainstream.

What can we learn from the phenomenon of chiropractic about the history of medicine and its evolution as a social institution? How similar and how different was it from that of other dissident groups of practitioners that challenged orthodox medicine in the 19th century? If different, what were the important differences and their consequences? If medicine responded to chiropractic differently than it did to other dissenting groups, why did it do so? What has been the relative significance of economic, political, cultural, and scientific factors in the creation and survival of chiropractic, in the contention between it and organized medicine, and in the current problematic relationships between them? What has been the relative importance of idiosyncratic factors, such as the charismatic leadership of particular individuals vs.

societal factors such as changing levels of technology, market forces, and political hegemony? These questions will guide the investigation as I review the evolution of chiropractic over the past century within the dynamically evolving U.S. society and culture.

Chapter 2

Unorthodox Practitioners in the 19th Century

In 19th century America, medicine was, at best,
practiced in a way that in Europe would have been
considered more typical of the 18th century.

Pierre-Louis Gaucher-Peslherbe (1992)

Section 1

Religious and Psychologic Factors in Healing

Probably the most important trend in Western culture since Darwin published his theory of biologic evolution in 1859 has been our increasing reliance on science and technology rather than religion to explain the mysteries of the biologic and social world. Progress is believed to derive from a scientific understanding of phenomena based on empirical study and logical reasoning. Our secularized society reveres science as a means of deciding between conflicting theories of why the world functions as it does, and this is what we also expect in the area of human health. We look to science for an understanding of illness, for relief from pain, and for a cure whenever possible. Although religion still is important in many people's lives, it is not expected to compete with science in teaching us how to prevent or cure illness. If a physician confronted with a serious illness were to intone, "Let us pray!," those present would be shocked and disheartened. (One recalls the Harvard surgeon who began using Lord Lister's carbolic acid as an antiseptic who would pun before surgery, "Let us spray.")

The differences between religion and science are fundamental. Religion is based on revealed truth, eternal verities, and supernatural authority rather than on the slow frustrating approximations of empirical and experimental science. When dissenters, heretics, or the founders of new religions challenge established authority, there is no agreed-on rational basis for resolving differences between them, as is expected in the case of contending scientific opinions. Note that the word "opinion" is appropriate

15

here, whereas nothing less than "conviction" is required when religious belief is at stake. Notice also that the same terms are applied to dissenting healers and dissenting religious believers. Chief among these is the word "cult," long used to describe chiropractic by its critics, while the slightly less pejorative term "sect" often has been used to characterize osteopathy and sometimes homeopathy.

It is surely no accident that these terms from the religious sphere have been used freely to describe dissident or alternative healing groups. I suggest that the reason for this parallel usage is not merely historical but substantial. Religion and healing have always been closely identified; the terms "witch doctor" and "medicine man" come immediately to mind. In preliterate cultures there is often an intimate connection between sickness and sin. Especially in the case of a mysterious illness (and how many illnesses were not at some time mysterious?), a supernatural spirit or deity often is believed to be inflicting punishment. The belief that illness is punishment for an offense against God, another person, or social norms provides a solid basis for what sociologists call "social control," encouraging conformity to approved standards of conduct. The anthropologist William Howells (1948, p 105) wrote: "Illness is . . . the teeth in the law, . . . the reason for observing tabus, . . . and so it helps give them the force they exert in society." When an illness is believed to be supernaturally caused, then logically so must be the therapy. It often requires placating the offended spirit or person, usually through some act of ritual expiation, often combined with the more concrete symbolism of using the hands, as Howells (1948, p 95) explains:

> The most direct system is simply to manhandle the disease, treating it as though it were tangible and manipulating it out. Sucking out a definite disease object I have described. Another practice is to scrape the illness off, as though it were outside the man, and throw it away. Similarly, according to some people, it may be sponged off. Or it may be moved around by massage until it is forced down one leg, into the foot, and out entirely.

Appeals to magical powers and sacrifices to gods or saints have been prevalent in all societies. Jesus and Mahomed healed by laying on their hands, as did the Mormon leader Joseph Smith (Homola, 1963, p 21), Mary Baker Eddy when she first began healing, and several other 19th century American religious leaders (Gevitz, 1982, p 13).

When the medieval Church monopolized science and learning and medicine was hardly recognized as a specialized field, a doctor (the word in Latin means "teacher") routinely took minor orders in the Church (Carr-Saunders and Wilson 1933, p 66). The surgeon was a mere technician operating under the supervision of the learned physician, who would not deign to soil his hands with manual (i.e., bloody) labor. While medicine owed much to the ancient Greeks, it was so fused with theological principles that practitioners labored to be doctrinally correct even if it limited their effectiveness; for example, the religious taboo on human dissection severely impeded the study of anatomy. Like theological heresy, innovative ideas in medicine were suspect. Later when such radical notions as microbes that could be seen only with microscopes, and methods to achieve asepsis and antisepsis were proposed, the medical establishment only gradually accepted them. Throughout the 19th century it regularly applied the terms "cult" and "sect" to groups holding a different healing philosophy.

Dissenting healing groups should not be confused with religious groups that incorporate healing practices into primarily religious rituals. The foremost example in America is Christian Science, best known for religious healing sought through prayer. Strictly speaking, Christian Scientists do not use prayer but repetitive reading from Mary Baker Eddy's *Science and Health With Key to the Scriptures* (1875; Wardwell, 1964, 1973). Indeed, their leaders and practitioners are also known as "readers." Based on the principle that God, goodness, love, light, mind, and such, are the basic realities and that their opposites, evil, death, and sickness, exist only in the mind, treatment consists in repeated denial of the latter and repeated affirmation of the former. Health and the correct view of the world are to be obtained by thinking correct thoughts. However, because thoughts can be evil as well as good, guided training and practice are needed to ward off evil thoughts. Mary Baker Eddy formulated her ideas at a time when "animal magnetism" was believed to account for hypnotic and other psychic influences, and she applied the phrase "malicious animal magnetism" (which she called "MAM") to the evil thoughts that pursued her personally and which she constantly warned others about as a source of disease. During her last illnesses she posted guardians at each corner of her sickbed, requiring them to think good thoughts so as to ward off the evil thoughts of her enemies! She even organized weekly meetings of specially chosen followers to study ways of coping with MAM. (It is interesting that her pursuing devil, MAM, is an anagram of the devil that the chiropractors believed pursued them, the AMA!)

Our secularized culture has not fully escaped the complex interrelationships between religion and healing, but they should be kept conceptually separate. Patients facing the crises of illness, disability, and death want emotional support beyond what science can offer. Such crises involve the conditions of uncertainty and impossibility that Bronislaw Malinowski (1948, pp 67–68) identified as the occasions when magic and religion arise to fill the psychic need to do something meaningful even though the facts of death, disability, and pain cannot be predicted or evaded. Religious ritual fills this need, especially when a group shares in praying, chanting, marching, or other rite, as at Lourdes (Cranston, 1955). Such practices do not preclude the simultaneous use of scientific methods of healing, and indeed often may assist them, but the two must be distinguished analytically.

Similarly, the importance of ritual and symbolism in modern medical practice, whether in office or hospital setting, cannot be underestimated. Our hospitals have been called, not without reason, "temples" in which physicians are the "high priests." They wear vestments befitting their status, have their own acolytes, their aseptically sterile (sacred!) places and practices, and their symbols of power (lancet, x-ray, computed tomography, magnetic resonance imaging), and they perform in highly ritualized ways using a language mysterious to outsiders. It is no wonder that lay persons are impressed (whether terrified or reassured) by the rituals and trappings of science, which indeed can be worshipped as the highest good, or God.

This discussion of religion and symbolism is relevant to some of the criticisms directed toward chiropractors and their successes. Often mentioned is the religious and psychologic significance of the "laying on of hands," which is obviously central to spinal manipulative therapy. There is no doubt that manual contact in itself conveys powerful psychologic suggestion, especially when accompanied by a forceful movement of vertebrae and a noticeable pop or click. And sometimes it causes pain, which also can have significant meaning for the patient; however, there probably is less pain and less symbolic meaning in a chiropractic adjustment than in the surgery or inoculations (shots) that MDs use.

The related criticism that chiropractic benefits are due mainly to a placebo effect ignores the fact that such effects can be considered relatively constant across professional boundaries. Many observers have noted that chiropractors are very solicitous in caring for their patients, take time to listen to them, respond to their needs, and develop especially good doctor-patient relationships. MDs often imply that they could do as well but that they simply don't have the time. The fact that the chiropractic patient lies prone (on a couch?), where relaxation is promoted, also can produce an important effect. One criticism is that chiropractic patients may be neurasthenic or neurotic or have imaginary illnesses that cause exasperated MDs to rebuff them, or that they have psychosomatic or stress-related complaints that benefit from the kind of psychologic support that chiropractors provide. The implication of these criticisms is that chiropractic's principal benefit is psychologic.

Other critics have implied that chiropractic is based on religious belief, although D.D. Palmer clearly stated that it is not. In *The Chiropractor* (1914, p 6) he emphasized that chiropractic is not a religion but a science and that the "art" (practice) of adjusting is based on chiropractic science. He was crystal clear on this point. More difficult is his concept of "Innate," or "Innate Intelligence." Some of the language he used when discussing it suggests a kind of mysticism, because he also wrote about God as Universal Intelligence. But it is clear that his Innate is really little more than vix medicatrix naturae, that is, the ability of the body to heal itself. That phrase was for Palmer not merely a simple observation but a profound insight and a cardinal principle of his philosophy of healing. For him it certainly was God-given, but that did not make chiropractic a religion. Although D.D. sought the *causes* of illness and health, he based chiropractic on evidence from the empirical world of science rather than on religion.

Section 2

Bonesetters

Before turning to medical dissent in the 19th century we will examine the ancient tradition of bonesetting (see also Wardwell, 1987). The word itself can be misleading because it has encompassed setting broken bones and reducing dislocations as well as manipulating minor "subluxations," a term used, incidentally, long before Palmer and with exactly his meaning. Similarly, the word "manipulation" encompasses different meanings: reduction of a fracture or dislocation, mobilization to increase the range of motion of a joint, to break adhesions, or to promote circulation, as well as to stimulate or inhibit neural transmission. Gaucher-Peslherbe (1992) notes: "All through the 19th century the generic term 'therapeutic manipulation' included such varied practices as massage, friction, Swedish or German gymnastics, English-style pressures, percussion, and also, of course, manipulation in the sense that we understand it today, which restricts it to the joints." Haldeman (1983, p 63) distinguishes seven categories of manipulation: "long-lever, nonspecific manipulation; specific short-lever high velocity spinal adjustments; active or functional manipulation; mobilization; manual traction; soft tissue massage; and point pressure manipulation." Nineteen different definitions are listed in *The Glossary of Osteopathic Terminology* (Gunby 1983, p 3148). Even the word "nerve" meant different things at different times, according to Gaucher-Peslherbe (1992, p 74): "Aristotle . . . thought that nerves emerged from the heart. In this physiology, nerves were all the fibrous structures of the body: the tendons and ligaments as well as what we now call nerves."

According to the Kung Fou document, a form of manipulation was practiced in China as early as 2700 BC, a practice Junxue Li (1990) refers to as "CMT" ("Chinese manipulative therapy"). There is evidence of similar practices in Babylonia, Egypt, India, and elsewhere. Robert Anderson (1983b, pp 20–21) states: "Traditional Chinese medicine and chiropractic are remarkably alike in their underlying theories. . . . Through deep massage at the occiput, for example, (contemporary) Chinese practitioners find that they can bring down high blood pressure, a practice analogous to that of chiropractors."

Hippocrates (470–357 BC) wrote at least three books on bones and joints, and his aphorism "Look well to the spine for the cause of disease" often is cited by chiropractors. However, Albert Abrams (1912, p 4) commented: "Hippocrates must have anticipated sectarian practice with relation to the spine. . . . After enjoining the physician to know the spine as requisite in many diseases, he inveighs against the practice of attributing cure to the reduction of dislocated vertebrae thus profiting by the ignorance of others." Nevertheless, Ligeros, in *How Ancient Healing Governs Modern Therapeutics* (1937, pp 52, 65, 421ff) claimed that Hippocrates advocated spinal manipulation (Figure 2):

> He evidently studied very closely the mechanism of the spinal column and understood thoroughly its importance and significance. He appears to have known well its relation and application to and effects upon the nervous system, and also its influence upon the whole organism. He described its mechanical maleffects upon the soft tissues adjacent to the spine, as make them tense and taut and somewhat elevated to the touch. He insisted that the practitioner should become well acquainted with all these facts, and learn the mechanical relation of the spinal column to the nervous system and of the latter to the organism, so as to be ever ready to make proper correction in case of such skeletal and spinal displacements, and malformations or similar derangements, by means of re-

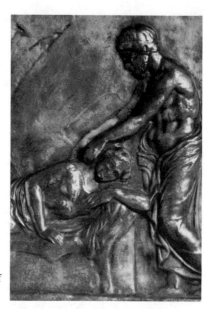

FIGURE 2.
Aesculapian manipulation. (Courtesy of
Christine Tamulaitis.)

duction, extension, counter-extension, succussion [sic], etc. . . . . Hippocrates and Galen
also made valid references to the intervertebral foramina. Both of them clearly point to
the fact that relative disturbance of the foramina and adjacent tissues within and around
the intervertebral opening takes place due to occlusion resulting from a minor spinal vertebral displacement or subluxation.

The medical historian of manipulation Elizabeth Lomax (1975, p 11) remains
somewhat unconvinced: "I hardly dare argue with a native but Ligeros does seem to
have read more into the Hippocratic writings than is obvious to the outsider using
translations." Later (1977, p 207) she states: "Only further scholarly research could
establish whether the Greeks merely attempted to reposition vertebrae displaced
through trauma, the conventional interpretation, or indeed frequently manipulated
spines as therapy for a wide variety of dysfunctions."

Samuel Homola (1963, p 8) agrees with Ligeros that Hippocrates "recognized
different degrees of displacement in the spinal joints and attempted correction accordingly." He found (1963, pp 2–3) that the use of massage and some form of manipulation have been a part of every culture:

> The art of massage and bonesetting are too closely allied to assume that those who prac-
> ticed massage did not apply forceful movement and pressure to the joints—especially
> when the joints seemed to be disturbed in their functions.

> Trying to trace the origin of joint manipulation and massage would probably be quite
> impossible, for both have undoubtedly existed in one form or another since the begin-

ning of man. It is a natural tendency for one to massage and manipulate an aching muscle or limb.

Julius Dintenfass (1970, p 29) agrees, saying: "The practice of manipulation is . . . close to being universal."

Villiers and Gahan (1971, pp 341–342; see also Schiotz and Cyriax, 1975, p 25) relate Captain Cook's account of the benefits received from the "pummeling and squeezing" by "twelve large, muscular Tahiti women" for his crippling rheumatism. The practice is called "romy" or "rumi." It also is documented that many of the early Indians of North, South, and Central America practiced spinal manipulation. The gauchos of South America performed "abrazo del ranchero" on one another, which "consisted of lifting an individual from behind after he had folded his arms across his chest" (Eisenberg, 1990, p 106). The custom of having children walk on troubled backs also has been reported from both Americas and from Polynesia, as well as being called a "peasant practice" known as "napravit" in Bohemia (Zarbuck, 1986). Homola (1963, p 4) writes: "My father, who grew up in Czechoslovakia, told me that, in his homeland, families had used spinal manipulation in the home for centuries. As a child he was regularly commissioned to walk barefoot up and down the spine of his father."

Robert Anderson, who first earned a Ph.D degree in anthropology, and then D.C. and M.D. degrees, has reported two personal encounters with folk practitioners of manipulation. In Hawaii he (1982) observed an elderly practitioner of traditional "lomilomi" who was licensed as a masseur but consulted medical books by James Cyriax (1951) and James Mennell (1952) and used the hard, deep kneading of lomilomi as well as backwalking aided by two canes. Anderson (1987) also made a limited but sophisticated analysis of 53 patients of a Mexican folk practitioner who preferred to be called an "arreglador de huesos" (bonesetter) but whose clients persisted in calling him a "sobador" (massager). Like the Hawaiian practitioner, he used some modern techniques he had learned by watching chiropractors. In the majority of 55 lesions treated involving bony articulations, he used massage, stretching and joint mobilization, and manipulation of the spine and extremities, with apparent benefit to his patients. Neither of these folk practitioners performed specific chiropractic adjustments, but they definitely manipulated vertebrae and stimulated spinal nerves.

Gaucher-Peslherbe (1992) describes the changing perceptions and symbolism of the human body in European culture:

> In the Middle Ages the only requirement for the spine was that it should be straight. This has a cultural explanation; a straight back was an attribute of nobility and a sign of valor: the knight had a duty to bear his armor with pride. . . . The cultural image of the Renaissance encouraged manipulation of the spine . . . but only in order to impose upon it the desired form.

(On bonesetting from late antiquity to the modern era, see Gaucher-Peslherbe [1991].) However, in the 17th century the classical theory of bodily humors brought a greater interest in the musculature of the body than in its bony frame, with the re-sult that "massages and frictions became the recommended treatment, and articular reductions were condemned" (Gaucher-Peslherbe, 1992). Lomax (1977, p 207) con-curs:

> Vertebral luxation was an acceptable explanation for back pain and deformity until the eighteenth century. Then, as surgeons delved deeper into pathological anatomy, alterna-tive interpretations came to the fore. Some argued that vertebral dislocation without con-comitant fracture was impossible, except at the atlantoaxial joint.

The earliest known English text on bonesetting was published by Friar Moulton in 1656, and republished by Robert Turner under the title *The Compleat Bone-Setter, Wherein the Method of Curing Broken Bones and Strains and Dislocated Joints, To-gether with Ruptures, Commonly Called Broken Bellyes, Is Fully Demonstrated, Re-vised, "Englished" and Enlarged, 1665 Edition* (Joy, 1954). Obviously it covered many more conditions and remedies than chiropractors ever claimed to treat. Ander-son (1983a, pp 13–14) doubts whether many of the mostly illiterate folk practitioners ever read *The Compleat Bone-Setter*, which in any case did not provide detailed in-structions regarding manipulative techniques; and he makes this sociologic observa-tion:

> Bonesetting became identified with the humble oral tradition of uneducated peasant and working people. That identification became a stigma. . . . Bonesetting became a symbol of low-level, non-professional status, and status alone blinded professional borrowers who might be tempted to bring it back to respectability.

Gaucher (1992) agrees: "Soon bone-setters were to be refused access to hospitals to treat cases relevant to their art." However, bonesetting continued as a folk practice well into the 19th century, when it again began to attract the attention of physicians. In Lincolnshire Dr. Edward Harrison (1827) found that bonesetters outnumbered phy-sicians nine to one (Lomax, 1975, p 16).

Lomax's two papers deal mainly with bonesetters in England, where they were also called "spine-menders." In France bonesetting was called "reboutage," and the practitioner "rebouteur," "renouveur," or "bailleul." In Germany the term was "Kno-cheneinrichter," "Knochenarzt," or "Wundarzt"; in Spain, "algebrista" or "ensalma-dor." In Czechoslovakia the term was "napravit" (Joy, 1954; Zarbuck, 1986). What is unclear because of ambiguous terminology is what the scope of practice of each was. Probably a lot depended on local custom or on whatever the individual practi-tioner felt competent to do (or perhaps to get away with!) Dintenfass (1970, pp 32) tells us:

> During the Middle Ages and the Renaissance the art of manipulation, often called "bonesetting," was handed down from father to son, or mother to daughter, and was practiced by at least one supposedly "gifted" person in most communities in Europe and Asia. . . . The results obtained by these individuals were so unusual that the people believed that they inherited a divine gift to heal the sick!

Gaucher-Peslherbe (1990) cites M. Eliade in *Le Chamanisme* as describing how "throughout history bones and joints have been invested with a symbolic and mystical significance." This link with the supernatural not only harks back to primitive cultures but continues in the persistent association between religion and healing.

Although spinal manipulation came to be feared as risky by orthodox physicians in the 19th century, the English Doctors A. Dods (1824), Edward Harrison (1827), W.J. Little (1868), James Paget (1871), and W. Hood (1871) all incorporated some variant of spinal manipulation into their practices, thereby upsetting their more orthodox colleagues. A French MD stated that he thought it necessary to pose as a bonesetter because: "If the people know I am a qualified doctor, I shall have no more customers" (Lovett, 1922). Gaucher (1992) states that of the four recognized medieval medical craftsmen—barber-surgeon, matron-midwife, toothpuller-dentist, and bonesetter—only the last survived until the modern era. James Cyriax (Schiotz and Cyriax 1975, p 72) tells us that it became unethical for MDs to collaborate with bonesetters in England after passage of the Medical Act in 1858.

The most disturbing bonesetter of all, and one of the most successful, was Mrs. Mapp, "Crazy Sally of Epsom," described as "an enormous, fat, ugly, drunken woman so much esteemed for skill in her craft that the authorities of the watering place of Epsom offered her $500 yearly to reside there," according to *JAMA* ("Osteopathy," 1897). She journeyed to London weekly "in a chariot drawn by four horses, with servants wearing splendid liveries," was caricatured by Hogarth, and was sung about at Lincoln Inn's Theatre in a comedy called "The Husband's Relief; or the Female Bone-Setter, and the Woman Doctor" (Bennett, 1884, pp 8–9):

> You surgeons of London, who puzzle your pates,
> To ride in your coaches and purchase estates,
> Give over for shame, for pride has a fall,
> And the doctress of Epsom has outdone you all.
>
> What signifies learning or going to school,
> When a woman can do, without learning a rule;
> What puts you to nonplus and baffles your art,
> For petticoat practice has now got the start.
>
> In physic, as well as in fashion, we find
> The newest has always its run with mankind;
> Forgot is the bustle 'bout Taylor and Ward,
> And Mapp's all the cry, and her fame's on record.
>
> Dame nature has given a doctor's degree,
> She gets all the patients and pockets the fee.
> So if you don't instantly prove her a cheat
> She'll loll in her carriage whilst you walk the street.

Gaucher-Peslherbe (1992) summarizes: "Toward the end of the nineteenth century, there were demands from all sides for more attention to be paid to the techniques of bonesetting. . . . In the last third of the nineteenth century bonesetters and their techniques became popular once more." The best known English bonesetter was Sir Herbert Barker (1927), knighted for his efforts in 1922. Anderson (1981, p S91) writes that by 1906 Barker was calling himself an osteopath, while Inglis (1964, pp 97, 108) tells us that he called himself a "manipulative surgeon." In 1925 the Andrew Taylor Still College of Osteopathy awarded him an honorary D.O. degree, which he referred to as his "American Knighthood" (Harris, 1985, pp 8–9). He was summoned out of retirement in 1936 to demonstrate manipulation before hundreds of orthopedic surgeons at St. Thomas Hospital in London, the only hospital using manipulation. James Mennell and James Cyriax were in attendance at that hospital, where it is claimed that manipulation was used "by every family doctor in the course of his daily round." Although Cyriax has written that he taught medical students only to "identify suitable lesions but not the actual maneuvers themselves," he also wrote (Schiotz and Cyriax 1975, p 69): "During my time at St. Thomas's Hospital, our medical and physiotherapy students were brought up to regard manipulation as an integral part of everyday treatment." The *Lancet* editorialized in 1925 (cited by Harris, 1985, p 9):

> The medical profession of the future will have to record that our profession has greatly neglected this important subject. . . . The fact must be faced, that the bonesetters had been curing multitudes of cases by movement . . . and that by our faulty methods we are largely responsible for their very existence.

In the United States the most famous were Bonesetter Reese of Western Pennsylvania and Eastern Ohio and members of the Sweet family, who practiced in Rhode Island, Massachusetts, Connecticut, and New York. The Sweets attracted clients from all over the East Coast and received many referrals from physicians. Joy (1954, p 427) tells us that because of their reputation for skill and not exploiting patients, there was " an open minded attitude among the medical profession," even though their broad scope of practice included open and closed fractures, and lacerations. Waterman Sweet (1933) recounts his visits as far south as Baltimore to treat thousands of patients. The last of the Sweets practiced in Rhode Island until 1917 and in Connecticut until 1929. While the following two generations of Sweets became orthopedists (one of whom I interviewed in Hartford), the Tieszen family of bonesetters in Marion, South Dakota, became chiropractors (Janse, 1976, p 75). So did the descendants of the Orton family in Canistota, South Dakota, who began studying at the National College of Chiropractic in Chicago in 1935 after two previous generations without formal training were so successful that they built a four-story, 72-room hotel with an attached clinic to accommodate their many patients from distant places (Orton, 1985, pp 27–28). Joy (1954, p 422) observes that bonesetters' reputations declined "as orthopedic knowledge became more and more a part of the armamentarium of the general physician."

Section 3

Early Dissent: Homeopaths

Most disputes over therapy in the 19th century involved much heat and little light. The quality of medical education was poor until the end of the century, because there was little scientific research on which to base sound judgments about illness and therapy. Earlier in the century the practice of "heroic medicine" was still in vogue: bloodletting, cupping (leeching), blistering, purging, and sweating, as well as heavy dosing with calomel (mercurous chloride) and other toxic chemicals. Inasmuch as these remedies were painful and could do more harm than good, patients not surprisingly often preferred the less obnoxious remedies of unorthodox healers. "Indian doctors" (herbalists) and other folk practitioners had been around for many years and were consulted when home remedies failed. Numbers (1977, p 68) states that "it is no exaggeration to say that home health care was the foundation upon which the American sects were built."

The most developed system of herbal treatment was that propounded by Samuel Thomson (1769–1843), an uneducated New Hampshire farmer. Following his successes he patented his remedies in 1813, marketed them widely, and published a compendium of his prescriptions (1822). His followers organized into "friendly societies" that later, in tune with jacksonian populism and the goal "to make every man his physician," lobbied legislatures against licensing laws administered by regular physicians. "By the 1840s almost all of these statutes were repealed, amended, or otherwise made ineffective" (Gevitz, 1982, p 8). Larson (1977, pp 19–20) summarizes the effects of the shift from licensure to school graduation as the basis for assuring competence:

> In America, the absence of restrictive corporate monopolies, such as that of the British Royal College of Physicians, permitted an unbridled expansion of the supply of physicians. Proprietary schools, with requirements as lax as their curricula were brief, proliferated in the first two-thirds of the nineteenth century, rapidly substituting their diplomas for the license which medical societies had granted in most states since the eighteenth century. After 1825, competition for students among these schools led to a general decline of standards and requirements, . . . on the basis of mostly ineffective therapies and unfounded pathological theories.

Two types of botanical medicine filiated from the thomsonians: the physiomedicalists and the eclectics. Although each had their own schools, journals, and associations, and the last of the physiomedicalist colleges closed only in 1911 and the last eclectic college only in 1939 (Rothstein, 1972, p 296), after 1900 their impact on health care was minimal.

Homeopathy posed a more serious challenge to orthodox medicine. First introduced in the United States by Dr. Hans B. Gram in 1825, it was based on two books by Samuel Christian Hahnemann (1755–1843), *The Homeopathic Medical Doctrine, or, Organon of the Healing Art* (1833) and *Materia Medica Pura* (1846), both translated from German into English in the early 1840s. Since homeopathic "provings" were based on controlled tests of the effects of drugs on healthy persons, it was perceived as more scientifically grounded than traditional medicine. Its doctrine of "similars," that is, treating a condition with a drug that produced the identical symptoms in a healthy person that the sick person experiences, was intended to assist the body in achieving its natural reaction to illness. However, its doctrine of "infinitessimals" so diluted the dosages as to produce only or mainly a placebo effect, a fact often noted by its critics (Kaufman, 1971, pp 30–41).

Many patients preferred homeopathy to the aggressive drugging of the "allopaths," as the homeopaths began calling orthodox MDs. The latter were even more disturbed when some of their colleagues began adopting homeopathic practices. Because there were few effective drugs at the time, and little scientific knowledge of their real effects, the homeopaths not only did less harm to patients, as even their critics noted, but made many of them well. Conceded even by its sharpest critics to be the "aristocracy of quackery," by mid-century homeopathy was being denounced generally. Oliver Wendell Holmes, anatomist and poet, in his classic lecture on "Homeopathy and Its Kindred Delusions" (1842) put homeopathy in the same category as tar water, Perkins' tractors, and the royal touch as a cure for scrofula. He devastatingly attacked infinitessimal dosages, the "psora" doctrine (that chronic disease is the result of allopathic suppression of the itch), drug provings that could not be reproduced, references to authorities that did not exist, and the unreliable statistics used to prove homeopathy (Kaufman, 1971, pp 40–42; see also Coulter, HL, 1975).

The state licensing laws authorizing medical societies to examine and register candidates, beginning in New Jersey in 1772 and in Massachusetts in 1781 (Shryock, 1967, pp 24–25), were repealed in the 1840s in all but two states (New Jersey and Louisiana) under attack as discriminatory by thomsonians and homeopaths and by jacksonian democrats opposed to all monopolistic legislation (Kaufman, 1971, p 23). Since their effect had been mainly to exclude all but orthodox practitioners, the counterargument prevailed that the average citizen should be able to select a doctor for himself from those claiming competence. The call for "medical freedom," that is, "equal rights" for patients as well as for practitioners (Shryock, 1967, p 29), later became the demand of osteopaths and chiropractors when the American Medical Association (AMA) tried to exclude them from licensure.

The purpose of the first National Medical Convention, called to organize the AMA in 1846 (2 years after that of the homeopaths), was to bring order and reason to the situation, but the move was interpreted by opponents, especially by homeopaths, as self-serving. Although an effective system of licensure was one of the AMA's goals, it was not until later in the century that state licensing boards were reintroduced, sometimes along with separate boards for homeopaths. Cooperation between homeopaths and allopaths in the matter of licensing had to wait until threats from the new dissenters (e.g., osteopaths, Christian Scientists, magnetists) forced acceptance of homeopaths as qualified, if not "regular," practitioners. The struggles over whether allopaths would accept homeopaths as professional colleagues foreshadowed later conflicts over accepting osteopaths and chiropractors.

Although Rothstein (1972, p 170) disagrees, historian Martin Kaufman (1971, p 56) maintains that the AMA was not organized primarily to exclude homeopaths but to raise the level of medical education and practice. Not until 1852 was there a discussion of homeopathy or other sectarian medicine, and not until 1855 did the AMA ask state and local societies to adopt the 1847 code of ethics that included the famous consultation clause: "No one can be considered as a regular practitioner, or a fit associate in consultation, whose practice is based upon an exclusive dogma, to the rejection of the accumulated experience of the profession." Kaufman (1971, p 56) concluded:

> The AMA, then, was not formed to destroy homeopathy. It was formed to raise the level of the medical practitioner so that the profession would regain its lost prestige and influence. Conversely, it was founded to improve orthodox medicine so that irregulars could no longer be able to attract patients.

Harris Coulter (1970, pp 17–18) is harsher on organized medicine, arguing that it dismissed homeopathy on a priori grounds, alleging that its patients were "not 'manly' enough to take the 'true' medication of the regulars" and that they were merely responding to the homeopath's placebos and his careful physical examination and willingness to listen to a long recital of symptoms. Similar allegations were later made against osteopaths and chiropractors. In any case, orthodox medicine "never conducted a controlled and supervised investigation" of homeopathy. However, Coulter notes that many homeopathic remedies were taken over by orthodox medicine, the best example being nitroglycerine for certain heart conditions, which was published by homeopath Constantine Hering in 1857 but not mentioned in an allopathic source until 1882.

The consultation clause was the basis for excluding irregulars. As a result, there developed two (and after the eclectics appeared, three) parallel sets of professional organizations, schools, and journals, each propounding its own theories and practices and disparaging the others.

Licensing and access to public hospitals were the critical issues. At first homeopaths were denied access to public hospitals in Chicago, New York, and Boston, but the New York City Commissioners of Charities and Correction in 1875 assigned Ward's Island Hospital to the homeopaths (Kaufman, 1971, p 148); and in 1881 the Chicago Commissioners gave the homeopaths control of one fifth of the wards in Cook County Hospital, thus making possible a unique study comparing the relative effectiveness of the two therapies. The homeopaths actually did slightly better: with one in four or one in five of 5,934 entering patients randomly assigned to homeopaths, 8.2% of the homeopaths' patients died, whereas the allopaths lost 8.6% (Kaufman, 1971, pp 150–151). However, since the homeopaths often also used some allopathic methods, the results could not be considered conclusive. Homeopaths, many of whom were former allopaths, often were better educated and commanded more respect, especially in the larger cities of the Northeast.

Proposals by the Medical Society of the State of New York in 1882 to revise the code of medical ethics so as to permit consultation with "legally qualified practitioners of medicine" (Kaufman, 1971, p 126) provoked the most violent controversy the AMA ever had experienced. Vitriolic debates and efforts to expel individuals and entire societies that refused to subscribe to the "old code" continued through the end of the century. However, in 1884 homeopaths and eclectics were appointed to the Massachusetts Medical Examining Board, and in 1888 the Massachusetts Medical Society voted to allow admission to homeopaths who recanted. But when the homeopathic Boston University School of Medicine in 1886 petitioned to use Boston City Hospital for clinical instruction, opposition from the allopathic Harvard Medical School forced rejection (Kaufman, 1971, pp 151–152).

Nevertheless, homeopaths and allopaths were drawing closer as they recognized the need to exclude not only incompetent MDs but also the more questionable types of practitioners, such as osteopaths, Christian Scientists, spiritualists, magnetic healers, and charlatans. Diploma mills were rife. Kaufman (1971, p 142) states that the most infamous salesman, John Buchanan, admitted on being arrested to having sold 60,000 diplomas at prices from $10 to $200, some to 2-year-old children!

Hostility between homeopaths and allopaths continued, with charges and maneuvers similar to those that recurred in the 1950s and 1960s in the debates over professional association with osteopaths. The same kinds of allegations of educational deficiencies and of adherence to an "exclusive and dogmatic" theory of practice would be made. And organizational splits developed within homeopathy like those that later occurred in osteopathy, that is, between "traditionalists," who insisted on original principles, and "modernists," who favored revision and openness toward newer practices based on later scientific findings. A similar split probably occurs in any new school of practice (and certainly it has in chiropractic!) as it broadens its educational base and is pressured to change by scientific, economic, and political developments.

According to William Rothstein (1972, p 246), "The zenith of homeopathy as a medical sect in the United States occurred around 1880." The principal obstacle to reunification was the sticky consultation clause on which professional interaction and acceptance on hospital staffs and in medical societies depended. Efforts to achieve cooperation and merge colleges began in 1894, but it was not until its 1903 annual meeting that the AMA House of Delegates modified the code of medical ethics with an "advisory document" that "paved the way for reunification of the orthodox medical profession, an event which took place during the next two years" (Kaufman, p 154). However, full acceptance led to the decline of homeopathy. By 1923 only two homeopathic colleges remained, and they were becoming ever more allopathic. According to Rothstein (1972, pp 296–297), Boston University dropped its homeopathic designation in 1919, the New York Homeopathic College did so in 1936, and Hahnemann Medical College in Philadelphia eliminated its required courses in homeopathy only in the 1950s and taught its last elective course into the 1960s. Kaufman (1971, p 173) concluded:

> Homeopathy had come full circle from its position as a minority in the 1840s, when it was universally condemned by the most prominent allopaths. During the 1880s and 1890s it had become respectable, and in 1903 the AMA even accepted homeopaths as members. Yet, by 1920 homeopathy had witnessed a dramatic decline. For the remaining years of the century, homeopathy, with its colleges disappearing and with fewer and fewer graduates, seemed to be heading for total extinction.

But it did not happen. In his more recent study Kaufman (1988, pp 115–127) reported on the revival of interest in homeopathic remedies and the increased teaching of homeopathy in the naturopathic colleges in Seattle and Portland. In Seattle, "about one third of the graduating class specializes in homeopathic practice, a total of about 150 each year in all." Even some chiropractic mixers are beginning to use homeopathic remedies. In 1983 a postdoctoral course was begun at the Arizona Homeopathic Medical University College of Medicine in Scottsdale, but its projected 4-year medical school has not opened. Arizona and Nevada have established homeopathic licensing boards for MDs and DOs who have taken a postgraduate course, but no homeopathic undergraduate medical school now exists in the United States, or for that matter anywhere in the world except India.

Because of the expanding interest in homeopathic remedies, the Food and Drug Administration (FDA) in 1981 threatened to classify them as prescription items. It later recanted and agreed to work with the American Association of Homeopathic Pharmacists to provide "legal muscle" if that organization would revise its pharmacopoeia and police its own membership. As a result, scientific "provings" of homeopathic remedies currently are being carried out with sophisticated laboratory equipment for the first time in history. Several universities and a French laboratory have participated in this research. Hence Kaufman (1988, p 123) revised his 1971 conclusion:

> Homeopathy has come full circle in the almost two centuries of its existence. It was born as an important response to the heroic medical therapies of the early nineteenth century; through conversion of allopathic physicians and then through education of homeopaths in their own medical colleges, it matured from the 1840s to the 1880s. It fell victim to the advancement of modern medical science and had almost disappeared from view by the 1960s, when the average age of America's homeopaths was over sixty. This author's book on the subject could fairly be subtitled *Rise and Fall of a Medical Heresy* when it was published in 1971. However, with the rise of the alternative health movement, homeopathy is once again on the upswing. Although it will never be the threat to orthodox medicine that it was in its earlier years, it seems clear that the movement will be here to offer its alternative to traditional medical treatment for some time to come.

Section 4

Osteopaths

The following discussion is not primarily concerned with the development of osteopathy but only with its relevance to the development of chiropractic. Osteopathy has always differed from chiropractic. Although initially both shared belief in the body's innate ability to maintain itself in good health if permitted to do so and emphasized manipulation of bones and joints as their principal technique, osteopathy's rationale for doing so was fundamentally different. Chiropractic focused from its beginning on specific spinal "adjustments" to release energy delivered through the nervous system, whereas osteopathy's focus was on the "rule of the artery" for the purpose of promoting better blood circulation through nonspecific manipulation of many joints of the body. It thus harked back to the ancient Greek doctrine of body humors, predominant until the 19th century, which underwent a kind of resurgence at the hands of the osteopaths and especially of those MDs early attracted to it. Examples would be the two Scots, Dr. James Littlejohn and Dr. William Smith, who became influential instructors in the school that Andrew Taylor Still (1828–1917) established in 1892 in Kirksville, Missouri, and chartered in 1894 as the American School of Osteopathy. The well-known editor of the *Journal of the American Osteopathic Association (JAOA)*, George Northup, in his *Osteopathic Medicine: An American Reformation* (1972, p 4) agreed: "Basically, osteopathic medicine and its physiological principles are supporters of the Hippocratic approach."

The son of a frontier preacher-doctor, Still (Figure 3) served in the Union Army as a hospital steward during the Civil War, entering the practice of medicine in Missouri soon thereafter. Though he claimed that he had pursued formal studies before the war at the College of Physicians and Surgeons in Kansas City, there is no documentation that he did, allegedly because the records were destroyed in a fire. Disheartened by the loss of his three children to spinal meningitis, in 1864 he began to experiment with manipulation of the musculoskeletal system, at first in combination with treatment by drugs. In 1874 he attempted to present his ideas to the faculty of Baker University in Baldwin, Kansas, but was rebuffed. It is documented that he also used at least two other healing techniques, for after moving in 1875 to Kirksville, Missouri, he advertised himself in the *North Missouri Register* as "A.T. Still, Magnetic Healer," and during the 1880s he advertised himself as a "lightning bonesetter" (Gevitz, 1982, pp 14, 16). Both practices lay outside the scope of orthodox medicine and reveal how medically unorthodox he really was. Gevitz summarizes (1985, p 17):

> Still would synthesize some of the major components of magnetic healing and bonesetting into one unified doctrine. The effects of disease, as the former said, were due to the obstruction or imbalance of the fluids, but this in turn was caused by misplaced bones, particularly of the spinal column. At this point, Still had given birth to his own distinctive system.

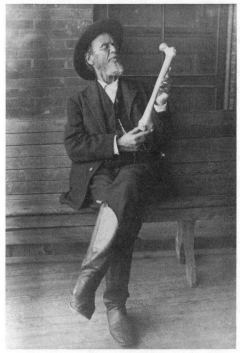

FIGURE 3.
Andrew Taylor Still, developer of osteopathy.
(Courtesy of Texas College of Osteopathic
Medicine.)

Nevertheless Francis Schiller (1971) states: "The genesis of osteopathy can best be understood, I think, on the contemporary background of spinal irritation." Although that term was always vaguely defined, it had been described in 1830 as "the greatest improvement in practical medicine," and remained a prominent topic throughout most of the century. Riadore's (1842) *Treatise on Irritation of the Spinal Nerves* seems even to have anticipated both Still and Palmer:

> If an organ is deficiently supplied with nervous energy or blood, its function is decreased, and sooner or later its structure becomes endangered. . . . When we reflect that every organ and muscle in the body is connected and dependent more or less upon the spinal nerves for the perfect performance of their individual functions, we cannot otherwise prepare to hear of a lengthened catalogue of maladies that are either engendered, continued, or the consequence of spinal irritation.

Schiotz and Cyriax (1975, p 71) concur: "The book that provided the inspiration for lay manipulation was in fact written by a doctor (Riadore)." Lomax (1977, p 214) also agrees:

> Andrew Taylor Still must have been influenced by the doctrine of spinal irritation, still prevalent in medical circles in the 1860s and indeed respectable until the end of the century. Yet, in his writings, the founder of osteopathy made no mention of being prompted by any such theory.

D.D. Palmer (e.g., 1910, p 206) offered several definitions of spinal irritation, but he treated it only as incidental to his other, more familiar concepts. Schiller (1971, p 266) concluded : "In the light of history Still's ideas appear neither as original as his admirers claim, nor as absurd as his detractors charge."

Osteopathy's early struggles paralleled those of chiropractic. Mark Twain's comments in this context are amusing (Shryock, 1967, p 59):

> I don't know that I cared much for these osteopaths until I heard you were going to drive them out of the State; but since I heard this I haven't been able to sleep. Now what I contend is that my body is my own, at least I have always so regarded it. If I do harm through my experimenting with it, it is I who suffer, not the State.

Similarities in the personalities and careers of A.T. Still and D.D. Palmer also are striking. Both were independent thinkers, charismatic, and contentious. Both had been magnetic healers, although Palmer not until 1886. And both combined magnetic healing with hands-on manipulation, especially of the spine. The fact that Still established his School of Osteopathy in Kirksville, Missouri, in 1892, less than 150 miles from Davenport, Iowa, raises the question of whether there was any direct influence of Still on Palmer, that is, of osteopathy on chiropractic. One also could and should ask whether there was any reverse influence of Palmer on Still, that is, of chiropractic on osteopathy. As early as 1897 the *Journal of Osteopathy* charged (Bayer, 1945, p 30):

> There is one fake magnetic healer in Iowa who issued a paper devoted to his alleged new system, and who until recently made up his entire publication from the contents of the *Journal of Osteopathy,* changing it only to insert the name of his own practice.

Whether this allegation, which we may presume was directed at Palmer, was true, it is clear that D.D. was fully aware of osteopathy, for he wrote in 1899 (Lerner, 1954, p 27):

> I have taken lessons and studied Christian Science, Faith Cure, Mind Cure, Metaphysics, Magnetic, and Osteopathy, therefore I am acquainted with each and know their differences.

Osteopath Arthur Grant Hildreth (1938, pp 44–45) tells us:

> During the summer of 1893 . . . there came . . . a man who said his name was Palmer. The person, probably in his fifties, was a large, heavy set man with a dark brown beard. He came to Kirksville, it was said, to take treatment from Dr. Still. Dr. Still's daughter Blanche, now Mrs. George M. Laughlin, told me that this man Palmer was not only treated by her father, but also sat at the family table upon the invitation of the old Doctor. . . . Palmer took treatments from Dr. Still for a few weeks. He also talked with Dr. Still's students and was treated by many of them. When we next heard of him, he had "discovered" a method of treating disease by the hands, which he called chiropractic.

Charles Still also claimed that D.D. had been a guest in his father's home, and several Missouri chiropractors reported seeing D.D.'s name in the guest book at the Still homestead on the Kirksville campus. However, B.J. Palmer disagreed (Gibbons, 1980b, p 13): "My father never was in Kirksville, never attended that or any other osteopathic school. It is true that he met and talked with Andrew T. Still at Clinton, Iowa, at the spiritualist camp meeting on several occasions."

Osteopathy's first text, *Osteopathy Illustrated* (1899), was written by Andrew P. Davis, a homeopathic MD who had taught at Still's Kirksville college and in 1898 studied under Palmer. He later circulated "a deposition that Palmer had not 'stolen' his chiropractic tenets from Still's osteopathy. . . . Davis affirmed that there was no basic similarity between the two schools" (Dzaman, 1980, p 273). However, Brantingham (1986, p 21) writes: "Although Davis swore under oath that chiropractic and osteopathy were applied differently, he felt they were philosophically the same."

Both Palmer and Still agreed that osteopathy and chiropractic were different. Gaucher-Peslherbe concurs, and documents that D.D., despite not being formally educated or trained in medicine, was not the bumbling incompetent that medical writers have alleged him to be, but a self-taught near-genius who was well-read in the medical and scientific literature of his day. Gaucher (1992) claims that D.D.'s contribution went far beyond anything that the osteopaths had advanced:

> It is not difficult to show that osteopathy in the early stages was based on concepts that were very different from Palmer's. The techniques employed were essentially bone-setting and massage, and at first these were mainly used to treat cysts, lumps, gummy eyes and wax in the ears. These techniques were supplemented by long lever manipulation, as in the Swedish system. Onto this were grafted Beveridge's methods, probably through the influence of Drs. Smith and Littlejohn. Finally, a practice was introduced that was similar to Prof. Vedder's lymphatic drainage or the kind of massage used locally by Thure Brandt, in the specialized field of gynaecology. The purpose of these techniques was to relieve congestion of the blood. It is clear that in all these examples the treatment is based on the system of humors. There appears to have been a return to the Hippocratic conception of the humors, as it was understood throughout the eighteenth century. Palmer had nothing to learn from this, though the converse is not true!

Among those referred to in the quotation are Per Henrik Ling (1853), who in 1813 established the Swedish system of medical gymnastics (Northup, 1972, p 48), known also as "movement cure," and the two early associates of Still at his Kirksville college (William Smith and James Littlejohn), physicians from Scotland.

Support for Gaucher's allegation is provided by George Northup (1987, pp 12–17, Fig 6.2). Writing on the history of osteopathic research, he provides dates for osteopathy's first use of the terms "mediation of the sympathetic nervous system" (1936), "muscle reflex activity" (1941), "neural basis for somatic dysfunction" (1947), and "neuromuscular system" (1951). Gaucher (1992) goes even farther, arguing that chiropractic not only is not osteopathy and did not filiate from it, but that osteopathy incorporated concepts and techniques from chiropractic:

> A.T. Still never spoke about subluxations before the turn of the century. . . . Subluxation (the concept we know of) has only been naturalized as an osteopathic catchword from 1903 onwards.

Of course, this was D.D.'s position, and as usual he was meticulous in his documentation (1910, p 145): "I find in A.T. Still's book on Osteopathy of 319 pages, only seven lines which refer to vertebral displacements, and these are called twisted vertebrae." In his typical confrontational style he directly contradicted Still (1910, p 29): "The circulation of the blood and its quality depend upon the condition of the nervous system." He could find confirmation of this in the earlier works of Claude Bernard (1861) in Paris, which Walter B. Cannon (1934, p 21) described as showing "the nice control of the circulating blood by nerves." Lerner (1954, pp 91–92) cites evidence that the "blood vs. nerves" controversy antedated Still and Palmer.

Alfred Walton (1915, pp 30–31), an 1879 graduate of Harvard Medical School and faculty member at the University of Pennsylvania Medical College, became a D.C. and wrote at length about the differences between osteopathy and chiropractic:

> The point the Author desires to especially emphasize is, that the Osteopath is doing work in a circuitous, roundabout and bungling manner, depending very largely upon manipulation, whereas the (chiropractic) physician, by employing specific adjustments, could accomplish infinitely better results, and in one-tenth of the time. . . . An Osteopath will take from thirty minutes to an hour in rubbing the affected joints of a patient suffering from rheumatoid deformens, giving three treatments a week, not infrequently for months, before there is any material improvement; by employing chiropractic it is rare the patient does not respond favorably as a result of a few adjustments, each consuming less than a moment of time. . . . The Osteopath has no method of adjusting a specific vertebra, below the vertebra prominens, excepting by the use of the knee as above described. He manipulates muscles and joints in much the same manner as employed by Swedish movement operators.

In the same year Arthur Forster (1915, p 3), a faculty member at the National School of Chiropractic, wrote:

> Osteopathy claims that chiropractic is but a branch of that science. A careful review of osteopathic literature fails to disclose the slightest reference to any mode of treatment resembling the chiropractic thrust. And while it is true that recent books on osteopathy dwell at some length on the application of the chiropractic thrust, it is nevertheless a fact that osteopathy took no notice of it until chiropractors had popularized spinal adjustment sufficiently to make its use "worthwhile."

Chiropractic academician Clarence W. Weiant (1941, p 6) agreed:

> Modern osteopathy is the old chiropractic concept slightly modified and renamed, as may be verified by comparing recent encyclopedia articles on osteopathy with the original treatises of Still and then with chiropractic fundamentals.

Gaucher (1992) makes the broadest claim:

> A well founded demonstration could be made asserting that *every one of the modern occidental approaches to manipulation* draws its conceptual origins either from chiropractic or from what chiropractic evolved in the first place. (Note: Except "manipulative surgery," due to the fact that the patient is anesthetized.) This is true even for osteopa-

thy, the basic concepts of which have literally been "recentered" by the definition of chiropractic as outlined by D.D. Palmer.

Osteopathic sports physician Frederick Lewerenz, speaking in Boston in 1990 to a seminar on hospital privileges for chiropractors, emphasized that chiropractic adjustments and osteopathic spinal manipulation do not duplicate each other: although both use some of the same techniques and achieve some of the same results, the intent and purpose are different; osteopaths' goal is to promote circulation, increase range of motion, break up fixations, or remove muscle spasm, while chiropractors' primary goal is to move bones so as to reduce pressure on or irritation of nerves, with resulting effects on distal organs or tissues.

Inasmuch as Gaucher is a chiropractor as well as the recipient of a doctorate in the history of science, his parting shot at Still is understandable (1983, p 13);

> Still was no regular doctor but a plain healer and bonesetter who happened during the Civil War to be employed as a hospital steward. He finally decided to register as a medical doctor when a Missouri law allowed him to do so in 1874.

If D.D. had commenced practicing magnetic healing a few years earlier than 1886, like Still he might have been entitled to register as a physician under the grandfathering provisions of the 1887 Iowa medical practice act (Gielow, 1981, p 105). Whether he would have done so is debatable, in view of his strong hostility and criticism toward orthodox medical practice. Perhaps if he had been able to do so, his hostility and criticism would not have been so intense.

The upshot was that the osteopathic and chiropractic professions went their separate ways. While individual osteopaths like Andrew P. Davis investigated chiropractic and some chiropractors became osteopaths (or even MDs), formal linkage between the two professions did not occur in the United States. In other parts of the world—England, Canada, Australia, New Zealand, and some European countries—osteopaths remained more like chiropractors (Baer, 1984, 1987, 1991; Bolton, 1987; Coburn, 1991; Willis E, 1991). Brian Inglis (1964, p 116) notes that the term "osteopractic" was invented by Parnell Bradbury (1957, p 43) in England "to describe the synthesis of the two methods he employed," although the word actually had been used much earlier (Lewis CA, 1902).

Osteopathic colleges in the United States soon began adding standard medical subjects to the curriculum, despite Still's opposition expressed in his *Autobiography* (1897):

> No system of allopathy with its fatal drugs should enter our doors. No orificial surgery with its torture and disappointments to the afflicted, can possibly find an abiding place in the mind of the tried, true, and qualified osteopath.

For the noncognoscenti, Gaucher (1992) explains that orificial surgery involved "the anal introduction of a bougie and dilation until a vagotonic reaction was obtained, the strength of which had a direct relation to the benefit anticipated."

Surgery and obstetrics were incorporated into the Kirksville College curriculum in 1897, and the other colleges quickly followed suit (Gevitz, 1982, p 62). Far more controversial was inclusion of materia medica, which took much longer to achieve. While parts of the pharmacopoeia had long been taught in the more liberal schools under different topical headings, the issue divided the profession until 1929, when the AOA House of Delegates decided that a thoroughgoing course in comparative therapeutics, including pharmacology, would be offered by all schools. A compelling consideration was the desire for a broader scope of licensed practice, for which qualification in pharmacology was required.

Going this far set osteopathy on a course that would move it farther and farther from chiropractic and from reliance on osteopathic manipulative treatment (OMT) as its primary therapy. Yet as late as 1921 the American Osteopathic Association (AOA) convention resolved "that all osteopathic colleges be opened to those . . . with a high school diploma and eighteen months or more of chiropractic training, these individuals to be given nine or more months of advanced standing" (Gibbons, 1980b, pp 13–14). Since the standard osteopathic course at that time was 4 years of 9 months each (Gevitz, 1982b, p 52), while most chiropractors graduated after 18 months, that was not a very great concession to make; probably few chiropractors took advantage of it. Osteopathy continued to become more and more medical in its orientation, much to the dismay of the so-called "10-finger" or "lesion" osteopaths. Gevitz (1988, p 291) notes that "by the 1920s, spinal manipulation was associated more with chiropractic than with osteopathy, and there were more chiropractors legally and illegally in practice than DOs."

In the 1950s began the process leading to nearly complete acceptance of osteopaths into organized medicine, which included dropping restrictions on their scope of practice in all states, authorization in 1968 to enter medical internships and residencies (Blackstone, 1977; Osteopathy: Special Report of the Judicial Council to the AMA House of Delegates, 1961) and merger of some medical and osteopathic hospitals (Biggs, 1975). In 1953 Nelson Rockefeller's personal osteopath persuaded him to have the first osteopath commissioned in the U.S. Public Health Service and the uniformed services. According to *Time* magazine (July 28, 1958) the annual convention of the AOA voted to drop from its constitution the following adulatory sentence: "The evolution of osteopathic principles shall be an ever-growing tribute to Andrew Taylor Still."

Blackstone (1977) shows how the strategy of organized medicine shifted from a primarily economically motivated effort to exclude competitors to a more realistic concern with the quality of care and efforts to upgrade osteopathic education and practice. In 1961 a comprehensive "deal" resulted in merger of the California medical and osteopathic associations, transformation of the California College of Osteopathic Physicians and Surgeons into the University of California College of Medicine at Irvine, and the option for California DOs to be relicensed as MDs following a few hours of weekend "reeducation"; some 2,000 DOs did so, for a fee of $65. In 1963 a specially created College of Physicians and Surgeons in Washington State awarded M.D. degrees to 54 DOs after 12 Saturday afternoons of instruction, but the court quickly ended the subterfuge (Blackstone, 1977, p 420).

Osteopaths reacted strongly to medicine's efforts to eliminate them as a profession, and rebounded. Currently there are 15 osteopathic colleges, five of them in state-supported universities; several have both a medical school and an osteopathic school. By 1972, 128 osteopathic graduates were in medical residencies, and 1,108 osteopaths were in 229 medical hospitals (Blackstone, 1977, p 424). In 1987 there were 551 osteopaths in 3-year allopathic family medical programs, compared with 243 in the second year of an AOA-approved program; after 1989 the post-internship osteopathic residency requirement was increased from 1 to 2 years (Aquilina, 1990, p 161). By 1988, 2,150 osteopaths were in allopathic residencies (Etzel et al, 1990, p 1036). Consequently "many of the osteopathic physicians who took allopathic residencies have drifted away and dropped their affiliation with the AOA" (Cummings, 1990, p 356). In 1990 a proposal that the American Osteopathic Hospital Association (AOHA), which represents about 100 osteopathic hospitals, become part of the American Hospital Association (AHA) failed before it could be presented to the general meeting of the Association. However, osteopaths differ from allopaths today in name only, and osteopathic manipulative therapy occupies only a relatively minor place in the osteopathic curriculum. The only remaining question is: How long will the word "osteopathy" continue to be used?

Section 5

Naturopaths

Finally, I shall discuss naturopaths briefly. Although the Austrian Vincent Priessnitz (1799–1851) has been called "the first nature doctor" (Boyle, 1989, p 8), the term "naturopathy" "was coined in 1895 by Dr. John Scheel of New York City. . . . Lust purchased the term from Scheel in 1902 to describe the eclectic compilation of doctrines of natural healing that he envisioned was to be the future of natural medicine." Benjamin Lust (1872–1945) arrived in New York City from Germany in 1892, commissioned by Father Sebastian Kneipp to bring to the United States the water-cure system (hydrotherapy) he had developed at his Institute in Woershofen (*National Cyclopedia of American Biography,* 1945). Lust claimed that he had earned a D.O. degree in 1897 from Universal Osteopathic College, an M.D. degree in 1913 from Homeopathic Medical College, and another M.D. degree from Eclectic Medical College, all in New York City, but Fishbein (1932, p 122) wrote that he failed to produce any evidence of them on the witness stand. In 1905 he established the American School of Naturopathy, later the cooperating American School of Chiropractic, and still later schools of physiotherapy and massage. He founded the American Naturopathic Association, was president until 1921, and for many years published *Naturopath and the Herald of Health,* the official organ of the Naturopathic Association. Clearly he deserved his title, Father of Naturopathy. Other terms used somewhat interchangeably with naturopath were "drugless healer," "sanipractor," and "mechanotherapist," a term derived from Per Ling's (1853) Swedish system of exercises and health maintenance.

Today naturopathy emphasizes prevention, health maintenance, and treatment using methods and substances that encourage the body's natural self-healing processes, specifically, nutritional substances, botanical medicines, homeopathic remedies, manipulative therapy, acupuncture, minor surgery, and counseling. However, the naturopathic historian George Cody (1985, p I-1) states that "even in the halcyon days of the 1920's and 30's the profession was never able to agree upon a concise philosophy," and that there is a "lack of a definitive definition of the philosophical basis of natural medicine." Furthermore, naturopathic authors Joseph E. Pizzorno and Michael T. Murray (1985, pp I-1, V-1) admit that "no technical reference books currently exist in the English language on the pharmacology of natural medicines." Nevertheless, a principal attraction of naturopathy has been its emphasis on natural methods of eating, living, staying healthy, and treating disease, which for more than 150 years have been major themes in American popular culture. Reed (1932, p 62) found only about 1,500 naturopaths in the United States. Two remaining naturopathic colleges in Oregon and Washington award the N.D. degree after a 4-year course preceded by at least 2 years of preprofessional college credits.

Fishbein (1932, p 122) charged: "Naturopathy has been developed as an effort to give chiropractic something more to sell than adjustments of the spine." It is easy to see why chiropractic mixers often were accused of being naturopaths even when they were not. Certainly some chiropractors preferred an N.D. license, because it permitted them a broader scope of practice. That was also true in Canada (Coburn, 1991). The National School of Chiropractic in Chicago began offering the N.D. degree in 1920 (Evans HW, 1978), at which time it changed its name to the National School of Drugless Therapy. Later renamed the National College of Chiropractic, it granted its last N.D. and D.D.T. (Doctor of Drugless Therapy) degrees in 1952. Homola (1963, p 75) states that at least four chiropractic colleges were then offering the N.D. degree and that when the National Chiropractic Association prohibited this it was "a death-dealing blow to the profession of naturopathy."

"Naturopathy has had a stormy existence from the legal and legislative point of view," according to materials prepared for the Department of Health, Education, and Welfare study for Congress of whether they should be included under Medicare (Cohen WJ, 1968). At that time naturopaths could practice legally in only eight states plus the District of Columbia; licensing laws had been repealed in six other states. The study found only 553 licensed naturopaths in the United States, although others were known to be practicing unlicensed. The Cohen report recommended to Congress that naturopathy not be included under Medicare, and it never has been. Only one small college was then in operation, in Portland, Oregon. There has been a small resurgence of interest in the field, but since the two small colleges in Seattle and Portland produce fewer than a hundred new graduates each year, it is clear that naturopathy has lost out in competition with chiropractic.

Chapter 3

SOME BASIC CONCEPTS

When the medical profession practices spinal ma-
nipulation, they call it specialization. When chiro-
practors do it, it's called quackery. We've lived
with that "bad rap" for years.

Joseph Janse (Hartford Courant, Sept. 8, 1976)

A conceptual framework is needed for any analytic study. Mine is frankly sociological. But that does not require the introduction of difficult esoteric concepts. Sociology jargon is not used. The concepts I use are explained in simple language, which
does not make the ideas expressed less meaningful.

It is both an advantage and a disadvantage that sociology deals with the everyday
events of everyday people as well as with crises and catastrophes such as wars, rev-
olutions, economic depressions, strikes, crime, drugs, divorce, and such. For that
reason lay persons often accuse sociology of being nothing more than common sense
that all people know or could figure out for themselves. On the other hand, they frequently misconstrue some of the terminology that sociologists use for precise conceptual analysis (e.g., "role," "status," "class," "organization"), because they do not understand or they forget their precise definitions, with the result that for them the ideas
being advanced may seem trivial or meaningless. Several basic concepts are used
throughout this book; their specific relevance for my analysis are covered in the remainder of this chapter.

Section 1

Medical Establishment

In every complex society an established elite dominates. In the political sphere it may
be the royal family, aristocracy, oligarchy, bourgeoisie, military, state bureaucracy,
or the entrenched politicians of a republic. In the fields of science and education it is

the prestigious universities, scientists, scholars, writers, and the public and private institutions that fund them. In that branch of science concerned with health there is the *medical establishment* with its multifaceted political and economic affiliations. Politically it is represented by such organizations as the American Medical Association (AMA) with its many affiliated organizations and associations, the Joint Commission on Accreditation of Hospitals (JCAH), the United States Public Health Service (USPHS), the National Institutes of Health (NIH), the medical departments of the military and the Veterans Administration, and the public health departments of cities and states. It is closely allied politically with associations of other health professionals (e.g., osteopaths, dentists, nurses, podiatrists, optometrists, physical therapists), although sometimes these groups find themselves in conflict with the AMA (which is the "point" of the medical establishment) and ally themselves with each other and sometimes even with chiropractors against it. When legislative bodies, courts, or elected officials seek expert opinion regarding health care they automatically turn to representatives of the medical establishment.

Much has been written about medical dominance, both over other providers and organizations and over the entire society, when questions of health care are raised. In the economic sphere organized medicine is integrated with profitable and powerful pharmaceutical and biotechnology corporations. And it receives substantial financial support from public funds and wealthy charitable foundations, as well as from the many voluntary associations (e.g., American Heart Association, American Cancer Society, American Kidney Association, Arthritis Foundation), whose effective marketing strategies persuade those affected by these diseases and others to donate funds. NIH provides the major financial support for medical research. Hospitals receive and spend the largest share of health care dollars in the United States and along with the AMA and insurance companies drive the health care market. Every employer bemoans the increasing costs of employee health insurance and of accident and pollution prevention. The expenses and profits of health and liability insurance dominate the insurance industry, which seeks ever more effective strategies to market group health plans, Health Maintenance Organizations (HMOs), and Preferred Provider Organizations (PPOs) to employers, employees, and union officials. Since money talks, these economic linkages further strengthen the political power and dominance of the medical establishment.

Many researchers have studied these linkages (Baer, 1989b; Berlant, 1975; Blackstone, 1977; Freidson, 1970a; Hyde and Wolff, 1954 pp 963–967; Raayack, 1967; Starr, 1982; Willis E, 1983). It would be important to learn who really calls the shots. It is certainly no longer so simple as Dr. J.F. Baldwin's statement, "The hand that rocks the vaccine factory is the hand that rocks the medical profession," which caused his ouster from the presidency of the Ohio State Medical Society in the 1920s (Turner, 1931, p 74). But that is not the topic of this book. Nor is the increasing tendency for health professionals to become "bureaucratized," that is, salaried and subordinate to nonmedical administrators, which Gilb (1966, p 231) sees as a reversion to a society based more on fixed status than on free contract, calling it "neo-medievalism." Suffice it to know that a medical establishment exists in the United States and that it dominates health care politically and economically. This incontrovertible fact has to be taken into account by other health care providers, government officials, insurance companies, employers, unions, ordinary citizens, and particularly by those who attempt to confront it, change it, or survive under it.

The definitive sociologic study of interacting professions as a system is that by Andrew Abbott (1988, pp 135–139), who analyzes the origin, growth, division, and fusion of professions as they compete with each other over "workplace jurisdictions." Although he mentions chiropractic only briefly, his analysis is appropriate to understanding chiropractic's relationships with other professions, especially medicine. He defines professional power as "the ability to retain jurisdiction when system forces imply that a profession ought to have lost it," and he argues that "jurisdictional invasion generally begins in the workplace, then moves to the public mind, and then into the law." He even notes how long it usually takes for the system to equilibrate after a jurisdictional challenge:

> Jurisdictions are renegotiated in workplaces over two- to three-year periods, in (the public's mind) over ten- to twenty-year periods, in the law over twenty- to fifty-year periods.

His time frame fits chiropractic quite well.

Dr. Benjamin Rush, signer of the Declaration of Independence, wrote (cited by Booth, 1905, p 313):

> The Constitution of this Republic should make specific provision for medical freedom as well as for religious freedom. To restrict the practice of the art of healing to one class of physicians and deny to others equal privileges constitutes the Bastilles of our science. All such laws are un-American and despotic. They are vestiges of monarchy and have no place in a republic.

Historian Richard Shryock (1966) sarcastically commented that this principle gave every American the "inalienable right to life, liberty, and quackery."

Chiropractors have been acutely aware of the medical establishment and have been forced to design strategies, both as individual practitioners and in association, to cope with it. It is impossible to understand chiropractors' behavior or the evolution of their movement without recognizing its overwhelming influence. Furthermore, interactions between MDs and chiropractors continue to occur within the context of the legal, political, economic, and scientific dominance of the medical establishment.

Section 2

A Marginal Profession

The sociologist Robert Park (1928) introduced the term "marginal man" to characterize the plight of a second-generation immigrant caught between American culture and
his culture of origin. He described him as "a cultural hybrid, a man living and sharing intimately in the cultural life and traditions of two distinct peoples." Everett
Stonequist further developed the concept in his book *The Marginal Man: A Study in
Personality and Culture Conflict* (1937), when he asserted that "in looking at himself
from the standpoint of each group he experiences the conflict as a personal problem."
However, a later writer (Goldberg, 1941) pointed out that marginal cultures often fur-
nish psychologic security and "adequate facilities for participating in group life."

In my doctoral dissertation (Wardwell, 1951), using interviews with Massachusetts chiropractors, I adapted this concept to the chiropractic profession. I contended
that marginality results not only from being located *between* two cultures, but occurs
whenever the occupants of any social role are denied rights and responsibilities attrib-
utable to it. I used as an example the plight of the southern black, whose rights as a
citizen were then more often denied him, sometimes de facto, as when it was difficult
for him to register to vote or receive equal treatment from the police and the courts,
and sometimes legally, as with segregation in public schools and laws prohibiting racial intermarriage. I argued that southern blacks clearly were "marginal" in their cit-
izenship role at that time. They were not in conflict over whether they wanted to be
full members of American society or of a lower class subculture. Their marginality
was yet real and oppressed them. Numerous studies have documented the deleterious
psychologic effects of such marginality, even when legal (Brown vs. Topeka Board
of Education, 1954, 347 U.S. 483; Myrdal, 1944).

I argued that chiropractors could similarly be characterized as occupying a *marginal professional role* vis-a-vis the medical profession. They were not in conflict
over whether they wanted to be fully accepted as autonomous health care providers.
Nor were they attracted to any other health care role that they conceivably might have
filled, and certainly not subordinate to the MD, like a nurse. And they suffered frustration and other psychologic problems in coping with their marginal role.

When I interviewed chiropractors in Massachusetts in the late 1940s they had not
yet obtained licensure. Because the Massachusetts Supreme Court had ruled in 1915
that chiropractic is the practice of medicine and therefore falls under the medical
practice acts, they were subject to arrest and prosecution at any time for "practicing
medicine without a license." It was clear that they occupied a marginal professional
status in that state, even though they may not then have been representative of most
of the rest of the country, where chiropractors' legal and social standing often were
better. I considered them marginal in five ways: (1) professional education and training, less than that of MDs, (2) scope of practice, more restricted than that of an MD,
(3) legal status, which was nil, (4) income, sometimes so low that it forced them out

of practice or into other part-time employment, and (5) overall social standing, which, due to the preceding disadvantages, was inferior to that of MDs.

I have been criticized by some writers for applying the word "marginal" to chiropractors, usually by those researchers who found chiropractors to be fully or nearly fully accepted and without serious problems (e.g., Coulter I, 1983, 1991; Rosenthal S, 1981). However, I still insist that at the time and place I did my initial research it was an appropriate designation. I was aware that Massachusetts could be considered an extreme case and that chiropractors in other states were usually better off. But I also knew that in some other parts of the country, and especially in earlier years, the plight of chiropractors had been just as bad. Furthermore, it is often an effective research strategy to focus on extreme cases, as psychologists do when studying psychopathology. I still believe my original study illuminated the difficulties faced by the profession as a whole because of its marginality and the opposition it faced in seeking full recognition. Obviously, "marginality" is a matter of degree and therefore is better used as a dimension of analysis rather than as a black-or-white appellation.

Section 3

Classification of Health Professions

In my next major piece on chiropractors (Wardwell, 1963) I placed marginal professions in a larger classificatory scheme that included all of the health-related professions. Using the medical professions as the touchstone, I placed each of them in one of four categories:

1. *Ancillary professions,* called "auxiliary professions" by Brian Inglis (1964), are dependent on physician direction, prescription, or supervision. The prototype is the nurse; others include pharmacists, physical therapists, occupational therapists, laboratory technicians, and the many other aides to physicians. As long as ancillaries remain "in their place" subservient to MDs, the AMA remains content with the unequal relationship. Typically trained only to the bachelor degree level (lower in the case of most nurses and some others), several of these professionals (especially nurses and physical therapists) recently have expanded their scope of practice, lengthening and strengthening their college curricula, winning legal rights to more autonomous practice, and hence encroaching on MDs' turf. Despite predictable resistance and hostility from the AMA, they usually have succeeded. What is important for the purpose of any classification, however, is that categories be clearly defined, not that there be no intermediate or doubtful placement in them of particular cases.

2. *Limited* (or *limited medical*) *professions* (called Limited License Practitioners in Medicare regulations) are autonomous health-related professions that restrict their practices to part of the human body and, compared with MDs, limit the range of pro-

cedures, instruments, or techniques they use in treatment. The best examples are dentists, podiatrists, optometrists, psychologists, speech therapists, and audiologists. Referral by an MD is not required, but each profession needs to be able to screen patients for conditions beyond its scope of practice so that patients can be referred to another profession when necessary.

Although historically there have been conflicts between dentists and surgeons, optometrists and ophthalmologists, psychologists and psychiatrists over the precise boundaries defining scopes of practice, medicine has no basic conflicts of interest (except economic) with limited medical professions. Unlike marginal professions (see below), limited professions do not challenge medicine's fundamental principles. They do not advance a different or contradictory theory of disease and therapy, as chiropractors have done. And they accept the superiority of the MD in treating systemic conditions or major complications. Hence limited professions have established a reasonably stable modus vivendi with the dominant medical profession.

3. *Marginal professions,* of which chiropractic has been the prime example, neither accept the right of MDs to supervise their practice, as ancillary professions do, nor, like limited professions, limit their treatments to one body part or system of the body. Chiropractors, naturopaths, and originally osteopaths historically claimed the right to use nearly all therapies except drugs and surgery for a broad range of illnesses. Furthermore, they originally denied the validity of orthodox medicine's theories of illness and therapy and propounded contrasting theories. Therefore relationships between them and orthodox medicine have been full of conflict and rancor. On the defensive and decried as "outsiders," marginal professionals have had to persuade potential patients that they offer a different or better service than MDs; and they always have attracted patients who were unable to obtain cure or relief from orthodox medicine. Osteopathy has evolved into something quite different over the past few decades. It now could be called a *parallel* profession to medicine, in that osteopaths still insist on their distinctiveness, although they are the formal equals of allopaths.

4. *Quasi professions* comprise a variety of healers whose methods cannot be empirically validated and whose benefits therefore are presumed to be primarily due to suggestion. My intent is not to demean suggestion (e.g., hypnosis, placebos) as a therapeutic technique but to create a residual category for faith healers (e.g., Christian Scientists), shamans (primitive healers who rely on magic), and quacks. Quacks differ from the others in that they *pretend* to be scientific and use *natural* forces (e.g., drugs or electronic devices) rather than *supernatural* forces to effect cures (Holbrook, 1959). Caplan (1987) notes that "in 1986 alone Americans paid over $10 billion to unscrupulous providers of fraudulent medical therapies, remedies, and gadgets. I mention the category of quasi professions primarily to exclude it from further consideration. Although these healers are of great interest to social scientists, they are tangential to my concerns here. Certainly all therapy involves suggestion, especially inoculation, surgery, and vigorous or painful manipulation. And all clinicians and researchers recognize the effectiveness of placebos. While the benefits of chiropractic

adjustments have sometimes been alleged by its critics to be due *solely* to suggestion, no chiropractic, osteopathic, or medical manipulator would agree. Nor do I. Manipulators belong in an entirely different category from the quasi professionals whose benefits are due *only* to suggestion.

Section 4

Solidarity vs. Group Conflict

All social groups, families, gangs, clubs, communities, societies, and political pressure groups exhibit cohesiveness, or solidarity; that is, they are to some degree "solidary" (not "solid"). Sharing common values, beliefs, and practices, they normally also possess internal organization involving differences in power and influence (i.e., leaders and followers). The "we-feeling" of a solidary group coexists with "they-feeling" toward outsiders. Although it is not inevitable that there be overt hostility between groups, the we-feeling sensitizes the members of both groups to differences between them, so that whenever there are goods, benefits, or other advantages at stake, competition or even violent conflict often follows. As a general rule, group solidarity increases when external threats must be faced. When outside challenges diminish, group solidarity may decrease. Far from claiming, as some theorists have, that conflict is the original basis of all group cohesion ("war created society"), it is nevertheless true that one of the "functions of social conflict" is to promote the solidarity and sometimes even the survival of a group. The sociologist Lewis Coser used that phrase as the title of his book (1956), no doubt unaware that B.J. Palmer had anticipated some of his ideas in an essay titled *Conflicts Clarify* (1951b).

Chiropractors have always been in conflict with the medical establishment. D.D. Palmer was arrested and convicted in 1906 for practicing medicine without a license. Chiropractors' early efforts to obtain licensure were opposed by medical authorities, who by 1922 had adopted the slogan "Chiropractic must die" (Reed, 1932, p 35). In 1987 Judge Susan Getzendanner found in the Wilk (1976) case:

> As early as September 1963, the AMA's objective was the complete elimination of the chiropractic profession. In November of 1963, the AMA authorized the formation of the Committee on Quackery under the AMA's Department of Investigation.

> In 1964, the Committee's primary goal was to contain and eliminate chiropractic . . . The Committee worked aggressively to achieve its goals in several areas. It conducted nationwide conferences on chiropractic; prepared and distributed numerous publications critical of chiropractic; assisted others in the preparation and distribution of anti-chiropractic literature; regularly communicated with medical boards and associations, warning that professional association between medical physicians and chiropractors was unethical; and attempted to discourage colleges, universities, and faculty members from cooperating with chiropractic schools.

In 1967 the AMA Judicial Council issued an opinion under Principle 3 specifically holding that it was unethical for a physician to associate professionally with chiropractors. "Associating professionally" would include making referrals of patients to chiropractors, providing diagnostic, laboratory, or radiology services for chiropractors, teaching chiropractors, or practicing together in any form. This opinion was published in the 1969 Opinions and Reports of the Judicial Council of the AMA ("1969 Opinions"), which was widely circulated to members of the AMA. The opinion on chiropractic was also sent by the AMA to 56 medical specialty boards and associations.

In 1973, the AMA drafted Standard X, which incorporated the unscientific practitioners ethics bar into the JCAH hospital accrediting standards. The AMA urged JCAH to adopt Standard X, and JCAH complied.

There were also many conflicts *within* the chiropractic profession, beginning in 1903 when Solon Langworthy opened his American School of Chiropractic and Nature Cure, in Cedar Rapids, Iowa, disagreeing with the Palmers over chiropractic philosophy and competing with them for students (Gibbons, 1981b). Disputes between father D.D. and son B.J. culminated in B.J.'s purchase of the school in 1906 and his father's humiliating departure from Davenport. Hostilities between rival schools and rival professional associations have always plagued the chiropractic profession. B.J. fostered both tremendous loyalty among his followers and an equal amount of hostility between himself and many other chiropractors.

Despite the rivalry between the followers of B.J. and those of his rivals, which weakened the profession, there usually was enough solidarity to unite it against the medical "enemy." If there had not been, it would have been nearly impossible to obtain any licensing legislation. The chiropractors who predominated in a particular state often obtained legislation favoring their preferred scope of chiropractic practice. As a result, even today some states are known as "straight" states and permit only a narrow scope of practice, whereas other states, historically dominated by "mixers," permit a broad scope of practice. For example, the adjacent states of Oregon and Washington differ considerably in their legislated scope of chiropractic practice: Washington is straight; Oregon permits chiropractors to perform minor surgery, cast simple fractures, deliver babies, and prescribe homeopathic medicines. From a national perspective the profession remains divided and sometimes in bitter conflict over what its proper scope of practice should be.

Section 5

Charismatic Leadership

The word "charisma" comes from ancient Greek and means "gift of grace" or "touch of the divine." Jesus was the prime example of one so gifted. His personal qualities inspired others to follow him and abide by his will. Max Weber (1947), the great

German sociologist of religion and of political structures, popularized using the concept for leaders of all types who garner authority to themselves. He contrasted it with two other types of authority: "traditional," that of parents over their children or of a king over his subjects, and "official," that wielded by a bureaucrat holding an office in an organization of appointed officials. Today the attribution of personal charisma often is made when a leader exhibits personal qualities that enable him to persuade others to follow him into new paths, especially in new social movements.

Chiropractic can be conceptualized as a social movement, now no longer new, in the health field. Obviously it did not spring from the head of Zeus already formed, but incorporated some preexisting elements from diverse sources. But it probably would not have been begun, developed, or survived had it not been for the charisma of its leaders. First was D.D. himself. Although involved in the Davenport scene only until 1906, during that period he was a true pioneer. From very little he created an original theory of illness and treatment, founded an infirmary and school, attracted students, many from other health fields, and published a sizable treatise on his new therapy (Palmer D.D., and Palmer B.J., 1906). After leaving Davenport he founded other chiropractic schools in California, Oklahoma, and Oregon. Like many other charismatic leaders, he was not an effective administrator, and possessed of a fiery temper and a contentious disposition, he frequently clashed with those (especially MDs) with whom he established schools.

B.J. was far more effective than his father in strengthening the Palmer School and leading the movement. He not only had the charismatic personal qualities that attracted others and inspired them to devote time, money, and energy to the cause, but also had the administrative talents required to build and ensure the survival of chiropractic. In some ways he was as difficult a personality as his father, often crude and insensitive; but history documents that he built Palmer School of Chiropractic (PSC) into the largest training institution for health practitioners in the United States and that he motivated thousands of chiropractors, most of them PSC alumni, to support and perpetuate chiropractic. Without him chiropractic might well not have survived. The assumption that if there had not been a B.J. someone else would have appeared to do what he did cannot, of course, be tested.

The fate of naturopathy provides a contrasting example. For many years it was taught alongside chiropractic, often in the same schools. The word "naturopathy" itself would have been, it seems to me, a more appealing name for the new profession than "chiropractic," a cumbersome term that so upset chiropodists that they changed their name to "podiatrists." The broader scope of naturopathic practice, incorporating all the "natural" remedies (heat, cold, water, exercise, whole-grain foods, and herbal remedies), would seem to have been a more attractive designation to both patients and practitioners. But it was not to be. D.D.'s conception persisted and defined what chiropractic was. Although mixers have always existed in large numbers, without B.J. there almost certainly would not be any straight chiropractic today, and perhaps not any chiropractic at all. B.J. made the difference because he was such an effective charismatic leader. His devoted followers awaited his most recent pronouncements at

PSC Lyceums, or "homecomings" (reunions of alumni), in Davenport with bated breath, and they dutifully adopted the newest devices and techniques he proposed (e.g., improved adjusting tables and x-ray machines, new diagnostic instruments, and his controversial HIO ["hole-in-one"] cervical adjusting technique). Only with his introduction in 1924 of an instrument called a neurocalometer (NCM), intended for diagnosing vertebral subluxations, did he seriously misjudge the extent of his authority over his followers. Nor could his opponents ignore him. They always had to explain where, how, and why they differed from B.J. He was the dominant figure in chiropractic throughout his lifetime. Although he amassed the greater part of his wealth from investments in land and the communications industry (radio and later television), his involvement in chiropractic was all-consuming for him and decisive for it.

Section 6

Chiropractic Theory and "Philosophy"

The phrase "chiropractic philosophy" is a misnomer. Not only most chiropractors but also most laypersons are unfamiliar with the precise distinction between philosophy and scientific theory. The mysteries of epistemology (i.e., the theory of knowledge, including science) are only beginning to be understood by chiropractic writers (see, however, Keating, 1989a). Most basic scientists teaching at chiropractic colleges know what empirical science is, but there has been such a complete division of labor between them and the teachers of chiropractic principles and philosophy that students often have not learned the essential difference between philosophy and scientific theory.

The words "theory" and "fact" also are misunderstood by most laypersons. An example is the debate over whether gravity is a theory or a fact. Phrasing the question that way reveals gross ignorance of the nature of scientific theory. A fact can only be a discrete "event" observable by one of the bodily senses, ideally quantifiable, and, it is hoped, agreed on by observers (Henderson, 1932; Whitehead, 1925). For example, an object of a certain mass falling from a certain height will attain a certain velocity at Earth's sea level. Many such events, or facts, permitted scientists to formulate a *theory* of gravitation, which was modified later by other theorists, such as Einstein. When the falling body is that of a human falling from a high bridge into the water, a different set of concepts is required for scientific analysis of the event: Was the fall accidental? Was the person pushed? Or did he jump? If so, why? And was the falling body alive or dead when it hit the water? The "fact" of falling must now be conceptualized in physiologic or psychologic terms rather than in those of physics (mass, velocity, acceleration).

Yet D.D. (1910, p 407) and Dye (1939, p 301) talk about the transition of chiropractic from a "logical theory" to proved "scientific facts." Even the well-educated chiropractor Willard Carver showed his ignorance of proper usage in a letter he wrote to Dr. H.K. Maxwell in 1940, a copy of which is in my possession:

> The fundamental of Chiropractic has never been disproved for the good and sufficient reason that it is an ultimate fact, and ultimate facts are not capable of proof "beyond a doubt," and are always incapable of disproof, because they are beyond the realm of empirical test . . . A science must be based upon a *primary ultimate fact,* and the systematization and classification that constitutes the science, must be deduced from that ultimate principle or fact.

He was, of course, confusing knowledge based on faith or intuition with scientific theory validated by empirical data, or facts.

A theoretical statement always postulates in hypothetical terms (usually in "if . . . then . . ." form) a consistent relationship between two variables such as mass and velocity, or depression and suicide, which can be verified or invalidated by systematic observation and evaluation of the relationships between facts (events). This constitutes research. Repeated validation under experimentally controlled conditions is required before a new scientific theory can be accepted as well-established. It does not then become a "fact," but forever remains a theoretical proposition capable of being rejected or modified later, as Albert Einstein did for Sir Isaac Newton. The process must conform to the rules of inductive logic, typified by the controlled experiment and approximations of it. There is a role for deductive reasoning from scientific principles that already have been established, as when predicting what later experiments or observations may be expected to reveal, but in science *not* for deduction from "first principles," such as God or the presumed certainty that subluxations exist.

The oft-heard injunction that research should be done to "prove chiropractic" offends scientific sensibilities. Research done to "prove" something is always suspect because the researcher's bias is clear. Most researchers usually *hope* to validate their hypotheses, and some intentionally or unintentionally improperly find what they seek, but the only legitimate scientific stance is an open mind and absolute objectivity regarding findings.

Philosophy, on the other hand, goes beyond observable facts and seeks answers to the most fundamental questions underlying science itself. Leaving aside its popular meaning as one's view of the world or personal *Weltanschauung,* technically philosophy asks: What is the nature of truth (epistemology), reality (metaphysics), the good (ethics), and the beautiful (aesthetics)? None of these is susceptible to empirical scientific inquiry. They are *meta-scientific;* that is, they go beyond empirical science. Logic is a special technique for reasoning deductively or inductively, but does not by itself add to empirical knowledge. A scientist needs to be aware of the philosophic assumptions underlying his conceptions of reality and truth, especially those of science itself, but should not confuse them with his search for scientific truths, which are never absolute but remain forever tentative and approximate. I hope I have not insulted the sophistication of readers to whom these ideas are already familiar; they are intended only for those who may benefit.

My conception of chiropractic theory is that it is *a body of interrelated empirically verifiable propositions about the effects of inhibition or stimulation of nerves, especially spinal nerves, and of faulty spinal biomechanics on other body tissues or functioning*. I believe that statement is simple enough for laypersons like myself to comprehend. In principle every proposition comprising a scientific theory should be empirically testable, and the evidence for or against it should accumulate as appropriate laboratory and/or clinical observations/tests/experiments are conducted and reported to research peers in professional meetings and journals. Such specific propositions constitute the substance of what is taught in academic courses in chiropractic science and then applied in clinical practice (sometimes called "art"). They are not philosophy, and there should be no mystery about them. Both the philosophy and the scientific theory of chiropractic are discussed further in Chapter 9.

Scientific theorists use models and paradigms to integrate better the isolated propositions they establish. There is no reason why chiropractors, while accepting many of the paradigms used in modern medicine, should not develop and use their own different chiropractic paradigms. Among those that come to mind are paradigms emphasizing homeostasis (the body's tendency to cure itself), the greater importance of the healthy host vs. germs and bacteria, the crucial role played by nutrition and life-style in maintaining health and preventing illness—in sum, a much greater emphasis on disease prevention and health maintenance than is found in traditional medical paradigms. Chiropractor Joseph Janse (1976, p 18) was explicit about this last point: "The ultimate goal in any program toward public wellbeing should be prevention rather than cure." Unfortunately, the chiropractic paradigm regarding health maintenance and disease prevention has been generally misunderstood.

Chapter 4

THE PALMERS AND THEIR FOUNTAINHEAD SCHOOL

*Chiropractic will not be a properly constituted sci-
ence until it can disentangle itself from its history,
but neither last long as a science if it does not accept the truth about this history.*

Pierre-Louis Gaucher-Peslherbe (1992)

The early history of chiropractic centers around leaders who developed particular chiropractic theories and techniques. Usually they organized their own schools, wrote books, and acquired supporters. The most important of these were D.D. and B.J. Palmer.

Section 1

Daniel David Palmer (1845–1913)

Daniel David Palmer (D.D.) was born in 1845 in a frontier log cabin in Port Perry, Ontario. His father, Thomas, had been in turn a shoemaker, grocer, schoolteacher, and postmaster. D.D. wrote concerning his parents (1910, p 17):

> My ancestors were Scotch and Irish on my maternal and English and German on my paternal side . . . When I was a baby I was cradled in a piece of hemlock bark. My mother was as full of superstition as an egg is full of meat, but my father was disposed to reason on the subjects pertaining to life.

D.D. later did much reasoning on subjects pertaining to life. Vern Gielow (1981, p 4) wrote: "According to Thomas J. Palmer's autobiography, T.J. and D.D. were educated by a brutish country school taskmaster, John Black." Although D.D.'s formal education was limited and intermittent, apparently it continued into his teen years. When he was 20 he and Thomas emigrated penniless to the United States. (Thomas later edited several newspapers and produced an autobiography titled *Thomas J. Palmer, Frontier Publicist.*) Within a year D.D. became schoolmaster of a one-room school in Muscatine County, Iowa (which in those days often was an early occupation of future doctors, lawyers, and clergy [Abbott, 1991, p 132]), and continued teaching in several other schools through 1871. His journal reveals his developing personality and character (Gielow, 1981, pp 9–11):

> One difficulty at a time is enough for a child. . . . Proceed from the known to the unknown. . . . Never tell a child what he or she can discover for itself. [Note the nonsexist choice of words!]. . . . Do not ring or rap long when calling school. . . . Use persuasion to get large boys to quit using tobacco. . . . The best physicians are Dr. Diet, Dr. Quiet, and Dr. Merryman.

In 1871 D.D. married Abba Lord in Aledo, Illinois, a village near the Mississippi River port of New Boston. In the same year he purchased 10 acres of upland, planted dozens of fruit and evergreen trees, and became a commercial apiarist, increasing his hives to 209 by 1880. By 1874 he had developed a new variety of raspberry bushes, which he named "Sweet Home" after his homestead and which, with other bushes and fruit trees, he marketed from Massachusetts to California. His journal for 1881 indicates that the cold weather killed all his bees, and Mercer County land records show that he sold all his farm property for $1,000 in the same year.

D.D. next moved to What Cheer, Iowa, where his parents had migrated and where his brother Thomas was publishing the What Cheer *Patriot.* He opened a grocery store, and also sold both local and tropical fish, which is apparently why Morris Fishbein, editor of the *Journal of the American Medical Association,* denegrated him as a "fishmonger." He also continued to teach school during some of these years. He and Abba Lord divorced in 1873, and in 1874 he married Louvenia Landers, who died in 1884, 2 years after B.J. was born. Next he married Martha A. Henning, who died or left the marriage within 2 or 3 years. In 1888 he took his fourth wife, Villa Amanda Thomas, who became his active helpmate in caring for patients needing lodging or overnight care.

Simultaneously with his entrepreneurial activities he was investigating spiritualism, then becoming popular in New Boston. By 1880 he had already written a brochure on it, and characteristically warring with others, claimed that he would "expose the Mott swindle" (Gielow, 1981, p 24). Although he retained a lifetime interest in spiritualism, he soon shifted his attention to magnetic healing. Influenced perhaps by the outstandingly successful Paul Caster in nearby Ottumwa, he began intensive study of magnetic healing and of other areas of health care. Joseph Donahue (1987, p 23) concludes that D.D.'s involvement in spiritualism in the 1870s led him into magnetic healing in the 1880s. In 1886 he went into practice in Burlington, Iowa, where the City Directory listed him as "D.D. Palmer, Vital Healer." He soon moved to the bustling Mississippi River port of Davenport, Iowa, and in 1887 placed the following advertisement in the Davenport Directory:

D.D. Palmer
Cures without Medicine
Ryan Block Building
Publisher of *The Educator*

In the following year he expanded his advertisement to read (Gielow, 1981, pp, 47–48):

> Where can you get cured quicker or for less money, and without making a drugstore of yourself? It may not be popular to be cured without medicine, so who cares so the sick will get well? . . . Consultations and treatment for the deserving poor are free. Price of treatment $1 each at my rooms; $2 to $5 at patient's residence.

In 1888 D.D. listed his expenses for 30,000 circulars and cards, $75; five signs, $26.50, including three to be put on boats; and 100 photos (of what, he does not record), $9. In addition to *The Educator,* in 1889 he printed at least 15,000 copies of his brochure *The Sick Get Well by Magnetism.* By 1991 he had changed his advertisement to read: "Dr. Palmer: Cures with His Magnetic Hands" (Lerner, 1954, p 26).

His practice flourished. He kept hours from 1:00 to 6:00 PM, and it is reported that he saw 90 to 100 patients daily. He records that he had possessed the gift of magnetic healing for 17 years, and in the "last three years he has given his whole attention to the curing of the sick" (Gielow, 1981, p 52). His grandson Daniel David Palmer II (usually referred to in the profession as Dave) described D.D.'s method of healing as follows (cited in Gielow, 1981, p 57):

> He would develop a sense of being positive within his own body; sickness being negative. He would draw his hands over the area of the pain and with a sweeping motion stand aside, shaking his hand and fingers vigorously, taking away the pain as if it were drops of water.

However, a textbook on magnetic healing discovered by Gielow (1981, p 53) in D.D.'s library clearly recommends more than mere "passes" over the patient's body; here are some examples:

1. Make passes from *heated or inflamed parts,* toward the extremities or cold parts.
2. Give a new tide of life to *cold negative parts, by holding, rubbing or spatting* [patting?] *them. Place the right hand,* which is positive, on the hot part, and the *left, or negative hand,* on the cool, on the principle that forces flow from positive to negative. Reverse this order in thoroughly lefthanded persons. . . .
7. If there is *Inflammation at the Lungs, Heart, Kidneys,* etc., do not manipulate directly over the place, but at a little distance off. . . .
10. *To tone up the muscular system,* rub thoroughly the upper back head, and just below the neck over the brachial plexus. . . . *To quicken a dull intellect, rub the forehead, brows, and temples. To animate the moral powers,* rub the top and front head. *To scatter heat in the passional region,* pass from the back head and neck, down the shoulders and arms. . . .
12. For *Convulsions, Apoplexy, Sunstroke,* etc., rub the back head and neck and spine

powerfully, heat the feet, pour water hot as can be borne for five minutes or more on the back head and neck, etc.

His brother Thomas described D.D.'s practice about 1891 in his What Cheer *Patriot* as follows (Gielow, 1981, pp 57–58):

> Dr. Palmer is making some money at least. His income from his treatments alone is from $15 to $30 per day, and he often turns off some, as he has all he can treat from 8 AM to 10 or 11 PM. He sets a ten foot table full of patients and now runs seventeen beds which are usually full. He has fourteen rooms which are crowded. . . . He has been in Davenport over four years and must be making some cures to work up such a practice. His cures are made by the use of his hands only. He treats the cause of disease and not the effects. . . . He wants cases which other doctors cannot cure, and judging by the ones I saw there, he certainly gets them. His rooms look like a hospital. He actually cures tumors and cancers without the use of the knife or medicine, some of which I saw cured while I was there. Female weakness he cures in a few days, at least so his patients state. Rheumatism, neuralgia, lame backs, sprains and the like are daily cures. Diseases of the stomach, heart and kidneys are found among his patients any day and as they testify are being cured. . . . His patients are mostly from the three cities, but many are from a distance, who board and sleep at the Infirmary. . . . His patients are of all classes, rich and poor, doctors, druggists, preachers and all classes, who cannot be cured by their family physicians. He does not cure all kinds of diseases, nor all persons, but the most of his patients are cured.

D.D.'s offices were decorated with an elaborate collection of mounted heads, antlers, and a set of ram's horns measuring 10 feet tip to tip. According to his grandson David Daniel Palmer (1967, pp 12–13), D.D. characterized this period of his life as follows:

> In 1886 I began healing as a business. Although I practiced under the name of magnetic, I did not slap or rub, as others. I questioned many MDs as to the cause of disease. I desired to know why such a person had asthma, rheumatism, or other afflictions. I wished to know what differences there were in two persons that caused one to have certain symptoms called disease, which his neighbor living under the same conditions did not have. . . . In my practice of the first 10 years which I named magnetic, I treated nerves, followed and relieved them of inflammation. I made many good cures, as many are doing today under a similar method.

Dye (1939, p 14) tells us that during this period D.D. sometimes also wrote prescriptions for drugs that were filled at local pharmacies, although he may not have had the legal right to do so. Although he minimized his knowledge of bonesetting, he clearly was familiar with it (Palmer, 1910, p 203). According to Lerner (1954, pp 27, 49), D.D. claimed in an 1899 publication that he had studied "Christian Science, Faith Cure, Mind Cure, Metaphysics, Magnetic, and Osteopathy" and also that he had earlier studied and lectured on phrenology, which helped him develop a keen sense of touch. Gielow (1981, pp 80–82) relates instances where D.D. even replaced a dislocated femur and ankle. Regarding this period D.D. (1910, p 17) wrote: "I was a magnetic healer for nine years previous to discovering the principles which comprise the method known as Chiropractic. During this period much of that which was necessary to complete the science was worked out." He also stated (1910, p 38) that in 1888 he "discovered that hemiplegia could be relieved by adjusting the fifth dorsal vertebra," which was 7 years before he claimed to have given his first chiropractic adjustment, an example of his famed inconsistency.

In 1895 D.D. successfully sued a patient for nonpayment of a contracted fee of $20, which Gielow (1981, p 66) suggests was done "to establish Palmer's right to practice in Moline without a physician's certificate." According to Gielow (1981, p 105), under state law if D.D. had "started his career of magnetic healing five years before he did in 1886, he would have been eligible for a certificate granting legal right to practice" presumably any kind of healing.

D.D. wrote that he administered the first chiropractic adjustment in 1895, to Harvey Lillard (Figure 4). Here is his often repeated account from *The Chiropractor's Adjustor* (1910, p 18):

> Harvey Lillard a janitor in the Ryan Block, where I had my office, had been so deaf for 17 years that he could not hear the racket of a wagon on the street or the ticking of a watch. I made inquiry as to the cause of his deafness and was informed that when he was exerting himself in a cramped, stooping position, he felt something give way in his back and immediately became deaf. An examination showed a vertebra racked from its normal position. I reasoned that if that vertebra was replaced, the man's hearing should be restored. With this object in view, a half-hour's talk persuaded Mr. Lillard to allow me to replace it. I racked it into position by using the spinous process as a lever and soon the man could hear as before. There was nothing "accidental" about this, as it was accomplished with an object in view, and the result expected was obtained. There was nothing "crude" about this adjustment; it was specific, so much so that no Chiropractor has equalled it.

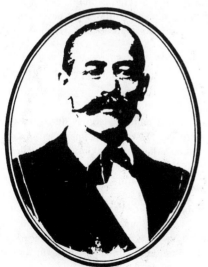

FIGURE 4.
Harvey Lillard, first chiropractic patient, 1895.
(Courtesy of Palmer College of Chiropractic Archives.)

Gielow (1981, p 79) offers two other versions of the story, one that the treatments extended over a longer period of time with D.D. using ever more direct approaches, and another version that D.D.'s "success" followed an earlier incident in which his clap on Lillard's back with a book produced partial improvement of the deafness. D.D. himself writes (1910, p 702) that he gave Lillard two adjustments. Carver (1936, p 5) relates a still different version:

> Harvey Lillard, a Spanish Creole West Indian Octoroon . . . came to Dr. Daniel David Palmer for general restoration; but particularly because some seventeen years before he had been lifting in a stooped and cramped position, in the room of a mine, when he suddenly felt the sensation of something giving away in his back, from which moment he ceased to hear out of his left ear. Dr. Palmer gave him the manipulations of the magnetic healer called the long passes of the spine or back. Incident to these he observed that there was an area near the fourth thoracic vertebra that when undisturbed was too light colored, and when manipulated became excessively red, and he noticed that either color changed slowly. . . . At the expense of a good deal of effort, and the study of the situation for more than a week, Dr. Palmer reached the conclusion that the fourth thoracic vertebra was disrelated in a certain direction, and the segment should be moved in the reverse direction to restore relationship.

> However, the distortion stubbornly resisted all his efforts to correct it. He performed all of the manipulations known to his system but failed to make apparent correction of the situation.

> Finally, on the 18th day of September, 1895, Dr. Daniel David Palmer, becoming impatient, struck the vertebra a short, sharp blow, with the ulnar side of his fist or closed hand, with the happy result that, although it hurt considerably, there was a snap and the bump changed appearance markedly, with the startling, but nevertheless true, result that the left ear was almost instantly unstopped, and remained so permanently.

Black chiropractor Bobby Westbrooks (1982, p 48), who interviewed Lillard's daughter Valdeenia Simons, gives us another story:

> According to Mrs. Simons, her father and a friend were telling humorous stories outside of the open doorway leading to D.D. Palmer's office. D.D. was reading a book in his favorite chair. Overhearing the loud conversation which was taking place, Palmer decided to join the two men and walked into the hall where they were standing. Obviously enjoying the story's climax, D.D., laughing heartily, struck Harvey on the back with the book he had carried with him. Several days later, Lillard commented to Palmer that he thought he could hear a bit better following the merriment of the story-telling and the back slapping incident. D.D. commented, "We'll try to do something about that." Shortly he began working with Lillard to restore his hearing. Valdeenia's explanation of the background of circumstances becomes most supportive

of Palmer's comment that the first adjustment was "accomplished with an object in view."

Although Mrs. Simons also remembered her father as always "stone deaf," she was, after all, born only in 1895, the year when Lillard's deafness was allegedly cured or at least improved. According to Lerner (1954, p 618), as late as 1899 D.D. had not fixed on a precise date for his "discovery" of chiropractic. Like most folklore, chiropractic's comes in several versions.

Although anatomists and neurologists have questioned whether D.D.'s treatment possibly could have cured deafness, such cases have been reported in the medical literature, beginning with an account by Paullini in 1698 (Gaucher-Peslherbe, 1992; see also Bechgaard and Bentzen, 1963; Christensen, 1981, 1983; Leach, 1986, pp 114–117). The medical manipulator John Bourdillon (1987, p 5) reported "dramatic and lasting relief of . . . deafness . . . after treatment of the thoracic joint," and remarked that Palmer's claim "may not be quite as fantastic as it sounds."

D.D.'s evolution from magnetic healer to chiropractor was gradual (Beck, 1991). He continued to experiment with specific adjustments, and developed a theory to explain the results (1910, pp 18–20):

> Shortly after this relief from deafness, I had a case of heart trouble which was not improving. I examined the spine and found a displaced vertebra pressing against the nerves which innervate the heart. I adjusted the vertebra and gave immediate relief—nothing "accidental" or "crude" about this. Then I began to reason if two diseases, so dissimilar as deafness and heart trouble, came from impingement, a pressure on nerves, were not other diseases due to a similar cause? Thus the science (knowledge) and art (adjusting) of Chiropractic were formed at that time. I then began a systematic investigation for the cause of all diseases and have been amply rewarded . . . .

> The amount of nerve tension determines health or disease. In health there is normal tension, known as tone, the normal activity, strength and excitability of the various organs and functions as observed in a state of health. The kind of disease depends on what nerves are too tense or too slack. . . .

> Nerves carry impulses outward and sensations inward. The activity of these nerves, or rather their fibers, may become excited or allayed by impingement, the result being a modification of functioning—too much or not enough action—which is disease.

Gaucher-Peslherbe (1992) remarks: "It was the 'tonos' of the Stoics on which Palmer founded chiropractic." D.D. added:

> Ninety-five percent of all deranged nerves are made by subluxations of vertebrae which pinch nerves in some one of the 51 joint articulations of the spinal column. Therefore, to relieve the pressure upon these nerves means to restore normal action—hence normal functions, perfect health.

That was written in 1910. Ten years earlier, when he was struggling to explain how the body functions and the benefits of manipulation, he was using a more mechanical analogy and giving some credit also to blood circulation. According to Lerner (1954, pp 123–128), quoting from D.D.'s 1899 *The Chiropractic* [sic]:

> A human being is a human machine and, like a machine, would run smoothly, without any friction, if every part was in its proper place. If every bone, every nerve, and all the blood vessels, muscles, etc., were just right, there would be nothing wrong. . . . Disease is the effect or result of some part of the body being disarranged. . . .

> The human body is a bundle of fine sensitive nerves, passing over, under and in between the 200 bones and the many muscles and ligaments. These nerves are liable to be pinched, strained, stretched, or pulled out of place by the displacement of any one of the bones, muscles, or ligaments causing any one of the nerve diseases. . . . Why not remove the pressure, adjust the framework, and take the strain off those sensitive nerves?

By 1908, according to Lerner (1954, p 684), D.D. had ceased referring to the body as a machine and was talking more about nerves. However, he contributed more to the theory of disease than the simplistic "pressure on nerves"; in fact, he sometimes sounds thoroughly modern (1910, pp 833–834):

> The science of Chiropractic has modified our views concerning life, death, health and disease. We no longer believe that disease is an entity, something foreign to the body, which may enter from without, and with which we have to grasp, struggle, fight and conquer, or submit and succumb to its ravages. Disease is a disturbed condition, not a thing of enmity. Disease is abnormal performance of certain functions, . . . a change in the amount of energy and function performed. The body in disease does not develop any new form of energy; what it already possesses is diminished or increased, perverted or abolished.

Seeking a name for his new method of healing he consulted one of his patients, the Reverend Samuel H. Weed, who helped him coin the word "chiropractic" (from the Greek cheir, "hand," and praxis, "practice," meaning "done by hand") (1910, p 12). He tells us that this did not happen until the following year, in 1896 (1910, p 105). However, Lerner (1954, p 79) found a letter dated December 18, 1896, in the 1899 issue of D.D.'s *The Chiropractic,* in which Weed stated that he took 15 treatments from D.D. in July 1894 and that D.D. then called his "most practical mode of diagnosing and treating the diseases . . . 'chiropraxis.' " Yet Lerner concludes from his study of original sources in the PSC archives that D.D. actually began considering himself a chiropractor (or rather a "chiropractic") only in 1897. (I presume that he at first called himself a chiropractic because he was accustomed to calling himself a "magnetic" rather than a "magnetist.") Other early variants on the word chiropractic were "chiropractics," "chiropractice," "chiropraxis," "chiropraxy," "chiropracty," "chiropractry," and even "chiropath" (obviously coordinate with allopath, homeopath, and osteopath).

Although D.D. practiced chiropractic secretively at first, an accident that nearly killed him persuaded him he should not risk the loss to the world of his important discovery. Hence in 1898 he took on his first student. In 1896 he had legally incorporated Palmer's School of Magnetic Cure. (Note that he was still using the familiar word magnetic.) He renamed it Palmer School and Cure in 1897, but introduced the word "chiropractic" into the title only in 1902, when it became Palmer Infirmary and Chiropractic Institute. In 1907 the school was incorporated for a second time, after B.J. had purchased it from his father in the previous year, as the Palmer School and Infirmary of Chiropractic ("New Questions: Why Did D.D. Not Use 'Chiropractic' in His 1896 Charter?," 1986). From then on it customarily was referred to simply as the Palmer School of Chiropractic (or PSC). The course of instruction lasted 6 months and cost $500. D.D. (1910, p 468) tells us: "There was one student in 1898, three in 1899, two in 1900, five in 1901, and four in 1902; among the latter was B.J. Palmer," D.D.'s son, who was then 20 years old. According to Lerner, B.J.'s *The Chiropractor* reported in 1920: "In 1901 there was one student; in 1903, three; in 1904, nine; in 1905, thirty; in 1906, seventy-five; in 1907, ninety-six; in 1908, 130; in 1909, 318; in 1910, 505," but no later writer seems to have taken these figures at face value. Probably PSC's true enrollment figures are lost to history. Worth noting, however, is that five of D.D.'s first 15 graduates were MDs or DOs (Gibbons, 1981a).

Oakley Smith's (1932, pp 5–6) critique of the instruction he received from D.D. in 1899 is severe and historically revealing, though one should keep in mind that when he wrote it he had already helped found the competing American School of Chiropractic in 1906, and later his competing school of naprapathy:

> The first thing I learned was that there was no instruction to be given. There were no blackboards, no text books, no notes, not a single lecture. For six days I witnessed the giving of a number of treatments. That was the sum total of information that was transferred in exchange for the tuition paid. The diagnosis as I witnessed it consisted of a quick gliding pressure from upper dorsal to middle lumbar to detect the position of posterior apical prominences. That was the sum total of examination that was given to any patient. The treatment consisted of giving a single forceful lunge on that prominent apex, using the flat of the hand as a contact. That was the sum total of the treatment. Nothing else was done. The patient's treatment for that day was finished. These treatments were given daily. There were no charts made, no histories taken, and no records made. After being permitted to watch this identical form of treatment on a number of patients for six days I was told that I knew all that was necessary for me to know, and that I should do the treating myself thereafter.

B.J. soon began working in the clinic and helping to run the school. He became solely responsible for its management, calling himself Secretary of the school and Adjuster-in-Chief (Lerner, 1954, p 53) in 1902–1903, when D.D. fled west to California to avoid prosecution for false arrest and defrauding a student who sued to get his tuition money returned (Lerner, 1954, pp 261–262). According to Gielow (1981, p 97), although B.J. was indicted in court in 1903 for "publicly professing to cure and heal without having procured and filed a certificate of the Board of Medical Examiners, the records at the Scott County Courthouse indicate there was no final disposition of the case." Lerner (1954, pp 275, 375), writes that the case was finally withdrawn in 1905; also that B.J. reopened the school in 1904, and held its first formal graduation in 1905, having discovered that although he was prevented by the indictment from practicing chiropractic, he was not legally forbidden to teach it!

In 1902 D.D. was in Pasadena, California (Zarbuck and Hayes, 1990), where he was arrested for practicing medicine without a license (later dismissed because of a faultily drawn paper), and in 1903 he was listed in the Santa Barbara City Directory as a physician. He also started a school with Oakley Smith and Minora Paxson, two former PSC students. In 1904 he returned to Davenport in time for B.J.'s marriage to Mabel Heath, who immediately took his course of instruction. In 1905 they all moved PSC to a large Victorian mansion on Brady Street, near which the college remains today.

In 1905 D.D. signed a death certificate for a patient, apparently the first one to die under his care (Lerner, 1954, pp 523–529), and a coroner's jury was convened:

> The records reveal that nearly 100 questions were asked of Palmer before he would admit that he had been working to heal and cure patients, . . . insisting that the terms "heal" and "cure" did not have the same meaning to him as they would have to the ordinary practitioner. . . . He had refused to take the oath required of witnesses, saying he was opposed to the idea of "swearing to tell the truth." The Coroner kept repeating, asking Palmer to say, "So help me God," and Palmer only answered, "I don't want any help from God." . . .
>
> When the Coroner asked Palmer, "What is Chiropractic?" the reply was: "Now, Dr. Lambach, you are seeking to learn from a 60¢ witness, for which my students pay me $500." . . . The jury voted to exonerate Palmer. The evidence was clearly established that the deceased girl had died from tuberculosis and that the care Palmer had given to her was not the primary cause of her death.

Several important things happened to D.D. in 1906. In January he married his fifth wife, Mary Hudler, his fourth wife having died the previous year. In the same year his grandson was born, christened Daniel David Palmer but later changed to David Daniel Palmer (1967, pp 24–25; Figure 5). He published with B.J. *The Science of Chiropractic: Its Principles and Adjustments* (1906). In April he was convicted of practicing medicine without a license, served 23 days in jail, and was released after his wife paid his fine of $350 plus $39.50 in costs (Gielow, 1981, p 114).

Carver (1936, pp 49–50) states that, contrary to his legal advice, D.D. had earlier transferred all PSC property to B.J.'s wife, Mabel, to protect it from the court. This gave B.J. the right to refuse further association with his father and to deny him admission to the school. No doubt D.D.'s mismanagement and irascible temper influenced B.J.'s rejection of his father. Neutral parties were called in to negotiate a settlement. Under its terms D.D. transferred his entire interest in PSC to B.J. for $2,196.79, plus a dozen books of his choosing from the library and "one normal and one abnormal spinal column and six individual vertebrae" (Dye, 1939, p 19). Heart-

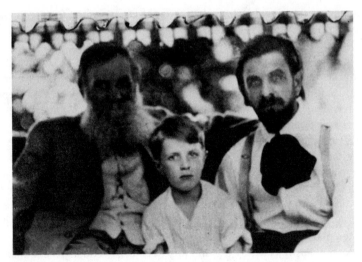

FIGURE 5.
Three generations of Palmers: D.D., Dave, and B.J., circa 1913. (Courtesy of Palmer College of Chiropractic Archives.)

broken, in 1906 D.D. traveled with his new wife to Oklahoma, where he started two other schools.

From then the historical record is confused. Homewood (1982, p 12) writes in his history of Western States Chiropractic College (WSCC) that D.D. founded the D.D. Palmer College of Chiropractic in Portland, Oregon, in 1907 and that it "had a life span of about two years." A diploma signed by D.D. was awarded to John E. LaValley in 1909, and D.D. (1910, p 420) indicates that the school was still functioning when he wrote. He also implies (1910, p 134) that it taught a 10-month course. After "the majority, if not all, of the students walked out on the founder" (Homewood, 1982, p 8), LaValley organized in 1910 the Peerless College of Chiropractic and Naturopathy, the antecedent of the current WSCC.

According to Carver's history (1936, p 55), which I find not always accurate:

> In 1908 Dr. D.D. Palmer founded a school at Santa Barbara, California, which he soon left, and organized another one in San Diego. It will be noted that Dr. D.D. Palmer had a line of school centers substantially the length of the Pacific Coast.

In 1911 D.D. returned to practice in Los Angeles, where he also taught at Ratledge Chiropractic College for at least a year. Tullius Ratledge (1971, p 68) wrote:

> I contacted D.D. Palmer and finally persuaded him to join the faculty, in 1912. He withdrew from the faculty in the following winter . . . He grieved over the termination with the Palmer School in Davenport, and I believed that he was planning—or perhaps dreaming would be the proper wording—another school of his own.

D.D. continued to travel and lecture at other colleges, including Carver in Oklahoma City, Universal in Davenport, and PSC, but he always believed he had not received proper recognition for his discovery of chiropractic.

D.D. was in Davenport for the PSC homecoming parade on August 20, 1913. Refusing to ride in B.J.'s car, although invited to do so, he grabbed an American flag and tried to lead the parade on foot. In the confusion apparently he was hit by B.J.'s car. Carver writes (1936, p 112; see also Dye, 1939, Chapter 3) that D.D. told him that "the car had bumped him and knocked him over, and he was seriously injured, from which injury he never expected to recover." However, he was able the next day to leave by train for California. His death there on October 20, 1913, was recorded as due to typhoid fever. The executor of his estate (Joy Loban, former PSC instructor and later head of Universal College) filed a civil court suit against B.J., alleging that his action was "willful, reckless, wanton, malicious, intentional, grossly negligent and purposely" (Gielow, 1981, p 125) and asking for $20,000 actual damages, $20,000 exemplary damages, and costs. A criminal suit also was brought by the State against B.J., but was rejected by a grand jury. The civil action was continued until it was withdrawn in December 1914. Whether B.J. contributed to his father's death as alleged, there is little doubt that, although he always paid formal tribute to his father as the "discoverer of chiropractic," he could be considered as having "symbolically killed" his father by taking PSC away from him, removing D.D.'s name from the title page of later editions of their 1906 *Science of Chiropractic*, and taking full credit for himself as the "developer of chiropractic" in directions that D.D. rejected. B.J.'s action in reinterring D.D.'s ashes in a memorial bust at PSC in 1921 was more an effort to show ritual respect to an icon than genuine recognition of his father's contributions to chiropractic's development.

While in Portland D.D. had published his mammoth *The Chiropractor's Adjustor* (1910), a loosely organized compendium of earlier writings, correspondence, and debates with other chiropractors and osteopaths, and repetitive explanations of his theory of chiropractic and of its superiority over other systems of healing. Turner (1931, p 29) described it as:

> Mosaic in its dicta and Platonic in its thoroughness. Flaying allopathy in particular he denounced the use of drugs and discussed the cure of almost every disease from abasia to zymosis. The book teemed with maxims, controversy, satire, poetry and irrelevancies, but, withal, revealed a genius that must have impressed his most offended colleagues. Least of all was his son spared in the many pages of diatribe.

His diatribes against his son, after B.J. began calling PSC the "Fountain Head," reveal his resentment, especially in such phrases as "this barefaced falsehood" and "an innate desire of a rascal to rob his parental benefactor." In this connection D.D. recalls the story of the curator in the Holy Land "who exhibited two skulls of St. Paul: one when he was a boy of 13 and the other when advanced in age."

Donahue (1990, p 36) asserts: "The text indicates he was well read in the medical field. *The Adjuster* contains several hundred references to over fifty of the best medical textbooks of the time." Gaucher-Peslherbe (1992), in addition to document-ing convincingly the authenticity of D.D.'s citations from standard medical texts and vouching for his comprehension of them, even has words of praise for his often tur-gid prose, writing that D.D.

> . . . took his concern for language to Socratic heights rarely found in the English-speaking world. His style is carefully worked out, he makes excellent use of his refer-ences, and these references reveal wide reading. He was a cultivated man, able to present his discovery in simple terms, arranged in an almost architectural pattern which highlighted his meaning.

Gaucher-Peslherbe (1992) adds that D.D. "had what Claude Bernard calls 'a sense of organization,' that is, an ability to see phenomena in the light of an organizing prin-ciple," and that "chiropractic had a firm neurological foundation, and an excellent scientific basis for its time."

D.D. was megalomanic. In Donahue's (1986, p 32) words, D.D. "saw himself as 'destiny's child,' as the elected bringer of a revolutionary science and philoso-phy." Here is a sample paragraph from D.D. (1910, p 491):

> What is life, disease, death, and immortality? These questions have been propounded by savants of all ages and have remained unanswered until the advent of Chiropractic. This science and life are coexistent; it now answers the first three questions and in time will lift the veil which obstructs the view of the life beyond.

He (1910, p 975) attributed to himself 32 chiropractic "firsts," and added (1910, p 819):

> I am the Fountain Head of Chiropractic; it originated with me; it was my ingenious brain which discovered its first principle; I was its source; I gave it birth; to me all Chiroprac-tors trace their Chiropractic lineage.

Although D.D. repeatedly claimed that he was the first to use "vertebral processes as levers," and so stated on the title page of his magnum opus, that appears not to be strictly correct. Here is what he wrote (1910, p 11):

> I have, both in print and by word of mouth repeatedly stated, and now most emphati-cally repeat the statement, that I am not the first person to replace subluxated vertebrae, for this art has been practiced for thousands of years. I do claim, however, to be the first to replace displaced vertebrae by using the spinous and transverse processes as levers wherewith to rack subluxated vertebrae into normal position.

The evidence does not support him. The British surgeon Little (1868) referred to Ed-ward Harrison's (1827) technique of "endeavoring to press the rotated spinous and transverse processes into a more favorable position." And Gaucher-Peslherbe (1992) quotes an 1884 description of how to do it: "Where the deviation is not very ad-vanced a degree of correction can be obtained by grasping the spinous processes with the fingers." If D.D. had been aware of these earlier writings he might have referred to them. On the other hand, he might have consciously chosen not to! Clearly there was a lot more continuity between him and his predecessors than he chose to admit.

Although D.D. argued that chiropractic is not a religion, he insisted (1914, p 5) that chiropractors have a "moral and religious duty" to replace displaced bones, so that we all may enjoy health, happiness, and the full fruition of our earthly lives:

> I hold it to be self-evident that all men and women who have acquired sufficient knowl-
> edge and skill to remove the nerve tension which prevents physical, mental and spiritual
> development, are engaged in work of a higher order than that ordinarily required of, and
> performed by, the physician. They are practically the moral duties and obligations of
> religion and any attempt to prevent such acts by law is an unmitigated crime against
> humanity.

Contentious and stubborn, D.D. nevertheless had a truly "magnetic" personality in the modern sense, which helped him achieve cures in his patients, whether using magnetism or chiropractic, and enabled him to inspire others to take up his philoso-phy and technique of healing and go forth to do likewise. Many of his difficulties resulted from his cantankerous personality and his apparently total lack of ability to administer effectively any of the many schools he founded. To find that ability we must turn to his son, B.J. Here is B.J.'s (1959b, p 40) final tribute to his father:

> All [his] thinking was off the beaten path. He took the side roads, he wandered alone
> into the jungle, cut down virgin forests and beat out a new road. The price he paid was
> to be alone, followed by few, shunned by many, misunderstood by most, fought on all
> sides by most of those who profited from his labors. But the sum total of that life led
> eventually to the great accomplishment that history will know him best for.

Actually, this description of his father also could be applied to B.J. himself. Carver (1936, p 10) described D.D. as "a true aristocrat, although in other respects most definitely democratic." Here is Carver's summary evaluation of D.D. (1909, p 4):

> It is a pity that D.D. Palmer, the founder of the greatest science which has come to bless
> humanity, was not a man of patience and continuity, and endowed with the qualities of
> a leader. If he had been, the science of chiropractic would have been international and
> in general use today; but not having these qualities, he has insisted upon standing in his
> own light, and in the way of advancement of the science which he gave to the world.

Section 2

Bartlett Joshua Palmer (1882–1961)

Bartlett Joshua Palmer (B.J.) had a difficult childhood. With an unpredictable and tempestuous father and two different stepmothers, it is not surprising that he was an indifferent student. Expelled in the seventh grade for releasing two mice in class, he had to fend pretty much for himself. Forced to sleep at times in alleyways, he earned his living doing the odd jobs available to a teenager, which included making store deliveries to houses of prostitution. His devoted biographer, Joseph E. Maynard

(1959, p 17), says that he was repelled by them, but anecdotes about his fascination with pornography still abound. Among the unbelievable stories that B.J. later told (and there were many) was that he would collect scraps of paper his father had written on and tossed in a wastebasket, and put them in a scrapbook, which he kept hidden and would eventually release; no one has ever seen it. He also claimed to have witnessed D.D.'s first adjustment in 1895, which is most unlikely, inasmuch as he was only 14 years old at that time and D.D. habitually practiced secretively behind closed doors. However, he attended and graduated from his father's 1902 class.

B.J. was a consummate salesman and showman. Dye (1939, p 278) tells us that he "traveled as an assistant to a mesmerist and performer in the late 90's" who was known as Professor Hunt. Lerner (1954, pp 265, 280) confirms that B.J. joined the troupe of Professor Herbert L. Flint for a year as professional "hypnotic subject." He also worked in a circus, and ever after adored circus performers. He always treated them without charge, and encouraged his followers also to do so, by issuing "Palmergrams" to them for free chiropractic treatments wherever they went. Grateful performers helped spread the word about chiropractic. He was the proud owner of reputedly the largest circus bandwagon ever built, and was instrumental in creating the Circus Hall of Fame in Sarasota, Florida, where the bandwagon can be seen.

Challenges to B.J. were not long in coming. First he had to solve the school's financial problems. How he was able at such a young age to persuade Davenport bankers to extend him the credit he needed remains a mystery. How was he able to make PSC into such a successful school, starting with practically nothing? It is, however, a simple historic fact that he was successful in building up the school and through it the profession of chiropractic. Although there were other leaders, most of whom he considered rivals and competitors, he became the unquestioned leader of what he chose to call "pure, straight and unadulterated chiropractic." Lerner (1954, p 368) noted that although a license is required to practice a profession, all that is required to teach it is gall, especially when one is only 21 years old and without any formal education whatsoever.

In 1907 a crisis befell the fledgling profession that thrust B.J. into the limelight and had major implications for chiropractic's future. A PSC graduate named Shegataro Morikubo was arrested in La Crosse, Wisconsin, charged with practicing medicine, surgery, and osteopathy without a license (Mawhiney, 1984, pp 33–36). He appealed to B.J. for help. Known as "the Jap," in the racist fashion of the day, he was the subject on whom adjustive techniques were demonstrated in the photographic illustrations of the first Palmer text (Palmer and Palmer, 1906; Figure 6). Fortuitously, they chose an attorney with an excellent reputation and good political connections, Thomas Morris (1861–1928), of the law firm of Morris and Hartwell, later elected Lieutenant Governor of Wisconsin. Perhaps the fact that Morris had studied medicine at McGill University for 3 years before dropping out for unknown reasons predisposed him to defend chiropractic enthusiastically against the medical establishment.

William S. Rehm (1986) has argued that Morris's successful defense strategy was based mainly on *A Textbook: Modernized Chiropractic*, published in 1906 by

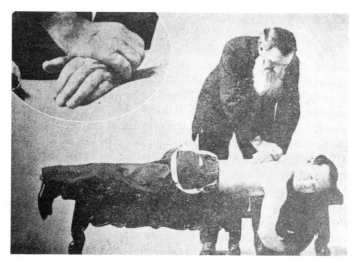

FIGURE 6.
D.D. Palmer performing an adjustment on Shegataro Morikubo, 1906. (Courtesy of Palmer College of Chiropractic Archives.)

Solon M. Langworthy, Oakley, G. Smith, and Minora C. Paxson, all former students of D.D. They had established the American School of Chiropractic and Nature Cure in Cedar Rapids, Iowa, in 1903, which taught a 6-week course for $250, had published the first serious chiropractic journal, titled *Backbone,* and by so doing implied, contrary to D.D., a narrowing of the field of chiropractic to the spine; had introduced a device called an "anatomical adjuster" designed to stretch the spinal column; and had organized the first national association, the American Chiropractic Association. Perhaps because the Langworthy volume failed even to mention Palmer, crediting instead the "Bohemian thrust" tradition (Gromala, 1986, p 60), D.D. and B.J. quickly published their own 1906 text and organized the competing Universal Chiropractors Association (UCA). Lerner (1954, p 339) designated Langworthy the "Columbus of Chiropractic," observing that he

> . . . first made use of the term subluxation in chiropractic; the first reference to the expression *intervertebral foramina;* the first reference to the shape and design of the *intervertebral openings;* the first reference to the *brain* as the *source of all nerve force;* the first reference to the *erect posture in man;* the first reference to the *laws of gravity* affecting the stature of the human being; the first reference to the *date of discovery* of Chiropractic; and the first reference to the *supremacy of the nerves* as distinguished from the Osteopathic claim concerning the "supremacy of the blood."

Langworthy also theorized that aging is due to the decreasing size of the intervertebral foramina as the spinal discs become thinner, with consequent reduction of nerve force from the "dynamo" (the brain) to "all parts of the body" (Lerner, 1954, pp

346–350). Hence, instead of D.D.'s emphasis on thrusts to adjust the spine, Langworthy emphasized stretching the spine to widen the intervertebral foramina.

Langworthy's point about the supremacy of nerves was the most important point for the defense. Rehm (1986, pp 53–54)) tells us that it was Tom Morris, rather than B.J., who grasped the significant legal advantage that Langworthy's innovative chiropractic philosophy offered:

> In Langworthy, Tom Morris had discovered gold. *Chiropractic* had defined the difference between chiropractic and osteopathy in terms of both philosophy and technique. Because of Langworthy, Morris could present evidence that the brain was the source of the "unseen power" in the body, not the blood, as the osteopath and medical doctor preached. In his book, Langworthy exhaustively and convincingly demonstrated spinal mechanics, the "spinal windows" (foramina), the interconnections of the autonomic system, and the possible aberrations of the health and well being of the human body. Just as convincingly, it demonstrated the effects of the "chiropractic thrust" as opposed to other spinal techniques. . . .
>
> Morris asked the court to amend the charge to "practicing osteopathy without a license" since the defendant was only using manipulation. Not suspecting a trap, the prosecution agreed. By this maneuver, Morris showed that osteopathy and chiropractic were not the same thing, as the state contended, and, therefore, his client could not be prevented from practicing.

B.J. and Marikubo were excellent witnesses, and the jury rendered a unanimous acquittal. The trial had two major consequences: B.J. retained Morris as national counsel for the UCA, which undertook to defend chiropractors everywhere who faced legal problems arising from practice; the other consequence was that B.J. began adapting Langworthy's philosophy to his own purposes, as Rehm explains (1986, p 54):

> For the first time, B.J. laid claim to the designation as chiropractic's "developer." The original Palmer book published by B.J. in 1906 giving D.D. and himself authorship credit was withdrawn from further circulation and would never again be mentioned in a publication from the PSC printery. . . . He adopted Langworthy's term "subluxation" and the expression "intervertebral foramina," and began to address the brain as the "unseen power," the origin of the "life force," just as Langworthy had been doing since 1903. Chiropractic had entered the realm of philosophy where, now, all phenomena could be explained. This, B.J. introduced in a ponderous definition: "Chiropractic is a philosophy of biology, theology, health, disease, death, the cause of disease . . ." not as speculation but as absolute truth. Whereas D.D. Palmer had originally dealt in the realities of life—the structure of the body—the new chiropractic could explain the mysteries of life. No one had yet explored the invisible world of chiropractic philosophy. For B.J., it became an opportunity that he had not ever imagined. Soon, he would portray himself in terms that left little room for role-sharing and no doubt at all as to his self-perceived authority when he wrote this:
>
>> Dr. B.J. Palmer, D.C., Ph.C., is the student, author, lecturer, teacher and defender of any phase of Chiropractic philosophy, science and art—anywhere—at any time.

> He is the Developer of the Philosophy, Science and Art of Chiropractic.
>
> He is the Secretary and Philosophical Counsel of the Chiropractors Association.

Lerner (1954, p 641), however, argues that it was really Tom Morris who was the philosophical counsel to chiropractic.

While the 1906 book with D.D. as the first author and B.J. second was titled *The Science of Chiropractic: Its Principles and Adjustments,* the 1910 second edition, which carried B.J. as sole author and the title *The Science of Chiropractic: Its Principles and Philosophies,* was actually a quite different book, incorporating much of the new thinking that Tom Morris had adapted from Langworthy's text. Narrowing the scope of chiropractic to the spine, B.J. maintained that he invented "specific" chiropractic adjustment of single vertebrae, even though D.D. (1910, p 171) had claimed essentially the same thing:

> In my fifteen years of teaching the science, principles and art of Chiropractic, I have found but few who are capable of learning it as a science. I cannot, at present, remember a Chiropractor whom I have seen analyze a case, correctly locate the displaced vertebra and adjust it for the ailment from which the patient desired to be free. All invariably adjust from two to two dozen vertebrae. There are very few who comprehend Chiropractic as a science, making it specific, adjusting definitely for a certain ailment.

However, D.D. (1910, p 37) also wrote: "I have found it better to give regional locations for adjusting rather than the number of the vertebra." Dye (1939, pp 115, 273), however, remained B.J.'s loyal biographer:

> I do not believe that the Founder meant the statement that Chiropractic is the science of adjusting by hand any or all luxations of the 300 articular joints of the human body. . . . Personally, I believe that B.J. Palmer takes precedence over his father.

B.J. adopted the term "mixer" from D.D.'s injunction that chiropractic not be "mixed" with other therapies. Ratledge (1971, p 70) wrote that D.D. "was opposed to the term 'mixer' because he held that what the doctor did was either chiropractic or was *not* chiropractic and that opposite principles could no more be mixed than could opposite directions."

B.J. insisted on new terminology to maximize chiropractic's differences from medicine and osteopathy. Instead of a diagnosis chiropractors made an analysis. Instead of a treatment chiropractors made an adjustment. The word manipulation became anathema because MDs, DOs, and physical therapists used it. X-rays became spinographs. Chiropractors later became diplomates in roentgenology, not radiology. His faculty published and taught from their own texts. Wife Mabel Heath Palmer wrote and taught from her *Chiropractic Anatomy* (1918), which allegedly contained several errors.

After acquiring PSC from his father in 1906, B.J. gradually paid off its debts, purchased more land and buildings, and recruited a faculty that always included several MDs. Gibbons (1987, p 10) summarizes his early achievements as follows:

By 1910 B.J. was a man of property, owner of one of the finest mansions on the top of Brady Street hill. He was the president of an institution with more than 300 students, called himself a doctor and was already an editor and an author. He had married the daughter of a respected family, wore a Van Dyke beard and dressed in a fitting role for the leader of a professional body, a scholar and an academic.

PSC grew slowly at first, then more rapidly. Exact figures are unknown. Dye (1939, pp 64–66) states: "The student body of the PSC from 1904–05 to 1908 averaged from a couple dozen or so to less than fifty." In 1910 he writes that it was approximately 250, by which time the course had been lengthened to a year. After 8 months the degree of Chiropractor was awarded, which permitted the "student who was short of funds and wanted to go out to practice for a time to recuperate his finances so he could continue with the remaining four months and get his D.C.—Doctor of Chiropractic degree." The degree of Chiropractor was discontinued in 1921. Dye (1939, p 103) claims that "by 1910 the free public clinics at the Palmer School were giving adjustments to approximately a thousand patients daily," which may be doubted, although in 1990 the school clinic was attracting 800 patients a day (*ICA Review* 1990, p 28). By 1915 PSC enrollment was 600 to 800; it rose to 1882 in 1919, to 2,300 in 1921 (Turner, 1931, p 34), and at one time neared the 3,000 mark, according to Dye (1939, p 137). In 1921 PSC graduated a class of more than 1,000 (classes were admitted several times a year). According to a medical source (Thewlis, 1923), B.J. once said, "I look to see the time when this institution will graduate 25,000 students a year." By 1920 the standard course was 3 years of 6 months each, normally taken continuously over 18 months. After the PSC student body and faculty voted to award B.J. the Ph.C. (Philosopher of Chiropractic) degree in 1908, it was regularly awarded to those who made high grades; later it was awarded more rarely as a postgraduate degree to those who did additional work or submitted a thesis, and sometimes as an honorary degree (Stout, 1988). It was discontinued after 1968 when the Council on Chiropractic Education ruled it should be considered honorary.

B.J. pioneered using communications media for advertising chiropractic. He once claimed that he developed chiropractic with printer's ink. By 1916 he owned what he called the "prettiest little print shop in America," decorated with busts of literary greats and caged singing birds. It produced thousands of advertising brochures describing for patients what chiropractic could do for various diseases (Gromala, 1984); these he sold at a profit to practicing chiropractors (Figure 7). He had a corner on the market for such literature because so few others had the resources to compete with him. By 1920 he had added business and marketing courses to the curriculum (Brennan, 1983a, p 27). Fishbein (1925, p 89) quotes B.J. as saying in 1920:

> Our school is established on a business and not a professional basis. It is a business where we manufacture chiropractors. They have got to work just like machinery. A course of salesmanship goes along with their training. We teach them the idea and then we show them how to sell it.

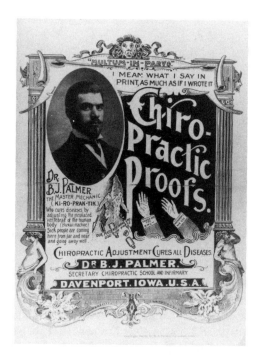

FIGURE 7.
Palmer poster, circa 1903. (Courtesy of Palmer
College of Chiropractic Archives.)

In 1922 B.J. began broadcasting from his powerful Davenport radio station,
WOC, alleged to be the second commercial radio station in the United States. In
1930 one of its sportscasters was President-to-be Ronald Reagan, who wrote in his
autobiography, *Where Is the Rest of Me?* (1965, p 47), that WOC stood for " 'World
of Chiropractic.' . . . Founded by Colonel B.J. Palmer of the Palmer School of Chiropractic, it was located in the top floor of the school." (B.J. had gotten himself appointed to the governor's staff as a lieutenant colonel, and characteristically relished
wearing his uniform.) However, WOC was more popularly believed to stand for
"Wonders of Chiropractic." (Frank Elliott, formerly B.J.'s business manager, told
me in 1974 that the letters actually had been assigned by the Federal Communications
Commission.) B.J. often used WOC for late-evening soliloquies, in which he would
introduce comments on the benefits of chiropractic. He also authored an innovative
text, *Radio Salesmanship* (1942). As a salesman he was like some of the early medical deans that Flexner (1910, p 19) criticized: "The deans of these institutions occasionally know more about modern advertising than about modern medical teaching."

B.J.'s personal and stage showmanship captivated audiences, whether students,
alumni, or the general public. He regarded the public as a source of new students as
well as of new patients for chiropractors. With a flair for publicity much like his father (who had sported two thoroughbred horses, Nip and Tuck), B.J. "had the first
auto in the area and, as with everything in the rest of his life, he was properly attired
for the occasion with the big khaki duster, cap, gloves and goggles" (Palmer DD,
1977, p 103). Of short physical stature, he early cultivated a distinctive beard that not

only diverted attention from his youthfulness but gave him a quite distinguished appearance (Figure 8). In response to the question of why he wore his hair long, he replied, "That's your answer." Some of his portraits reminded me of Jesus Christ. When the three key figures were portrayed as a group—D.D. with his bushy white beard, B.J. as the central focus, and wife Mabel, often styled the "Mother (or "Sweetheart") of Chiropractic" (Ferguson, 1984), looking very much like a madonna—the total effect was that of the Holy Family. Adoration flowed. Followers frequently displayed prominently in their waiting rooms that picture of the "first family of chiropractic." It was not unusual for students to name their daughters Palmera or to use Palmer as the middle name for their sons (Lerner, 1954, p 632). Critic Charles Warner (1930, p 97) stated: "Chiropractic is a religion, it is the worship of B.J. Palmer. Palmer encourages the idea by wearing his hair and beard to resemble Christ; and by having his pictures taken in a pose to imitate Christ in the painting 'Christ Before Pilate.' " Arthur Seyse, M.D. (1924) cites "B.J.'s favorite quote of 1916, 'The first man that cured by laying on of hands they crucified.' "

Napoleon Hill, author of the popular *Think and Grow Rich* (1937), visited PSC in 1920 and penned the following glowing impressions (Linhart, 1988, pp 28–29):

> Here I found the most inspiring institution of any kind—bar none!—in America. Here I found MY teacher! A man who not only teaches about things, but how to do things. A man who embodies in his life and work the principles of living and doing, the fine "Art of selling Yourself." . . .

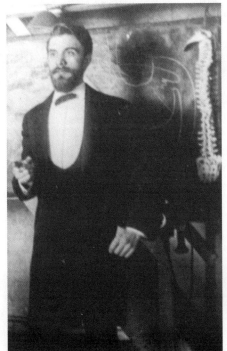

FIGURE 8.
B.J. Palmer, "Developer of Chiropractic,"
lecturing. (Courtesy of Palmer College of
Chiropractic Archives.)

Those students reminded me of scores of newly charged electric batteries. They were vibrating—and "vibrating" is the word—with enthusiasm that reached out and enmeshed me. . . .

The graduates of The Palmer School receive more than a training in Chiropractic: more than a knowledge of the human anatomy; they receive the best of training in the art of loving humanity: in good cheer, enthusiasm and self-confidence.

Here is how B.J. addressed his followers in 1935 (Dye, 1939, p 320):

I have made it my aim in my life to impart this message to the world through you, to teach this message of Chiropractic and its possibilities to you, that you could carry the message and the vision into those highways and byways for me.

B.J.'s influence on his students was impressed on me in my interview with Massachusetts chiropractor Harry Runge, who grew up in La Crosse, Wisconsin, made deliveries from the grocery store owned by Tom Morris's father, and was influenced by both Tom Morris and Shegataro Morikubo to study chiropractic. Incidentally, Runge described Morikubo as a well-educated man who fitted well into the La Crosse community. After graduating from PSC in 1912 Runge became one of the first chiropractors in Boston. Here is how he described in 1948 the atmosphere at PSC in 1912:

B.J. had the students so they could hardly wait until they could get out into practice, to carry chiropractic to the world, and to get sick people well. He filled us with enthusiasm and self-confidence. We knew that we had the power to do these things right in the palms of our hands. We were "miracle men." . . . I wanted to be a pioneer, a leader, a martyr if necessary. I wanted to be B.J.'s representative in Boston.

Regarding "martyrs," on the walls of the B.J. Palmer Chiropractic Clinic at PSC were 75 plaques dedicated to the "Early Martyrs" of chiropractic who had been convicted and sent to jail (Dye, 1939, p 91).

A distinguished 1956 graduate, Sid Williams (1990a), offered this confirmatory testimony:

[BJ] spoke as if he were *The One* in authority, as if he had been given the torch and the message straight from the source. . . . When the full impact of B.J.'s 'Big idea' hit me, I was more excited than I have ever been before. I felt I had full authority. I knew I was right. It was as if I'd entered a new age. I could see the light.

B.J.'s dominant presence at PSC is revealed in the following account of a 1948 graduation ceremony recalled in a commencement address by Dr. Christopher J. Klaes (1980):

Thirty-two years ago I sat where you are now sitting, as a new graduate of the Palmer College, only in those days we didn't have this beautiful auditorium to hold our commencement exercises in.

The commencement program for the class of March 1948 was held in the facilities of the Masonic Temple, down Brady Street a few blocks, and I will never forget as our class marched into that vast auditorium to the provocative and stirring cadence of "Pomp and Circumstance," took our seats, looked up at the keyboard of that massive and challenging theatrical organ, and there sat—B.J. Palmer.

At the invocation we bowed our heads in silent meditation, gave thanks for the spiritual blessings of the past, and asked for divine guidance to our professional futures, and the invocation was delivered by —B.J. Palmer.

We listened to the inspirational commencement address, which commissioned us to administer the Wonders of Chiropractic, to go out into the sick and suffering world and to be known as chiropractors and not physicians, and the commencement address was delivered by—B.J. Palmer.

At the conclusion of the ceremony, we all marched across that great stage and one by one proudly received our diplomas as a doctor of chiropractic, and the diplomas were handed to us personally by the President of Palmer College—B.J. Palmer.

B.J. was fond of aphorisms, for example: "The more you tell the quicker you sell"; "Early to bed, early to rise; work like hell—and advertise; makes a man healthy, wealthy and wise"; "Is life worth living? It depends on the liver"; and "Be a 100 percent American; keep your tonsils and your appendix." He loved to ridicule the medical profession, and would say: "DC = disease conquered; MD = more dope— more death." He boasted: "The distinctividuality portrays the personality of B.J. Palmer." He would pun: "My analysis is better than urinalysis." In an early publication he derisively defined x-ray as a technique used by surgeons to retrieve instruments left in patients after surgery. The only opportunity I had personally to hear him lecture was in 1950 in the Grand Ballroom of the Waldorf-Astoria Hotel in New York City, where he derisively explicated the medical etymology of the word "diagnosis" as based on two roots: "agnosis," meaning we don't know what's wrong with the patient, and "di," meaning let's divide him between us. One of his more tasteless remarks (and there were many!) was that there wasn't enough chiropracTIC in some chiropracTORS, making them chiropracTOIDS. He also made the following outrageous statements (Brennan, 1983a, pp 27–28): "All cancers, tumors, asthma, appendicitis, deafness, . . . have a common cause, namely impinged nerves," and "Bacteriology was the greatest of all gigantic farces ever invented for ignorance and incompetency." Here is a choice bit of invective penned by B.J. (1916, pp 42–43, 359–360):

I want to talk to you on the American Mendicants' Association, otherwise known as the medical octopus, the medical trust, and this phraseology is not merely a convenient term used to express our disgust and contempt for a certain small body of political medical men who control a much larger body of sincere scientific medical men; it is in truth all that we call it, a trust using constructive methods. First organized as an educational and protective association, it has spread its tentacles out over the entire country like a vampire. It controls the surroundings of your birth, milk supply, water supply, food supply, the sanitation in your house. . . . The AMA controls the time you are born and the time you die. They help both. . . . There is no trust like it in existence. Of late years it has degenerated into a vast political machine, the biggest dam to medical progress the world has ever seen. It condemns every method, every procedure, every theory, idea or help to humanity that does not originate within and financially help to fill the pockets of its own ranks. It cares not what you, as a patient, think; they will ride over your wishes and respects without an ask-you. It uses its vast wealth and political power to smother everything but its own inefficient methods. For ten years or more this octopus has tried to get legal and political control of every method of healing, maintaining paid lobbies in every state capitol of the country, and just so long as the people send doctors to the legislature, just so long will we be burdened with such confiscatory, unconstitutional, and unjust, inhuman and inhumane laws.

B.J.'s big ego revealed itself in the titles of his later publications: *The Subluxation Specific; The Adjustment Specific; An exposition of the Cause of All Disease* (1934), *The Bigness of the Fellow Within* (1949), *Up from Below the Bottom* (1950a), *Fight to Climb* (1950b), *Upside Down and Right Side Up with B.J.; Including the Greatest Mystery of History* (1953), *Fame and Fortune and the Know-How and Show-How to Attain It* (1955), *Palmer's Law of Life* (1958b), *Giant Versus Pygmy* (1959a), and *The Glory of Going On* (1961). When he said "History is *his* story," I interpreted it to mean B.J.'s story. He named one of his instruments, designed to measure mental impulses, the electroencephaloneuromentympograph (1951a, pp 241–252). Even after B.J.'s eclipse and loss of leadership resulting from the neurocalometer debacle in 1924 (see Section 3, below), the generally unsympathetic Lerner (1954, p 302) described B.J. appreciatively:

> Here was a man at the top of his profession; regarded as a leader, as a teacher, as a scholar, as an impressive public speaker; as an author and as a writer of many books; as a lecturer; as a "philosopher of chiropractic"; as the developer; as a man who has appeared in courts all over the country for many years as an expert witness; who has been headmaster of the oldest school of chiropractic in the world; who has appeared on the platform to lecture before hosts of audiences.

He edited the monthly *The Chiropractor* from 1906 until his death, and the "erratic" *Fountain Head News* for about 47 years (Gibbons, 1987, p 11).

B.J. revealed his personal style in his comments on my doctoral dissertation (Wardwell, 1951), which he sent to me in a three-and-a-half-page, single-spaced letter dated August 9, 1951, presumably personally typed, as was his custom:

> I have now had the time to go over the thesis carefully, studying it in its every part. I take it that you want honest criticism. With that in view, the following are my comments:

What is the hidden purpose of this laborious production?

Are you a D.C.; if so, from what school? Evidently you are a law or medic student of Harvard.

You quote and misquote B.J. more than any other person. Why?

You interpret and misinterpret B.J. more than any other. Why?

Many of your statements are not true to fact, then or now.

It is excellent as a thesis, but rotten as history because much of it is unreliable and inaccurate.

You reiterate much on Massachusetts, which is not typical of all states. . . .

You have quoted more anti-Chiropractic sources than pro-Chiropractic.

Your manuscript shows you lean more to the concept of mixing than to straight.

Your legislative observations and quotations are in the main, but not entirely, reliable. Your comments are in the main biased against us.

You have not taken into consideration that we are a young movement, therefore are suffering with growing pains in personnel, professional, scientific, and legislative. . . .

You do not discuss whether the principle and practice of Chiropractic is right or wrong, from a constructive view, independent of people involved; but discuss, at great length, the weaknesses and strengths of people of our profession and how far wrong they may be as individuals. . . .

It is evident that you have not seen, read, or studied my writings. It appears evident you have deliberately ignored them. . . .

You quote mostly from anti-PSC sources and little from our pro's. . . . You were a reporter seeking controversial trash and sensational news to fill blank pages, hoping to give your story a thesis appearance, hoping it would please the prejudices of Harvard Faculty who are proverbially pro-medicine and anti-anything-else, so you could win the Doctor of Philosophy. . . .

Your thesis is based on your observations, like medicine men. You sought symptoms and pathologies and found them. You proceed to "treat" them the same as a medical man would. The subjective cause and its correct adjustment, to get [the] patient well, has been overlooked. . . .

I come to the conclusion that you have labored long and hard to "sell Chiropractic down the river." . . .

Your thesis is so full of inconsistencies, incongruities, misquotations, misinterpretations, wrong comments, that it would take me a couple of months to go over it page by page and cite and correct them. . . .

We thank you very much for sending the copy of the thesis to us, and trust you will take my criticism in the spirit of fairness in a desire to set you right.

(Note the royal or editorial "We") He must have had my entire dissertation retyped, because PSC archivist Glenda Wiese later found a newly typed copy in B.J.'s personal library. Perhaps his critical evaluation of it was partly influenced by his increasingly painful stomach ulcer (Quigley, 1989c), because in his August 9, 1955, letter reacting to my first *published* paper on chiropractic (Wardwell, 1952) he was far more gracious:

> From the viewpoint of "a man in the street" as "an innocent bystander" trying to evaluate the conflicts between medicine and Chiropractic, medical men and Chiropractors, the practice of medicine and the adjustment of cause by the Chiropractor, WE think you have done a creditable presentation.
>
> Of course we can't agree with you in ALL your conclusions, but we certainly CAN agree with many. Because of that we congratulate you.

It was obvious that he had spent considerable time on my thesis, even taking into account the speed with which he habitually worked. I felt flattered that he had done so; and although he didn't intend to compliment me, I felt that his remarks were evidence of the objectivity which I had sought in my thesis, especially since medical reviewers seemed to believe I was equally biased in the opposite direction.

He was certainly a survivor! A complex character, he acquired tremendous self-discipline despite a childhood deprived of loving care. He was abstemious in the extreme. He never touched intoxicating liquor. He went to bed promptly at nine o'clock at home no matter what distinguished guest was present, and he entertained, among others, Presidents Coolidge, Hoover, and Truman; Thomas Edison; William Jennings Bryan; and Elbert Hubbard, who wrote (1913) favorably about chiropractic. According to Lerner (1954, p 666), it was Hubbard who, through John D. Rockefeller's personal physician, homeopath Hamilton Biggars, persuaded Rockefeller to use chiropractic and "natural" remedies after he became ill and nearly unable to eat following stomach surgery and medical treatment. B.J. could also be generous and community oriented. Son Dave wrote (1977, p 151): "He had a standing invitation with the Iowa Parole Board to employ at least one parolee each year." Tullius Ratledge, president of a major college in California from 1911 to 1955, wrote: "From 1913 until the time of his passing, I regarded B.J. Palmer as the President of the Chiropractic World" (cited in Smallie, 1990a, p 44).

Willard Carver (1936, pp 42–43) relates sarcastically his impression of B.J. as an infant in 1881: "Mrs. Palmer came to the door . . . holding . . . B.J. . . . . He was talking quite extravagantly, not to say vociferously, but Willard says he does not know what he was saying, but that such talk has always been his habit, and that nobody has ever known what he was talking about." A medical writer who attended one of B.J.'s public lectures in Washington, D.C., described him as "egotistic as a Chinese God and as ignorant as an African cannibal" (Brennan, 1983a, p 29).

B.J. was not the well-read student that D.D. was. His most egregious error was to claim discovery of a "duct of Palmer connecting the spleen with the stomach" (Brennan 1983a, p 28; Meyer, 1925). In addition, D.D. (1910, p 800) quotes B.J. as saying, "When I saw there was no use for a Sympathetic Nervous System, I threw it out, and then just had to put something better in its place, so I discovered Direct Neural Impulse." Gaucher-Peslherbe (1992) states that B.J. "with one stroke of his pen obliterated the sympathetic nervous system and replaced it with a new system," which he called " 'mental influx'. . . that richly deserved the epistolary beating it got from his father. . . . [BJ] regularly plundered his father's lecture notes for material to use in his own publications: a habit to which Palmer took strong exception, especially in view of the use his son made of it." B.J.'s wife, Mabel, later wrote in her *Chiropractic Anatomy* (1918, pp 262–268) that B.J. discovered serous circulation in 1905 and that it "begins in the small intestine and absorbs serum and ends at the kidney and the skin, meanwhile going into and becoming a part of every structure of your body." But D.D. (1910, pp 274, 403) would have none of that:

> The author of "serous circulation" could have saved himself from committing a serious blunder and from misleading his students by referring to any dictionary where he could have learned the meaning of circulation. To circulate is to move in a circle, to move round and return to the same point; blood circulates but *serum does not*. Serum is transudated by the laws of vital osmosis—regulated by affinity. . . . I have cracked some of the paragraph shells and find that what is new is of no value and what is of worth is given in every book on anatomy, physiology and pathology. It is ridiculous for any one to state that "Serous Circulation has never been conceived before." It certainly never has been.

Often D.D. (1910, p 678) simply belittled B.J.:

> He writes of himself, "His every thought is a gem, and when compiled in this fashion are treasure houses of knowledge." It would be nearer the truth to say that his thoughts are frequently the outburst of egotistical ignorance, filling his cranium and others with a lot of rubbish that retards Chiropractic.

Perhaps it was because D.D. felt robbed and deprived by B.J. that he thought it necessary constantly to claim recognition for himself as the founder of chiropractic. He (1910, p 629) never hid his anger toward B.J.:

> Little did I think that B.J. Palmer, my only son, would prove to be the sneak thief who would try to appropriate the credit of originality and would desire to rob his father of the honor justly due him. Little did I think then that my only son would play the Judas, put me in prison, rob me financially and of credit justly due me.

However, B.J. had written the following about his father in 1907, according to D.D. (1910, p 820): "His actions and thoughts are sharp, alert, and ahead of the times. He holds an enviable and honored position because others are being taught to reach his intellectual level. His every thought was *Why?*"

Like his father, B.J. was an abrasive, opinionated autocrat who created many enemies as well as many devoted followers. It would take volumes to write his definitive biography, which ought to be written but never has been. Herbert Hender, PSC Dean after 1943, described B.J. as follows (cited by Gibbons, 1987, p 10:

> He was born into a family . . . with little wealth. His mother died when he was one and a half years old. From then on, he was at the mercy of three cruel stepmothers, each worse than the one before. The first 20 years of B.J.'s life were spent in being educated to hate people and everything they did. He was often forced to sleep in dry-goods boxes in alleys, sometimes with the weather below zero.

According to Fishbein (1925, p 80), B.J. testified in court in Milwaukee in 1910 while defending a chiropractor: "At the age of 11 I was kicked from home, . . . studied art some in Chicago, not very long, . . . landscape work, painting. I have studied music."

Schafer (1991c) reports an observation he made while living with his family across Brady Street from PSC:

> One day I saw B.J. approach and spit in the face of two students who were walking on the sidewalk near "Little Bit of Heaven." I could not understand this and asked my dad what could cause such behavior. I was told that B.J. vehemently hated Jews and so acted on occasion—yet he would accept their tuition. It was common knowledge that B.J., like Charles Lindbergh, openly supported Hitler in the 1930s.

Lerner (1954, pp 308–317) tried to probe the depths of B.J.'s personality on the basis of several face-to-face interviews, some tape-recorded but apparently now lost. He concluded that B.J. had been much influenced by spending a year as a professional hypnotic subject. He noted that B.J. customarily talked as though he were "on stage," acting a role, one of which was imitating his father, which he did word-for-word at first.

Finally, B.J.'s son Dave (1977, pp 95, 97, 134, 165) evaluated his father as follows:

> B.J. was the personification of originality. He . . . had the talent to be another P.T. Barnum. He also had the courtroom talent of a prosecutor or defending lawyer of the stature of Clarence Darrow or Melvin Belli. He did not live his life by the book and had no intention of trying to do so. He picked up the responsibility and torch from his father as the leader of the chiropractic profession. . . . Of all B.J.'s talents I would say the finest was his ability to speak before large audiences. . . . As a raconteur he was unbeatable. . . . No one but B.J. traveled so much, fought court battles so often successfully, introduced chiropractic legislation for the continuing betterment of the profession. As the "Developer," he deserves the heartfelt thanks of every Doctor of Chiropractic who serves in the interest of mankind.

Section 3

The Neurocalometer Debacle

A 1922 PSC graduate, Dossa D. Evins (1886–1932), also an electrical engineer, spent many months developing an instrument capable of registering heat differentials on the skin between the two sides of a vertebra. Called the neurocalometer, or NCM, it was designed to identify "hot boxes" that would reveal more scientifically the location of subluxations. B.J. decided that it was just what the profession needed to alter the course of its history, so with Evins and his business manager, Frank Elliott (1887–1976), he decided to patent it. Although it and copies were already being marketed, B.J. summoned his supporters for a startling new announcement at the August 1924 PSC annual homecoming (Lyceum) and convention of the Universal Chiropractors Association. William Heath ("Nip") Quigley, Mabel's nephew and reportedly closer to B.J. than was son Dave, had spent many days in his youth helping B.J. construct the famed botanical retreat behind the Palmer mansion that B.J. called "a little bit o' heaven." Although he was only 9 years old at the time, here is how Quigley (1989a) described the excitement and events as the day of the promised announcement, billed as "The Hour Has Struck," approached:

> B.J. appointed a faculty research committee whose first priority was to develop a standard technique for use of the instrument which was to be called the Neurocalometer, but it was usually referred to as the NCM. He also set the research goals for the team. Unfortunately, he snubbed the three major faculty members, Harry Vedder, Steve Burich, and James Firth. They were widely known throughout the field as the Big Three with a sizable following of their own. I don't know why he ignored them but he did. . . .

> He had met a few days previously with the faculty and staff. He gave them a summary of the research team's findings and what he planned to do. He demanded that everyone pledge support to the NCM program. He let everyone know that if they didn't subscribe fully he didn't want them on the faculty. He was surprised when Drs. Vedder, Burich, and Firth handed in their resignations. I'm sure they left Palmer with regret but, feeling as they did, there were no other options.

> B.J. made the presentation in the D.D. Palmer Auditorium on the morning of the 24th. The hall was jammed and the second floor fire escapes were overflowing with men clinging with whatever hold they could manage, hoping to catch a word or two of B.J.'s announcements. Inside, the densely packed throng sat on the edge of their seats, nearly breathless as B.J. extolled the NCM as capable of locating the exact location of subluxations in the spine. In the context of his philosophy he was saying the NCM will find the cause of dis-ease. . . .

> The next phase of the presentation cooled the ardor somewhat. . . . B.J. explained that the NCM would not be sold, but leased. The cost of the lease was $3,500 and the monthly rent was $5.00. This was bad enough, but what followed was even worse. He threatened that if the profession did not begin using the NCM in sufficient numbers he would turn it over to the barbers whom he predicted would replace chiropractors overnight.

> The Lyceum crowd immediately and later the field split into two factions: those who would lease and use the NCM and those who were unconvinced and felt exploited. The latter group broke away from Palmer, giving their support and loyalty to other chiropractic leaders including the Big Three. Whether this was a black day for Palmer and B.J. was difficult to assess. Predictably, the campus was in uproar for the rest of that historic Sunday. But by Monday the dissenters had left for home and those who remained were euphoric, eagerly waiting for delivery of their NCMs. We do know that the long term effect was that B.J. suffered a major loss of support and a partitioning of his power and leadership. Because the NCM was such a stunning financial success there was little evidence of this misadventure on campus. Years later Otto Schiernbeck, the

late head of the NCM Service Department, told me that more than 1000 instruments were leased at homecoming and another thousand during the next year. . . .

Characteristically, he rarely took an active part in the financial planning of the school or his broadcasting company. For example, when he built the B.J. Palmer Research Clinic he didn't ask how much it would cost. He presented an architect with what he wanted, then turned the negotiations over to Ralph Evans, his vice president. . . . His mode of operation was to promote his enterprises as he saw fit and Ralph would be expected to provide the wherewithall. Similarly, when the NCM contract was drawn, his attorneys dealt with the detail he disliked and I doubt if it ever occurred to him that the cost of the NCM might be beyond the average practitioner's means. As he did with those of us close to him, he assumed that like him, if we wanted something we would simply "get" it.

His threat to turn the NCM over to the barbers was preposterous. Nothing could have convinced him to do that because he was wed forever to chiropractic. This out-of-character episode was never discussed by the family in my presence, therefore it is difficult to place it in a realistic perspective. . . . There were a few Lyceums which generated anger and divisiveness. The Lyceum of 1924 was certainly one of them.

Frank Elliott confirmed to me in 1974 B.J.'s financial stance: "I made the money and B.J. spent it."

The initial fee to lease the NCM has been elsewhere variously reported as $1,200, $1,500, and $2,500. Without doubt the price fluctuated, and it soon fell to $150, plus $5 for the monthly rental charge. Within 5 years PSC suffered a 90% decline in enrollment. B.J.'s most decisive loss was that of the Big Three from his faculty (Fig 9): Stephen J. Burich (1887–1946), author of *A Textbook of Chiropractic Chemistry* (1919); Harry Vedder (1891–1949), author of *A Textbook on Chiropractic Physiology* (1916) and *A Textbook on Chiropractic Gynecology* (1919); and James Firth (1886–1964), author of *A Textbook on Chiropractic Symptomatology* (1914). Later Arthur G. Hendricks (1894–1962), coauthor with Earl A. Rich (1921–1967) of *X-Ray Technique and Spinal Misalignment Interpretation* (1947), joined them. They established Lincoln Chiropractic College in Indianapolis, which soon became recognized as one of the best colleges (Stowell, 1983). Among its presidents were Vedder (1926–1940), Firth (1940–1954), Hendricks (1954–1962), and Rich (1965–1967). Due to financial difficulties it merged into the National College of Chiropractic (NCC) in Chicago in 1971.

Unfortunately for chiropractic, two other near catastrophes coincided with the NCM episode. In 1923 Nellie Revell, a popular theatrical performer and columnist, after being treated by a New York City chiropractor for a serious spinal condition, "collapsed and had to be taken to the hospital immediatcly" (Lerner, 1954, pp 759–762). She then wrote a book, *Right Off the Chest,* relating her experience but graciously not naming the chiropractor (Revell, 1923, pp 74–75):

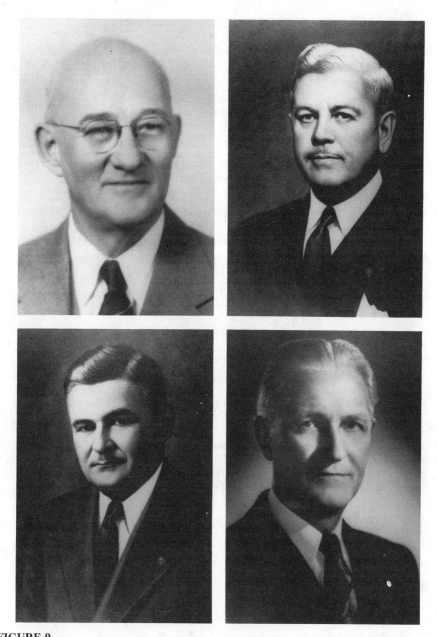

FIGURE 9.

"The Four Horsemen," professors who abandoned B.J. Palmer in 1924, because of his insistence on use of the neurocalometer, and subsequently established Lincoln Chiropractic College in Indianapolis in 1926. *Top left,* James Firth; *top right,* Harry Vedder; *bottom left,* Stephen J. Burich; *bottom right,* Arthur G. Hendricks. (Courtesy of National Chiropractic College.)

The breakdown which landed me in the hospital had been approaching a crisis for two years. . . . Three vertebrae had been caved in. In simple justice, I must say I do not believe the chiropractor's treatment would have injured them had they not already been affected. I should probably have broken down very soon in any case, with my spine in that condition, and I do not wish to lay the primary blame for my illness at this man's door. But I am convinced that no chiropractor should fail to preface his treatments with an X-ray examination to ascertain whether there are any diseased parts. . . . It is not reasonable to condemn the many for the faults of the few and I am not decrying the whole body of chiropractors because of this incident.

But her friends began ridiculing chiropractic from the stage.

Then in 1924 Morris Fishbein became Editor of *JAMA* and began his antichiropractic campaign in lectures and print. He might have drawn ideas from the disastrous legal brief prepared by B.J.'s lawyers to persuade the U.S. Patent Office to make an exception for the NCM application, because at that time its policy was not to grant patents for new methods of treating the sick. (Frank Elliott told me when I interviewed him in Denver in 1976 that it was only after he had threatened to appeal to then Secretary of Commerce Herbert Hoover that a "process patent" was granted.) Some of the damning words from the brief examined by Lerner (1954, pp 770–771) were:

Heretofore, attempted correction of subluxations or nerve impingements has been *guesswork, . . . the adjustment was uncertain, unscientific, and liable to cause injury rather than to correct the abnormal condition presented for correction.* Applicant's process has entirely obviated all these difficulties, and has changed that which has heretofore been *uncertain, unscientific,*— in fact *guesswork*— and even *dangerous*—and has now made it possible to produce scientifically correct and accurate adjustments of the spine.

After his Lyceum talk B.J. never regained his dominance of the profession; Lyceum attendance dropped from more than 8,000 in 1921 to 700 in 1926 (Crisp, 1984). Although B.J. remained its titular leader and continued to publish books and millions of copies of tracts and informational brochures, his future personal fortune came more from business ventures in radio and television broadcasting and land. However, one result of the NCM debacle, according to Turner (1931, p 45), was to create greater unity among the "fundamentalist element" loyal to B.J. and his principles.

Section 4

The Palmer School After 1925

PSC's enrollment shrank to fewer than 400 after the NCM debacle. Bank failure caused by the depression had wiped out school and personal accounts. B.J.'s son Dave, a 1929 graduate of the University of Pennsylvania Wharton School of Finance and Commerce, returned to PSC and was named Vice President and Business Manager. He later wrote (1977, p 33): "I found PSC virtually bankrupt and under the control of our First National Bank of Davenport." He also tells us (1977, p 55) that B.J. had never solicited donations from his graduates because "he didn't want the alumni to interfere with his management." Dave initiated cost-cutting and income-producing measures that he says rescued PSC from financial disaster. One of his schemes to raise money was to sell "Gold Bond" notes to alumni, regarding which he says B.J. later "wrote a letter pleading hardship and asking the notes be donated to the school," which brought in enough money to save the school.

Dave (1977, p 66) considered that his "first major campus improvement . . . was to get rid of 'the tent,' which had been for years our only means of housing Lyceum crowds, " and to attract sufficient donations to construct in 1970 an "Alumni Auditorium seating 5000 at a cost of over a million dollars." Although Dave suffered a (little known) nervous breakdown amidst all these financial difficulties, according to Frank Elliott, who preceded Dave as Business Manager, as a true Palmer Dave gave his own performance high marks, writing: "My accomplishments were achieved over almost overwhelming odds" (1977, pp 52–53).

B.J. had ceased active practice about 1912 (Dye, 1939, p 319) to devote full time to teaching and administration. Between 1925 and 1934 he spent much time traveling overseas. In 1931 he began scheduling Pre-Lyceum courses, at which he would announce new developments to the profession. In 1935 he announced stereo-scopic spinographic procedures, and established the B.J. Palmer Chiropractic Clinic, at a cost of $125,000 (Dye, 1939, p 334), primarily to carry out research on chiropractic. He described its objective as follows (Wilcher, 1989a, p 122):

> The fundamental of this clinic is to see how little we can do, at how few places, how rarely and how quickly it can be done, to accomplish the greatest changes in the shortest space of time at the least cost to the case, and to know what to do and why to do it before doing it.

In the early 1930s B.J. prescribed a new adjusting technique as controversial as the NCM, and insisted that all chiropractors adopt it. Montenegro (1988) quotes him as saying: "I have found the only cause of disease." It was an upper cervical specific adjustment that he called "hole-in-one" (HIO) because he had determined that the only vertebrae chiropractors should adjust were the atlas and the axis, that is, the first two cervical vertebrae. Students in the PSC clinic were not permitted to adjust below the axis, and even had to get permission to adjust it. Vertebrae below the axis were to be called "misaligned" rather than "subluxated" (Dye, 1939, p 305). "From September 1936 to August 1937, inclusive, Atlas was adjusted as Major 17,436 times and Axis but 379 times, or about 98% for Atlas as against 2% for Axis" (Dye, 1939, p 167). Surprisingly, Dye (1939, p 305) states that B.J. "accepted the generally accepted medical and anatomical theory that the subluxation of a spinal vertebra below the inferior surface of Axis is an impossibility." Hence he further narrowed the scope of practice for that segment of the profession that followed his leadership. Since his mandate was contrary to the training, reasoning, and clinical experience of most chiropractors, it was even less acceptable than the NCM. Nevertheless, it was the only technique taught at PSC until pressure from the field in 1949 persuaded B.J. to reinstate full-spine techniques and to extend the course of instruction to 4 years of 9 months (Quigley, 1989b).

Quigley (1989c) has given us a detailed account of the "Last Days of B.J. Palmer." He suffered intensely from a stomach ulcer for which he characteristically refused medical treatment (see his own account in 1951b, pp 700–705). However, he remained president of PSC until his death in 1961, giving his last Lyceum lecture in 1960, but leaving its day-to-day administration largely to others. Gibbons (1987, p 10) summarizes:

> For better than half of this century, B.J. was the center of much of the solar system of chiropractic, yet for the last 37 years of his life he was a setting sun in a profession founded by his father and largely developed by himself. He would become a prophet scorned, relegated to a philosophical Mecca that could no longer command annual pilgrimages of unquestioning followers.

After assuming the presidency Dave justified his chosen designation as "The Educator" by strengthening the academic program and changing PSC to PCC (Palmer *College* of Chiropractic) in 1965, thus bringing it into line with most other colleges. Although he had taken a nominal D.C. degree in 1938, Dave never practiced or became closely involved in the internal affairs of the college. He designated a series of "administrators" to manage it, among whom was his cousin "Nip" Quigley from 1974 to 1976. On Dave's death in 1978 the PCC Board of Trustees chose the first non-Palmer-family president, Jerome F. McAndrews, D.C., who had been Executive Vice President of the International Chiropractors Association since 1971. Under his leadership (1978–1987) PCC regained stature not only as the largest but also as one of the more progressive chiropractic colleges, especially in research. Palmer family control was again exerted in 1987 when Dave's daughter Vickie Palmer Miller persuaded the Board of Trustees to elect her as chairperson; Donald P. Kern then became president. PCC's educational and research momentum, its current size, and its more than 12,000 licensed graduates keep it still, symbolically at least, the fountainhead of the profession, although Life College in Atlanta announced in 1990 that, with 1,657 students, it had overtaken PCC's 1,622.

Chapter 5

Other Early Leaders, Schools, Associations

*The greatest problem facing the profession is the
quarrel among its teachers — and not among its
practitioners.*

Cyrus Lerner (1954, p 330)

D.D. and B.J. Palmer and the Palmer School of Chiropractic (PSC) did not comprise the entire history of early chiropractic. Other leaders wrote books, organized schools, and attracted followers. Without books how else could they establish a reputation? Joseph Janse (1976, pp 4–6) accounted for chiropractic sectarianism as follows:

> The great personalities of our early professional history . . . felt that survival resided in proselytism, indoctrination, and the maintenance of a crusading fervor. In fact, these methods represented much of the early chiropractic education; an educational process based upon the development of convictions through emotional promptings and the teaching of empirical conclusions. . . . Such a type and method of leadership . . . always leads to great hero worship. Possibly no professional group has afforded its early leader greater adulation than the peoples of our profession. Unfortunately, this did lead to an overemphasis of personalities. . . . For the first four decades of our existence we practiced professional feudalism.

However, for many years there was reasonable organizational unity in the field in the one professional association of any significance, the Universal Chiropractors Association (UCA), with B.J. as permanent Secretary and unquestioned leader.

Section 1

Other Leaders and Schools

The American School of Chiropractic and Nature Cure, founded by Solon M. Langworthy, Oakley G. Smith, and Minora C. Paxson in 1903 in Cedar Rapids, Iowa, has been mentioned. Both it and their American Chiropractic Association disappeared within a few years. Oakley Smith (Figure 10) later moved from Cedar Rapids to Chicago, and created a new field of health care, *naprapathy,* closely related to chiropractic but emphasizing damaged ligaments ("ligatites") rather than nerves. Gaucher-Peslherbe (1992) tells us that the word "naprapathy" is derived from a Scandinavian root meaning to repair or correct and that Smith said it means "to correct the cause," thus closely paralleling the Palmer theory. Smith later (1932, p 8) defined a ligatite as "partial immobility of a joint." He also stimulated the anatomist Harold Swanberg (1915) to undertake pioneering research on the intervertebral foramina, which allegedly supported the subluxation hypothesis. And he founded the Oakley Smith College of Naprapathy, which filiated eventually into the Chicago National College of Naprapathy. I assume that Smith was the principal author of *A Textbook of Modernized Chiropractic* (Langworthy, Smith, and Paxson, 1906), because he republished it with a prologue of only 16 pages as *Naprapathy Genetics* in 1932 with himself as sole author (Zarbuck, 1986). Although D.D. (1910, p 665) criticized the 1906 text for stating, "I know this, that every fundamental Chiropractic original idea (with meager exceptions) was gained—either borrowed or stolen—directly from the Bohemians"

FIGURE 10.
Oakley Smith, founder of naprapathy, circa 1920.
(Courtesy of National College of Chiropractic.)

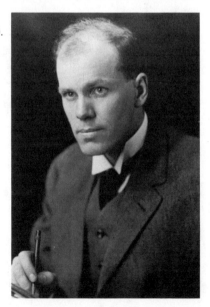

(referring to napravit), Gaucher-Peslherbe (1985, p 214) notes that D.D., usually "so quick to criticize the faults he saw in others, never really condemned Smith's work, which took a line of which he fundamentally approved." The similarity between naprapathy and chiropractic was attested to in an address by chiropractor John C. Lowe to the American Naprapathic Association ("Houston DC Addresses Naprapathic Convention," 1989):

> Lowe explains and teaches a chiropractic approach that both chiropractors and napra-paths accept. The bulk of Dr. Lowe's three-hour presentation was devoted to recent scientific findings that support the basic premise of naprapathy, as well as an important concept in chiropractic—that it is mainly excessive muscle and connective tissue constrictions that impair biomechanics and neural and vascular function.

Several hundred naprapaths still practice in Illinois (Semmes, 1978). However, in 1989 the Illinois Supreme Court denied to the Naprapathic College the right to continue. Its students who could qualify were admitted to study for a D.C. at the National College of Chiropractic (NCC), in Chicago.

Further complicating terminology, Andrew P. Davis (1835–1915), a graduate of Rush Medical College who also had studied and taught at Andrew T. Still's American School of Osteopathy in Kirksville, Missouri, before becoming D.D.'s second MD student in 1898, authored *Osteopathy Illustrated* (1899) and founded yet another variant of chiropractic and osteopathy called "neuropathy." Using "neurology" and "neuropathy" interchangeably, he published *Neurology* (1905) and *Neuropathy* (1909). His 1905 book appropriated D.D.'s chiropractic thrust as "neurologic manipulation," although in it he condemned both Still's and Palmer's techniques. He founded many schools of short duration, including (with Benson S. Bullis) in 1911 the School of Neuropathy, Ophthmology and Chiropractic, in Los Angeles (Zarbuck, 1988). Although naprapaths and neuropaths gained licensure in a few states, neither group could challenge chiropractic's dominance of the field.

Another offshoot from chiropractic was the "spondylotherapy" of Albert Abrams, M.D. (1863–1924), whose early work had gained him "an international reputation as a neurologist" before he was later "drummed out of the regular profession" (Gibbons, 1980a, p 22). He wrote several books on spondylotherapy (e.g., 1910, 1912), and in another (1914, p 103) wrote: "Spondylotherapy concerns itself only with the excitation of the functional centers of the spinal cord by different methods." According to the *National Cyclopedia of American Biography* (1945), Abrams "asserted that human blood is radioactive; that it gives off certain wave-like emanations through which diseases of the human body may be detected and cured." Although he had been a professor at Stanford University and vice president of the California State Medical Society, his venture into ERA (Electronic Reactions of Abrams), better known as "radionics," prompted *JAMA* to rank him "the dean of all twentieth century charlatans" (Coe, 1970, p 225). Gaucher-Peslherbe's (1992) more perceptive historical judgment is that Abrams was "a timely medical counterfire to the spreading of osteopathy and chiropractic" in that he "rediscovered" a mode of percussive treatment of "the spinous processes of the vertebrae" used in France by Recamier and Seguin 50 years earlier.

Willard Carver (1866–1943; Figure 11) tells us in his unpublished *History of Chiropractic* (1936, p 22) that he "had been an invalid from infancy until he received the application of the principles of Chiropractic." An 1891 graduate in law from Drake University, despite residing in Oskaloosa, Iowa, Carver was a long-time friend and performed various legal services for D.D. beginning in 1898. Having little affection for the young B.J., he chose to study at Charles Ray Parker's School of Chiropractic in Ottumwa, Iowa, graduating in 1906 (Dzaman, 1980, p 278). He wrote (1936, pp 32–34):

> By June of 1906 there were some six or seven Chiropractic schools and colleges scattered widely over the United States, and . . . each school had a different theory as to the art of Chiropractic, which it was attempting to teach and demonstrate. . . . Between 1905 and 1910 the system called "vertebral adjustment" was extending very rapidly; that is, many people were taking up the so-called study of Chiropractic, not according to a fixed science or system, and therefore a definite plan; but according to the peculiar ideas and experiences of many persons, clustered around the idea of "removing pressure from nerves," on the hypothesis that such pressure caused 95% of disease.". . .
>
> It therefore came about that the Chiropractic profession was constantly disturbed by "new adjustments," and every bizarre "movement," "every ridiculous application, even the most dangerous and absurd expedients; such, for instance, as a harness by which the patient was hung by the head to traction his neck, and various stretching apparatus, and other inexplicable things, too numerous for record. As a result of the flurrie there were

FIGURE 11.
Willard Carver, "Constructor of Chiropractic";
President of Carver Chiropractic College,
Oklahoma City, 1906–1943. (Courtesy of Logan
College of Chiropractic archives.)

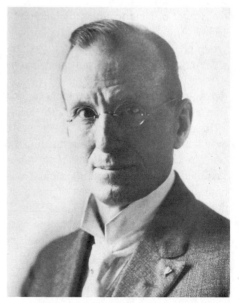

"The Parker Lumbar Discovery," "The Langworthy Method," "The Smith System," "The Howard System," and so on, throughout the list of all those who assumed to conduct schools.

With L.L. Denny, Carver opened the Carver-Denny School of Chiropractic in Oklahoma City in 1906, which in 1908 became Carver Chiropractic College, the first to receive a state charter. He designated his college the "Science Head," in contrast to B.J.'s "Fountain Head," and himself "the Constructor of Chiropractic," in contrast to B.J.'s self-designation as "the Developer." Carver's philosophy gave equal importance to any anatomically produced 'nerve occlusion,' whether or not related to the vertebral column" (Rosenthal, 1981, p 26), while his *structural* approach to spinal biomechanics became more "holistic" than B.J.'s segmental one-bone-out-of-place approach. According to Ratledge (1971, p 81), who graduated under Carver in 1907: "We were permitted to become good adjusters while in school because of an arrangement that allowed us to enter at any time and start in learning to adjust. Students attended adjusting classes every day." Carver published *Carver's Chiropractic Analysis* in 1909, one of 18 books he wrote, several of which dealt with psychology. His theories were later developed by Mortimer Levine (1917–1975) of his New York school in an influential book, *The Structural Approach to Chiropractic* (1964).

Carver established four chiropractic colleges in all: his college in Oklahoma City; Carver Chiropractic Institute, in New York City in 1919; Carver Chiropractic Research Institute, in Washington, D.C. in 1922; and Colorado Chiropractic University, in Denver in 1923. The Oklahoma City school remained strong until 1958, when it merged into Logan College of Chiropractic in St. Louis. The Washington school apparently soon disappeared. The Carver Chiropractic Institute in New York City was absorbed into the New York School of Chiropractic in 1934. Homer G. Beatty (1897–1951), who had graduated from Carver's Oklahoma school in 1922, became dean of the Colorado school in 1923 and its president in 1924, serving until his death in 1951. In 1939 Beatty published *Anatomical Adjustive Technique*. By 1935 the school was reorganized as the nonprofit University of the Natural Healing Arts, which offered three doctoral degrees, D.C., N.D., and D.P.T. (Doctor of Physical Therapy), the last requiring 3 years of study rather than the 4 required for the others. In 1965 the school closed and its charter and records were transferred to NCC in Chicago.

The first dissenter from B.J.'s own faculty was John Fitzalan Howard (1876–1953; Figure 12), a 1905 graduate who believed that the PSC curriculum was weak, especially in human dissection (Beideman, 1983; Howard, 1912). Howard wrote in his memoirs (cited in Beideman, 1990, p 7) that "a delegation [of students] called upon me and implored me to organize a school and teach chiropractic as it should be taught." In 1906 he founded the National School of Chiropractic in the same Ryan Building that D.D. had first occupied, moving the school to Chicago in 1908. Between 1910 and 1914 he brought five MDs onto its staff, and in 1914 sold it to one of them, William Charles Schulze (1870–1936; Figure 12), who was also president of the American College of Mechano-Therapy. A graduate of Rush Medical

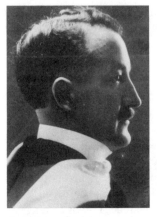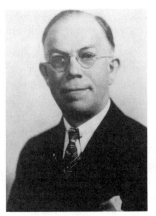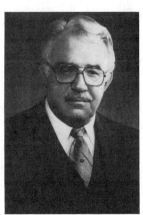

FIGURE 12.
Presidents of National College of Chiropractic, Chicago: *Left,* John Fitzalan Howard, 1906–1914; *middle,* William Charles Schulze, 1914–1936; *right,* Joseph Janse, 1945–1983. (Courtesy of National College of Chiropractic.)

College, Schulze placed stronger emphasis on the basic medical sciences, and by 1912 had added "physiological therapeutics" to the curriculum (before the terms "physiotherapy" and "physical therapy" had been invented!), which made National a strong mixer school and a particular target of B.J.'s venom (Ransom, 1984). However, the term physiological therapeutics had been used in the title of a book as early as 1902 (Cohen, 1902–1905) and was taught at the Cincinnati Post-Graduate School of Physiological Therapeutics by 1903. Although Dye (1939, p 136) claimed that it was the unsuccessful chiropractors that turned to mixing, that was hardly fair. Later renamed the National *College* of Chiropractic (NCC), it became and remains one of the strongest chiropractic colleges. Schulze was president until his death in 1936. From 1945 until 1983 it was vigorously led by Joseph Janse (1909–1985; Figure 12), to whom Gaucher-Peslherbe dedicated his book, calling him "the Old Dad Chiro of our time." A prolific author, Janse (1947; 1955; 1976, p 110) continued to emphasize physiological therapeutics, which as he explained "encompassed the clinical application of light, heat, water, traction, exercises, manipulation, pressure point therapy, etc. Certainly this would indicate that 'physiotherapy' found its initial emphasis and clinical phylogenesis in the chiropractic profession." There is a subtle terminologic distinction between "physiotherapy," the word used by chiropractors, and "physical therapy," preferred by physical therapists. Partial confirmation of chiropractors' chronologic priority in this field comes from the well-known physical therapy educator Frances Tappan, who states: "Between 1854 and 1918 the practice of massage developed from an obscure trade to a field of medical health care, and the profession of physical therapy began" (1988, p 6). It was only during and after World War II that physical therapy became a recognized profession. In 1986 James E. Winterstein became president of NCC.

The next schism at PSC occurred in 1910 when Joy M. Loban (1876–1939), who had been personally selected by B.J. to teach his beloved philosophy courses, broke with B.J., with the following result (Dye, 1939, p 71):

> In the middle of B.J.'s lecture on Philosophy one morning in mid-April, 1910, as if by a prearranged signal, forty or fifty of the students arose and marched out of the class-room, down the hill to Brady and Sixth Streets, and the next thing everybody knew a new school of Chiropractic was in operation in Davenport. That school was the Universal Chiropractic College.

In 1912 Loban published *Technic and Practice of Chiropractic*, and in 1929 his 500-page *Textbook of Neurology*. Universal College was merged into the Pittsburgh College of Chiropractic in 1918, which, with researcher Leo J. Steinbach (1886–1960) as dean and from 1927 president, was successful until 1944 when it merged into Lincoln Chiropractic College in Indianapolis.

Wiese and Ferguson (1988) identified 392 different chiropractic schools as having existed in the United States. When those for which there is no evidence of more than a year of operation are eliminated, the number is reduced to 188. Most of them probably produced few graduates. D.D.'s injunction to go forth to practice and teach impelled many chiropractors to do both. The number of schools increased rapidly to their largest total between 1910 and 1926, and then contracted, particularly during the depression of the 1930s and World War II. Although veterans' educational benefits after World War II attracted more students, the number of schools continued to decline through 1970, largely through mergers, as the costs of the improved curricula exceeded the tuition that fewer students could bring in.

Alva Gregory, M.D., D.C., with whom D.D. founded the Palmer-Gregory School of Chiropractic in Oklahoma City in 1907, kept the school going for a few years after D.D. left for Oregon. He authored two early classics, *Spinal Adjustment* (1912) and *Rational Therapy* (1913), in which he explicated chiropractic principles without using the word "chiropractic" or crediting D.D., but criticized "chiropractic spondylotherapy." Like D.D., he talked about "lung place," "stomach place," "liver place," and "kidney place" in the vertebral column. And like Smith, he gave much credit to the Bohemian tradition of napravit (Gromala, 1986, p 60).

Tullius F. Ratledge (1881–1967; Figure 13) earned a D.C. degree in 1907 from Carver College, and in 1908 opened schools, first in Tulsa, Oklahoma, and then in Kansas. In 1911 he moved to Los Angeles and founded Ratledge Chiropractic College which figured prominently in chiropractic education until its acquisition by Carl S. Cleveland, Sr., in 1955, at which time it had only 17 students. Ratledge had been as active in securing licensing legislation in California as Carver was in Kansas and Oklahoma. He wrote: "I thank God that I was permitted to know Dr. Willard Carver for the first impression of the science of chiropractic from him. Later, I was fortunate in knowing D.D. Palmer and having the fundamentals from Dr. Carver. I was in position to compare their thinking patterns. I believe their thinking was more similar than any of the other school men" (Smallie, 1990a, p 48). He was as insistent as B.J. that chiropractic remain straight, uncontaminated by medically oriented "therapies."

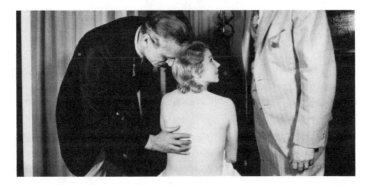

FIGURE 13.
Tullius F. Ratledge, President of Ratledge Chiropractic College, Los Angeles, 1911–1955. (Courtesy of Joseph C. Keating, Jr.)

Carl S. Cleveland, Sr. (1896–1982; Figure 14) and his wife Ruth founded the nonprofit Central College in Kansas City in 1922, and in 1924 renamed it Cleveland Chiropractic College. After they purchased Ratledge College for $40,000, renaming it in 1955 Cleveland Chiropractic College—Los Angeles (CCC-LA), Carl Sr. became its president also (1951–1981), with son Carl Jr. (Figure 14) as vice president of both schools. In 1967 Carl Jr. became president of CCC-KC. When Carl Sr. retired in 1981, Carl Jr. succeeded his father as President of CCC-LA, and in 1982 his son, Carl III (Figure 14), became president. This is only one example of many three-

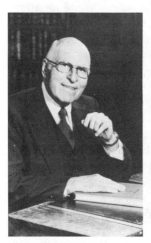 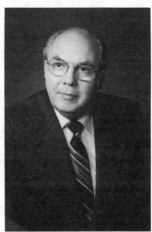 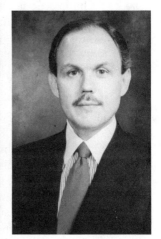

FIGURE 14.
Presidents of the Cleveland Colleges in Kansas City and Los Angeles, 1922–1991: *left,* Carl S. Cleveland, Sr.; *middle,* Carl S. Cleveland, Jr.; *right,* Carl S. Cleveland III. (Courtesy of Cleveland Chiropractic College.)

and four-generation chiropractic families. And Carl Sr.'s wife, Ruth, was herself the daughter of a pioneer chiropractor in Nebraska.

D.D.'s student John E. LaValley (1872–?) had established with others in 1910 in Portland a successor school to the D.D. Palmer College, the Peerless College of Chiropractic and Naturopathy, which in 1912 merged into the Pacific College of Chiropractic. By 1913 its course of instruction was 27 months long and included human dissection. In 1929 William Alfred Budden (1884–1954; Figure 15), a graduate and former dean at NCC, purchased Pacific College for $20,000, and reorganized it in 1932 as the nonprofit Western States Chiropractic College (WSCC). Author of *Physiotherapy, Technique and Treatment* (1928), he headed WSCC until his death; it continued to teach naturopathy until 1958. A strong advocate of high educational standards, by 1932 he extended instruction to a 4-year course of 9 months each, and by 1953 installed a 2-year preprofessional requirement for admission (Gatterman, 1982). During the 1956–1970 period WSCC's total enrollment never exceeded 38; it survived only because of the personal and financial sacrifices of dedicated board member Milton I. Higgins and Presidents Ralph M. Failor (1954–1956) and Robert E. Elliot (1956–1976). Herbert J. Vear was president from 1979 to 1986, followed by William H. Dallas.

Charles A. Cale established the Los Angeles College of Chiropractic (LACC) in 1911. He and his wife Linnie A. Cale, who had earned D.C. and D.O. degrees, developed LACC into one of the largest and strongest chiropractic colleges. In 1927 it offered an 18-month day course and a 36-month evening course for $750 per term ("Schools of Chiropractic and Naturopathy in the United States," 1928, p 1737). Over the years it absorbed no fewer than seven other colleges.

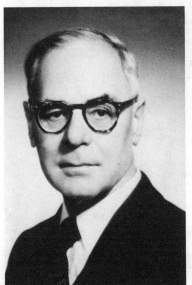

FIGURE 15.
William Alfred Budden, President of Western States Chiropractic College, Portland, Oregon, 1929–1954. (Courtesy of Western States Chiropractic College.)

James R. Drain (1891–1958) graduated from PSC in 1912. After practicing in Kansas until 1919, he moved to San Antonio, Texas, and became affiliated with Texas Chiropractic College (TCC), which had been founded by M.M. Stone in 1906. Drain was president from 1920 until his death. He authored *Chiropractic Thoughts* (1927) and *Man Tomorrow* (1949). During the 1930s he and his associate both lost their homes as a result of financial reverses but managed to keep TCC alive. An effective lobbyist as well as a prominent educator, he is also the only chiropractor known to be charged with being "about to practice medicine without a license," a charge later dropped.

Craig M. Kightlinger (1881–1958), a graduate of the New Jersey College of Chiropractic in Newark in 1917 and of PSC in 1919, founded Eastern Chiropractic College in Newark in 1919, moving it to New York City as Eastern Chiropractic Institute in 1923. The Carver Chiropractic Institute, of which Thure C. Peterson had been dean since 1928, had been absorbed by the New York School of Chiropractic in 1934. In 1944, through the leadership of Stephen E. Owens, the three remaining proprietary schools in New York City, that is, the New York School, Eastern Chiropractic Institute, and Standard Institute of Chiropractic, merged to become the professionally owned, nonprofit Chiropractic Institute of New York. At first Kightlinger was its president, and Peterson the dean; in 1953 Peterson became president, with Clarence W. Weiant (1897–1986; Figure 16), one of the most prolific and scholarly chiropractic authors (1945; 1947; 1958), as dean. It closed in 1968 and, like so many others, merged with NCC.

Frank E. Dean (1891–1958; Figure 17) had attended medical school at the Uni-

FIGURE 16.
Clarence W. Weiant, Dean of the Chiropractic Institute of New York, 1954–1962; author of *Medicine and Chiropractic* and *The Case for Chiropractic in the Literature of Medicine.* (Courtesy of Logan College of Chiropractic.)

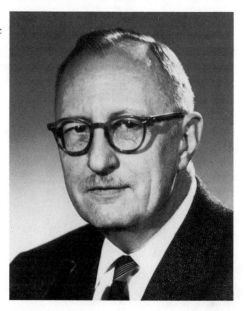

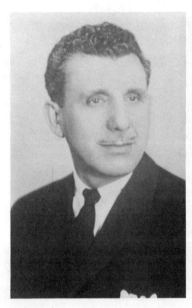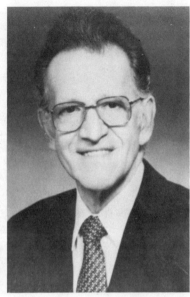

FIGURE 17.
First two presidents of Columbia Institute of Chiropractic, New York City (in 1977 renamed New York Chiropractic College): *left,* Frank E. Dean, 1916–1958; *right,* Ernest G. Napolitano, 1958–1985. (Courtesy of New York Chiropractic College.)

versity of Warsaw in Poland, and later earned a D.C. degree at the Standard Institute of Chiropractic. In 1919 he founded Columbia Institute of Chiropractic under a Delaware charter, but operated it in New York City. Claimed to be the first nonprofit chiropractic college, it was led by Dean until his death. His wife Lorraine Welch, D.C., who assisted him in administering the school, wrote her doctoral dissertation in education at New York University on *The History of Medical Organization and Counter-Organization in the United States* (1955). Ernest G. Napolitano (1911–1985; Figure 17) formerly president of the absorbed Atlantic States College of Chiropractic in Brooklyn, was president from 1958 until he died. In 1977 the college was renamed New York Chiropractic College (NYCC) at the insistence of the New York Board of Regents, which wanted no confusion with Columbia University. In 1989 NYCC purchased the former Dwight D. Eisenhower campus in Seneca Falls, New York, and moved there in 1991, with Kenneth W. Padgett as president.

Hugh B. Logan (1881–1944; Figure 18) established Logan Basic College of Chiropractic in St. Louis in 1935, and published *Logan Basic Technique* (1950). In 1944 his son Vinton F. Logan (1905–1961; Figure 18) became president, served until his death, and was succeeded by William N. Coggins, who served from 1961 to 1979. In 1955 it was renamed Logan College of Chiropractic (Figure 18). Very successful, in 1958 it absorbed Carver Chiropractic College in Oklahoma City, and in

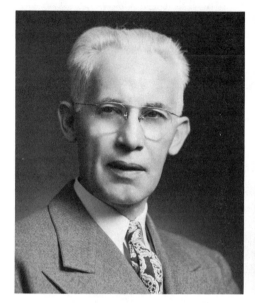
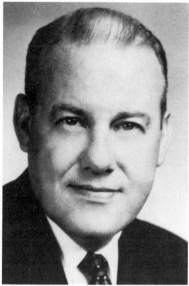
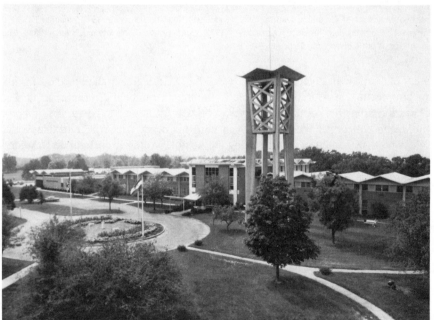

FIGURE 18.
Presidents of Logan College of Chiropractic from 1936–1961: *Left,* Hugh B. Logan; *right,* Vinton F. Logan. *Bottom,* campus in Chesterfield, Missouri. (Courtesy of Logan College of Chiropractic.)

1964 the Missouri Chiropractic College in St. Louis, which had been led by Henry C. Harring, D.C., M.D. (1888–1974) from its founding in 1920. Since 1981 Logan's president has been Beatrice B. Hagen, D.C.

The Minnesota Chiropractic College was founded in 1909 in Minneapolis by Robert Ramsey, and functioned with him as president until 1942. In 1941 John B. Wolfe (Figure 19) led a group that organized Northwestern College of Chiropractic (NWCC), also in Minneapolis. He served the third longest term, after B.J. Palmer and C.S. Cleveland, of any college president, from 1946 to 1986 (Fay, 1986; Hinz, 1987). NWCC quickly became one of the strongest colleges. For a few years it innovated having its basic medical science subjects taught by a local Catholic college, which attracted great hostility to it from organized medicine.

In 1945, exactly 50 years after D.D.'s first chiropractic adjustment, the Canadian Memorial Chiropractic College (CMCC; a memorial to Canada-born D.D.) was organized in Toronto as the professionally owned successor to several small private colleges. The mandate in its charter that it teach naturopathy was removed in 1964 (Coburn, 1991, pp 16, 18). After John Nugent, then NCA Director of Education, declined the office of dean (Lee, 1981), a charter faculty member, A. Earl Homewood (1916–1990; Figure 20) was appointed dean in 1952; the title was changed to president in 1958 (Lee, 1982). Author of the widely used *Neurodynamics of the Vertebral Subluxation,* (1962), he took time off to earn a law degree and publish *The Chiropractor and the Law* (1965) before retiring as president in 1970. With support from a unified profession CMCC rapidly became and remains one of the strongest chiropractic colleges, in part because each member of the Canadian Chiropractic As-

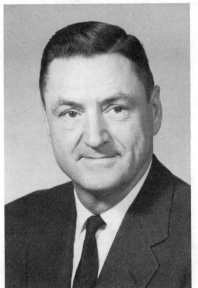

FIGURE 19.
John B. Wolfe, President of Northwestern College of Chiropractic, Minneapolis, 1946–1986.
(Courtesy of Northwestern College of Chiropractic.)

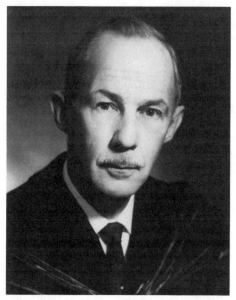

FIGURE 20.
Albert Earl Homewood, President of Canadian
Memorial Chiropractic College, Toronto,
1952–1970; author of *Neurodynamics of the
Vertebral Subluxation.* (Courtesy of Canadian
Memorial Chiropractic College.)

sociation is assessed $575 per year to support it. In 1974 the Ontario Council of
Health, senior advisory body to the Ontario Government, recommended "that the Canadian Memorial Chiropractic College, currently the only institution for chiropractic
education in Canada, be brought within the public education system of Ontario. To
this end it is desirable that the College be joined to a University." Following Herbert
J. Vear and Donald C. Sutherland as presidents, Ian D. Coulter, a New Zealand sociologist, became president (1983–1990), and immediately began negotiating for formal university affiliation, but without success.

Other colleges currently in existence, and dates of their founding, are Sherman
College of Straight Chiropractic (SCSC), in South Carolina (1973); Pasadena Chiro-
practic College, in California (1973), renamed Southern California Chiropractic Col-
lege (SCCC) in 1989; Life Chiropractic College, in Georgia (1974); Pacific States
Chiropractic College, in California (1976), which in 1981 became Life Chiropractic
College—West; Northern California Chiropractic College (1978), which in 1980 became Palmer Chiropractic College—West (PCC-W); Pennsylvania College of
Straight Chiropractic (PCSC), in Philadelphia (1978), previously known as ADIO
Chiropractic College (from the initials of B.J.'s well-known phrase "above
down–inside out"); Southwestern Chiropractic College, in Texas (1979), which in
1982 became the Parker College of Chiropractic; the University of Bridgeport College of Chiropractic (1991). The overseas colleges include Anglo-European College
of Chiropractic (AECC), in Bournmouth, England (1965), of which H.R.H. Princess
Diana became patron in 1990; International College of Chiropractic, near Melbourne,
Australia (1975), affiliated with the Preston (later Phillip) Institute of Technology,
which with its redesignated School of Chiropractic and Osteopathy was absorbed into

LaTrobe University near Melbourne in 1990; Centre for Chiropractic Studies of Macquarie University (1989), formerly Sydney College of Chiropractic and Osteopathy, earlier Sydney College of Osteopathy and Chiropractic, and before that Sydney College of Osteopathy; Institut Francais de Chiropractie, in Paris (1983); and the Chiropractic Faculty of Natal Technikon, in Durban, South Africa (1989). Other new colleges are in planning stages in Odense, Denmark; Brisbane, Australia; Trois Rivieres, Quebec; and Japan. The Commonwealth of Independent States, formerly the Soviet Union ("Soviet Medical School to Offer Chiropractic Degree," 1991) and Egypt are reported to be planning to teach chiropractic in medical settings. In Australia there is so little difference between chiropractic and osteopathy (and even physiotherapy) that the Australian Council on Chiropractic Education has been redesignated the Australian Council on Chiropractic and Osteopathic Education (Bolton, 1987; Sweaney, 1989).

Clearly chiropractic history has been dominated by charismatic personalities. Some of them (e.g., the Clevelands) adhered closely to B.J.'s philosophy of straight chiropractic; others early adopted a stronger, often more medical, curriculum including human dissection and sometimes physiological therapeutics (physiotherapy). Most were proprietary schools dependent on tuition and clinic fees for survival, which was always problematic. Little research was possible under these conditions, and except for some case studies little real research was carried out, but dozens of chiropractic texts were published by the early leaders, as noted. The legal status of chiropractic also was problematic in many jurisdictions despite the efforts of B.J., Tom Morris, and the UCA to obtain licensing legislation and defend chiropractors facing prosecution. The amazing thing is that chiropractors continued to practice, new schools opened, student enrollment increased, patients kept coming, and the profession survived.

Section 2

National Associations

Here I present a brief account of the various national associations that chiropractors have established. Already mentioned is Langworthy's short-lived American Chiropractic Association, which prompted B.J. to create his rival Universal Chiropractic Association (UCA) in 1906; both were composed initially of school alumni. With B.J. as permanent Secretary (and "Philosophical Counsel") and the law firm of Hartwell and Morris of La Crosse, Wisconsin, as legal counsel, the UCA prospered as it undertook to defend nationwide chiropractors arrested for practicing without a license, provided they practiced only straight chiropractic. The cost of membership initially was $5 a year, and UCA liability was limited to $5,000 per case. In 1909 the short-lived International Chiropractors Association was organized, with Colonel Sol Long as General Counsel (Carver, 1936, p 64). In 1913 the UCA began admitting mixers, which annoyed B.J. It had 900 members in 1913, and a few years later 2,500, the largest it ever became (Dye, 1939, pp 54–56). In 1912 a National Federation of State Chiropractic Associations was created by Carver, but was opposed by B.J., and, ineffective, it closed its books in 1920 (Carver, 1936, p 65; Turner, 1931, pp 188–189).

After the NCM was introduced, Morris broke with B.J. at the 1925 UCA convention in Chicago, but continued as its counsel until his death in 1928 (Turner, 1931, p 178). B.J. offered to retire and turn PSC over to the profession, but was dissuaded. However, in 1926 he withdrew from the UCA and organized a new national association with similar functions, the Chiropractic Health Bureau (CHB), which Turner (1931, p 182) tells us lost only one legal case in 22 months. It cost $10 to join, followed by similar assessments from members as needed. In 1941 it was renamed the International Chiropractors Association (ICA), which remains the primary national organization of straight chiropractors (for its history see "Vision to Action," 1986).

A new American Chiropractic Association was organized by chiropractic mixers, in 1920 according to Carver (1936, p 67) and in 1922 according to Turner (1931, p 288), with Frank R. Margetts (1871–1968), LL.B., D.D., D.C., as its only president (Dzamen, 1980, p 306). In 1930 it merged with the scattered remnants of the UCA to form the National Chiropractic Association (NCA), which soon became the largest chiropractic association as it moved to improve education, defend arrested chiropractors, and promote chiropractic through better licensing laws and public relations. Loran M. Rogers (1897–1976), who had been instrumental in organizing it, served as its executive director (1932–1963) in Webster City, Iowa, and then in Des Moines. Louis O. Gearhart, president of the University of the Natural Healing Arts in Denver until its demise in 1965, became executive director until the office was moved to Washington, D.C., in 1981. Gerald M. Brassard was Executive Vice President from 1981 to 1987, succeeded by Ronald Harris from 1987 to 1989, and then by J. Ray Morgan, a non-DC. The ICA moved its offices from Davenport to Washington in 1971, when Jerome F. McAndrews was Executive Vice President. He was succeeded by Bruce Nordstrom in 1978, and by non-DC Ron Hendrickson in 1989.

The Saunders (1954) survey of a 10% randomized sample of 20,000 chiropractors, 717 (31.4%) of whom returned questionnaires, reported that 87% were straight as far as analysis and diagnosis were concerned, and 59% were mixers when both analysis and treatment were considered. It also found that ICA members were straight 6:1, whereas NCA members were mixers 5:1. At that time the NCA had approximately two and a half times as many members as the ICA.

Merger of straight and mixer associations at the national level has not yet been achieved. After B.J.'s death, an effort in 1963 led by ICA Vice President Alan A. Adams to merge the ICA and NCA into a new American Chiropractic Association (ACA), based on a "unity definition of chiropractic and scope of practice" agreed to by 12 representatives from both associations, succeeded in persuading only about half of the ICA members to join NCA members in the new ACA. In the early 1970s Malcolm Macdonald of Falmouth, Massachusetts, attempted to use state associations as leverage for unification, but the effort failed, partly because the ACA and ICA leadership gave it only weak support (Macdonald ME, 1974). In the mid-1980s a new effort to merge was undertaken by ICA President Michael D. Pedigo and ACA Presidents Kenneth W. Padgett and Kenneth L. Luedtke. Amicable discussions over several years produced the first joint national convention of the two associations, in 1987, and high hopes for merger. There was almost no opposition within the ACA, which favors chiropractors' right to practice whatever state laws permit, but an opposition movement within the ICA, led by President Sid Williams of Life College, fought to preserve a separate ICA as the defender of traditional straight chiropractic. Despite two majority votes for merger by ICA members, the required two-thirds favorable was not obtained, so by 1989 it was clear that the attempt at merger had failed again. However, many of the most important ICA leaders and members moved to the ACA.

A third, even more conservative, national organization was left outside this merger attempt. Led by Thom Gelardi, founding president in 1973 of Sherman College of Straight Chiropractic, in Spartanburg, South Carolina, the group is called "superstraight" by its opponents. It wants the "P, S, and U" (pure, straight, and unadulterated) chiropractic taught and practiced as B.J. originally formulated it. Gelardi continues to maintain that chiropractors do not "treat disease," but "analyze" the spine for "subluxations," which they "adjust" to remove the cause of "dis-ease." He objects to use of the word "diagnosis," although he reluctantly teaches the courses in pathology and diagnostic techniques needed by his students to pass national board examinations. He also objects to chiropractors' use of physiotherapy and other adjunctive therapies. In 1977 his supporters acquired the failing ADIO College in Pennsylvania and renamed it Pennsylvania College of Straight Chiropractic (jocularly known as "Penn Straight").

Because most states require graduation from a chiropractic college accredited by CCE or by "a national accrediting agency" for licensing, and Sherman graduates were denied licenses in many states, Gelardi formed a new national association, the Federation of Straight Chiropractic Organizations (FSCO), in 1976, and a second national accrediting agency, the Straight Chiropractic Academic Standards Association (SCASA), in 1978. In 1988 President Reagan's outgoing Secretary of Education, William Bennett, much to everyone's surprise and contrary to the recommendation of his own staff, responded to political pressures and approved SCASA as the official accrediting agency for straight chiropractic on a 2-year provisional basis, as is customary with a new agency. Shortly thereafter SCASA provisionally accredited SCSC, PCSC, and the renamed Southern California College of Chiropractic (SCCC), which when it was Pasadena College of Chiropractic had been threatened by CCE with loss of accreditation. Hence the graduates of three small superstraight colleges now can be licensed in a dozen or so states. The struggle for chiropractic recognition thus continues in legislative halls, with chiropractors fighting chiropractors. Professional differences again become political differences (discussed in Chapters 6 and

13). At this writing the U.S. Office of Education staff again has recommended against approving SCASA, and final action by the Secretary of Education is awaited. Meanwhile, Sherman College faces declining enrollments and income, and SCASA and CCE have begun negotiations to see if they can reconcile their differences.

Each state has at least one, in some as many as *four,* chiropractic associations, further splintering the profession. Canadians have since 1943 benefited from being united in a single national Canadian Chiropractic Association. In Australia two national associations, one representing chiropractors educated overseas, the other consisting of those trained locally, united in 1990 after years of difficult negotiations.

Section 3

Numbers of U.S. Chiropractors

The following estimates and projections of the total number of chiropractors in the United States at various times are derived from the sources indicated:

1904	"Not more than 50" (Smallie and Evans, 1980)
1906	100 (Turner, 1931)
	500 (Gielow, 1981)
1908	400–600 (Turner, 1931)
	3,000 (Gielow, 1981, from D.D.'s lecture notes)
1910	2,000 (Evans HW, 1978)
	5,000–6,000 (Dye, 1939)
1916	7,000 (Palmer BJ, 1916)
1920	"Three times what they were in 1910" (Dye, 1939)
1922	20,000 ("Professional Mortality," 1949)
1923	24,000 (Evans HW, 1978)
1924	25,000 (Dye, 1939)
1930	12,000 (U.S. Census)
	16,000 (Reed, 1932)
1950	13,084 (U.S. Census)
1954	18,980 (Saunders Associates, 1954)
1960	13,873 (U.S. Census)
1967	23,000 (Evans HW, 1978)
1970	13,459 (U.S. Census)
1979	23,000 (Von Kuster, 1964)
1980	19,768 (U.S. Census)
1982	25,880 (*Supply and Characteristics of Chiropractors,* 1986)
1984	28,500 (*Annual Report of CCE,* 1984)
1988	39,000 (Bureau of Health Professions, Department of Health and Human Services, 1990)
1989	44,904 (Federation of Chiropractic Licensing Boards, 1990)

1990   49,000 (ICA, U.S. Census figures not yet available)
1991   50,000 (ACA)
2000   52,500 (Bureau of Health Professions, 1990)
2010   60,600 (Bureau of Health Professions, 1990)
2020   66,600 (Bureau of Health Professions, 1990)

As with other health professions, not all licensed chiropractors are in active practice. A few practice only parttime; some are partly or fully retired; others are engaged in teaching, research, or business; still others have given up practicing or never practiced. Those in practice sometimes hold licenses in more than one state or divide their practice between two states. Hence even for the most recent periods the best estimates are only approximations.

Chapter 6

STRUGGLE FOR LICENSING LEGISLATION

The chiropractors in this state think that as soon as they get a bill through it will be easy sailing, but it won't. Of course a lot of them have fought hard, and they want to die with a license even if it isn't as good a bill as it might be.

Massachusetts chiropractor, 1949

Section 1

Why Licensure?

The primary purpose of regulation by law of the activities of any profession is to protect the public and enhance its welfare. The greater the amount of knowledge and skill required for an occupation, the less widely distributed it is likely to be in the population and the more likely it is to be the monopoly of a group of "professionals" set apart from the general population. If in addition the group's services are vitally needed by the public, then monopolistic control brings considerable power to the group, because it then may be able to decide unilaterally the terms on which its services will be provided. This is particularly true when the professional group has exclusive responsibility for imparting instruction in the art or skill to newcomers to the profession, and the power to decide who the newcomers shall be.

The dilemma involved in public regulation of a highly educated and specialized group is that outsiders are ignorant of the technical aspects of the field of specialization. Although most laypersons can evaluate some phases of a profession's activity, and those who are trained in related professions can evaluate other phases, there always remain critically important aspects that no one but a member of the fraternity can evaluate. Hence what usually happens when a professional group is regulated is that the group in effect regulates itself, often with only the faintest of surveillance by disinterested representatives of the public. In some instances, for example, the medical profession both in England and in the American colonies, the power to license was turned over directly to the profession or to the academic institutions that "credentialed" them by conferring degrees. Even when a government agency is established, the majority of individuals appointed to it almost invariably come from the profession being regulated. In the nature of the case, this almost has to be.

A consequence is that the public interest may not be well served, especially where it conflicts with the interests of the profession. Hugh Cabot (1940) saw this possibility clearly:

> The supervision of a profession by the group itself always carries with it certain dangers and objections. There is always a chance that a group of this kind, licensed by the state and therefore a legal monopoly, will tend to take on the characteristics of the old Guild organizations. . . . The group is likely to confuse its personal benefits with the public interest. It is likely to be tempted to diminish the supply of capable members. It is likely to attempt to maintain prices at an unreasonable level by methods of scarcity production.

George Bernard Shaw expressed his opinion even more forcefully in a famous letter to the London *Times* (cited in Hale, 1926, pp 58–59):

> The Free State Government will, I hope, resolutely carry out its announced intention of rescuing Ireland from the disastrous control of that despised and self-disgraced trade-union—the British Medical Council. . . . The General Medical Council has about as much to do with Science as the Miners' Federation has to do with geology and mineralogy. . . . The medical profession in Ireland will lose no prestige by dissociating themselves from it. But now comes a serious question: Will an Irish Council prove any better? . . . President Cosgrove's sensible announcement contained one terrifying phrase—'self-controlled profession.' . . . A self-controlled profession is a conspiracy against the laity. And of all professions on earth, the medical profession, consisting mainly of private medical and surgical practitioners who have a direct pecuniary interest in making us ill, keeping us ill, and mutilating us, is one that needs the sternest disinterested control, not only in the common interest of the general body of citizens, but in that of science.

George McAndrews (1982, p 20), the chiropractors' attorney in the Wilk (1976) antitrust suit, phrased it: "The ermine glove of altruism frequently conceals the brass knuckles of greed."

In 1919 the American Medical Association (AMA) declared that the state should enact legislation to protect the public against incompetent or unscrupulous practitioners but should not infringe on a profession's right to decide technical questions (Green, 1919, p 16):

> The Supreme Courts hold without exception, from the Supreme Court of the United States to that of the youngest state, that the sole justification for the enactment of medical practice acts is the protection of the public from incompetent and unscrupulous persons; that the state has a right to enact laws creating any reasonable standards for this privilege; that the object of such laws is not the protection or the benefit of physicians but the protection of the public; that it is not the function of the state to decide scientific questions of the relative value of different forms of treatment or to determine the scientific value of one school or method of practice as compared with another; but to establish and enforce reasonable regulations for the protection of the public; that the qualifi-

cations and conditions enacted must be reasonable and must be the same for all those who desire the same privilege; and that the function of examining boards is to test the qualifications and knowledge of the applicant in order to determine whether he may be entrusted with the treatment of the sick without public danger.

The irony in this statement is that it leaves open the question of how the state is to ascertain competence when there is more than "one school or method of practice." The Illinois Supreme Court dodged the question when it ruled in 1921 (People vs. Love, 298 Illinois 304, 1921): "It is not the province of the courts to extol or belittle chiropractic, osteopathy or medicine and surgery. They are now all established as useful professions."

But can the state avoid deciding between competing claims? Is it not forced to "decide scientific questions of the relative value of different forms of treatment or to determine the scientific value of one school or method of practice as compared with another"? At the very least, legislative action is required to set up the regulatory agencies to be established, specifically in the case of the healing professions, whether one board shall license all health practitioners or whether there shall be several specialized boards. And someone has to decide which "schools" are to be represented on these boards and given the power to administer the licensing machinery. As an example, the United States Court of Appeals (U.S. vs. Hoxsey Cancer Clinic 198 F2nd 273, 1952, p 277) did this when it handed down the following decision in a case involving an unorthodox treatment for cancer:

> Despite the vast and continuous research which has been conducted into the cause of and possible cure for, cancer, the aggregate of medical experience and qualified experts recognize in the treatment of internal cancer only the method of surgery, X-ray, radium and some of the radio-active by-products of atomic bomb production.

However, the real danger of monopolistic control by one school of therapy, as Shaw indicated, is that scientific and technologic advance may be stultified by orthodoxy. Many of the major advances in medical science have historically come not from practitioners or even from medical researchers but from the laboratories of nonmedical scientists or observant laypersons. The distinctive contribution of chiropractic (and similarly of osteopathy) may represent another such forward stride that society cannot afford to lose. Only an open-minded judgment by disinterested persons over the long run can decide the question. In his remarkable *The Political Life of the American Medical Association* Oliver Garceau (1941, pp 169–170) observed:

> Little headway has been made in convincing the public that the present-day conflicts between orthodox and unorthodox medicine are not in any way comparable with the scholastic, philosophic rumpus of earlier times. The public notion of science is still in terms of an efficient magic; so there is no harm in encouraging lots of different magicians.

As a practical matter the resolution of scientific questions often lies in the political arena. Although in theory their resolution should be the responsibility of the scientific community, using its techniques of publication, replication, and critical review, at any given moment in time a political judgment must be made. It can be to dodge the question by making academic institutions responsible for deciding which candidates should receive degrees or certificates testifying to the adequacy of their training, as is the case in Great Britain, where medical doctors and chiropractors with degrees are authorized to practice under the doctrine called "prior arts right" and can be sued only after the fact if they turn out to be incompetent. Or the state can establish its own agency to examine and license (i.e., register) candidates. When that is the case, the scope of practice usually is defined in law, unless only use of the name is licensed, as is often the case when a field of practice, such as psychology, is difficult to define. The definition is inevitably subject to political pressures and lobbying activities of interested parties. The group wins that can corral the most political and public support, raise the most money (which can be used for either legal or illegal purposes), and persuade legislators to vote their way.

What are the advantages of licensure for a profession? New York's 1806 licensing law was amended in 1807 to impose a fine of $5 for each month of practice by an unlicensed practitioner, but the penalty did not apply to herbalists or to those who did not pretend to be physicians (Kaufman, 1971, p 22). "In New Jersey, acts of 1813 and 1818 required the suppression of 'all irregular bred contenders . . . under the names . . . of practicing botanists, root or Indian doctors . . . or any other quacks' " (Shryock, 1967, p 25). However, the Massachusetts and Connecticut laws providing that only licensed physicians could sue for payment of fees meant that the hazard of practicing without a license was merely to risk the loss of fees (Berlant, 1975, pp 209–214). When medical licensure became more firmly reestablished toward the end of the 19th century, all nonmedical (except religious) practitioners who sought remuneration for their services came under the medical acts and could be charged with practicing medicine without a license. The legal basis for licensure was secured in the 1888 *Dent vs. West Virginia* (129 U.S. 114) decision of the U.S. Supreme Court, which upheld the state's power "to exclude people without license from practicing medicine." States could "protect society by imposing conditions for the exercise of that right, as long as they were imposed on everyone and were reasonably related to the occupation in question" (Starr, 1982, p 106). Interpretation and enforcement of the laws was another story, allowing for great variability.

Section 2

Varieties of Chiropractic Legislation

Ever since the Flexner report in 1910, organized medicine has opposed any compromise of its high standards of professional training. For example, it only reluctantly approved advanced training for midwives. Since there have never been enough physicians willing to cut corns or fit glasses, two new professions arose outside medicine to fill those needs; the same was true of dentistry at an earlier date. Certainly physicians as a group are not prepared to do much bodily manipulation, spinal or otherwise, although the demand for such services is much greater than the specialists in neurology, orthopedics, and physiatry possibly can fill. It would be as unreasonable to expect the mass of American people to go to them for all their bodily strains and sprains as it would be to expect them to take all their mental and emotional problems to the relatively few psychiatrists available. And they don't. Whether physical therapists in the future will develop the educational background and manipulative skills needed to compete with chiropractors, and the qualifications in differential diagnosis needed to become true portal-of-entry practitioners, remains to be seen.

The client needs professional licensure to enable him or her to find a therapist who is both competent and ethical. Licensure enhances confidence in the therapy, thus facilitating recovery or rehabilitation from serious illness. Not only for psychiatric or psychosomatic disorders is the attitude and emotional state of the patient critical, but also for recovery from somatic illness, for the placebo effect of the therapist is a major component of any therapy.

The dilemma that medical authorities and policy makers have always faced was whether to bring chiropractors (or other new practitioners) under state regulation and help them raise their levels of education and training or to deny them any form of licensing at all. Almost invariably medicine has chosen the latter alternative. It strenuously fought every effort by chiropractors to obtain licensure, as it did with osteopaths until it made a policy shift around the middle of this century (Blackstone, 1977).

A new profession wants licensure primarily to legitimate its status. This not only helps attract clients, it confers legal standing on the profession with all the rights and privileges pertaining thereto. Furthermore, because licensure requires some definition of the field of practice, legislation can legitimate the definition favored by one subgroup of the profession at the expense of a less influential subgroup. That is what often happened in the case of chiropractic.

Of all institutional areas, the economic is least resistant to change. Under the common law, once a new way of earning a living is established, provided it is not illegal or nipped in the bud by authorities alert and zealous to protect vested interests, the right to continue in that occupation cannot easily be withdrawn. That right is recognized in the familiar grandfather clause of most initial professional licensing legislation.

Laws authorizing *medical* boards to license and regulate chiropractors were overturned in some states. For example, the Supreme Court of Tennessee ruled in 1920, according to Turner (1931, p 80), although I have not been able to verify his citation:

> Chiropractors cannot be classed along with charlatans and fakirs. It is a well developed system of healing, recognized in many jurisdictions, and many believe in its efficacy. . . .
> The requirement that [chiropractors] study and be examined on subjects in no way pertaining to their occupation is an arbitrary and unreasonable attempt to restrict their lib-

erties and the liberty of the people who wish to patronize them. Such reasoning has no reasonable tendency to promote the public safety and welfare. . . . An innocent business . . . cannot be prohibited under the guise of regulation.

The first effort to obtain a chiropractic licensing law was initiated in Minnesota in 1905 by Solon Langworthy and Dan Riesland, along with their plan to start a 20-month chiropractic school. Because D.D. Palmer disliked the broad-scope definition of chiropractic in the proposed law, he went to Minneapolis and persuaded Governor Johnson to veto it (Lerner, 1954, p 392). According to Martin (1978, pp 70–71), "B.J. Palmer even dismissed licensing in 1912, asserting that only the people could and should determine the fate of chiropractic" (*The Chiropractor,* VIII, Oct 1912).

Willard Carver submitted a proposal to license chiropractors to the Oklahoma legislature in 1907, but a law was not obtained there until 1921. The first state to pass such a law was Kansas, in 1913, but Arkansas, which passed its law, drafted by lawyer Carver, in 1915, was the first state to issue regular chiropractic licenses. Other states that passed early laws were North Dakota, Oregon, Ohio, North Carolina, and Connecticut (Table 1). It became almost a ritual for early chiropractic boards to award the first license (genuine or honorary) to B.J. By 1923, 27 states had established chiropractic licensing boards, and their legality had been upheld by 11 supreme courts. By 1950, 43 states had given chiropractors some form of legal recognition. The last states to license them were New York (1963), Massachusetts (1966), Mississippi (1973), and Louisiana (1974). Chiropractors also are licensed in Canada, Switzerland, Australia, New Zealand, South Africa, Scandinavian countries, and in a few other places.

Actually, the first two chiropractic licenses were issued on May 24, 1904, to Minora Paxson (license number 438) and Oakley Smith (license number 440) under the drugless practitioners provision of the Illinois Medical Practice Act of 1899 (Zarbuck, 1986, pp 79–80). Both were faculty members of Langworthy's school and coauthors of the Langworthy text (1906).

TABLE 1.

Year of First Licensing, by State

Region/Subregion/State	
Northeast	
New England	
Connecticut	1917
Maine	1924
Massachusetts	1966
New Hampshire	1921
Rhode Island	1923
Vermont	1919
Middle Atlantic	
New Jersey	1953
New York	1963
Pennsylvania	1951

South
  South Atlantic
    Delaware   1937

Region	Year
South	
South Atlantic	
Delaware	1937
District of Columbia	1929
Florida	1919
Georgia	1921
Maryland	1929
North Carolina	1917
South Carolina	1932
Virginia	1944
West Virginia	1925
East South Central	
Alabama	1959
Kentucky	1928
Mississippi	1973
Tennessee	1923
West South Central	
Arkansas	1915
Louisiana	1974
Oklahoma	1921
Texas	1949
North Central	
East North Central	
Illinois	1923
Indiana	1927
Michigan	1933
Ohio	1915
Wisconsin	1925
West North Central	
Iowa	1921
Kansas	1913
Minnesota	1919
Missouri	1927
Nebraska	1916
North Dakota	1913
South Dakota	1921
West	
Mountain	
Arizona	1921
Colorado	1933
Idaho	1919
Montana	1918
Nevada	1923
New Mexico	1921
Utah	1923
Wyoming	1929
Pacific	
Alaska	1939
California	1922
Hawaii	1925
Oregon	1915
Washington	1919

The following story of how Vermont's licensing law was obtained in 1919 was told to me by William A. Gage of St. Johnsbury in an interview in 1948:

> There were only twelve chiropractors in the state, but an important lawyer in the legislature was an enthusiastic chiropractic patient. He met with a committee of three chiropractors, which I was on. We sat down and copied the osteopathic law, inserting "chiropractic" wherever the word "osteopathy" appeared. That is why there is no definition of chiropractic in the law, because there was none of osteopathy. I didn't think we would get the bill through because none of the twelve chiropractors had been in the state more than three years. We didn't even tell the other chiropractors what we were doing until a week before the hearing, and then we all started sending letters in. The public health committee had more doctors on it than laymen, but instead of turning in an unfavorable report they put on nine crippling amendments and reported the bill out favorably. They would have done better not to do that. One speaker said: "This is worse than the Chinese Exclusion Act because occasionally a Chinese can get in, but if this law is passed no more chiropractors can come in and those that are here will have to get out." At one point the opposition introduced a "darkie" from Bellow's Falls as a chiropractor so as to discredit us. He bowed low and left. When someone asked why he was brought in the answer was: "So the legislators can see what a chiropractor looks like." One of the proponents of the bill said: "That darkie is the type of man we want to keep out of this state." That move lost the medics fifty votes. The chiropractic law was enacted during that session.

In other states chiropractors were not often so fortunate. Long hard fights were the rule. Opposition was particularly strong in California, Montana, Wyoming, and Indiana (Dye, 1939, p 91).

In Missouri a powerful MD from Carthage was Speaker of the House, and blocked passage of a chiropractic law for years until the mother of a chiropractor appealed to an undertaker friend in Carthage, who replied: "I know Dr. Parker very intimately, he is obligated to me and he will do most anything I ask him. . . . I shall phone him immediately." An hour later Dr. Parker was in the undertaker's office, and after hearing what the chiropractors wanted, he said: "I always admired the chiropractors for their sincerity. Not only will I cease opposing them legislatively but next year I will introduce and sponsor their bill!" It passed in 1927 (letter to me from Dr. Syl Walters, Dec 1973).

Where organized medicine could not prevent chiropractic licensure, it sought the narrowest possible definition of its scope and control of the licensing process through a medical board that sometimes included representatives of the other professions it licensed. In some states chiropractors accepted such control in return for a lenient grandfather clause, that is, one licensing without examination those already in practice. B.J. castigated such a compromise as "selling chiropractic down the river." In some states (e.g., Wisconsin) grandfather clauses were so lenient that even students were exempt from examinations, because of "experience in the clinic" (Mawhiney, 1984, p 98). One alternative to practicing without a license was to obtain a charter to start a school even though it might have only a couple of students.

California provided a striking example of ultimate chiropractic success. In 1916 President Tullius Ratledge (1971, p 81) of Ratledge College was sentenced to jail for 90 days for practicing without a license, and served 75 days. (After his release he went back into practice and was never bothered again.) In 1917 there were so many arrests that the Alameda County Chiropractic Association adopted the slogan "Go to jail for chiropractic," inspired according to Lerner (1954, p 230) by Tom Morris, and required its members to do so rather than pay a fine. In one year 450 chiropractors chose to go to jail, often singing "Onward Christian Soldiers" on the way (Reed, 1932, p 53). In jail they set up their portable adjusting tables and proceeded to treat the patients who came to show support. In Los Angeles Harry Gallagher "was arrested twenty-seven times between 1914 and 1919. He was the only chiropractor who succeeded in remaining in the state for such a period of time" (Turner, 1931, p 99). According to Turner (1931, p 132):

> The Reverend Emil Meyer of Sacramento wrote in *The California Telegram* of April 27, 1922: "To our knowledge not one accusation, as a matter of record in California, has been brought against any chiropractor by any patient. Charges and convictions were based upon decoy evidence. . . . If chiropractic is criminal, is it not a crime to incite the practice of chiropractic?"

When Dr. Minnie Leach collapsed in jail after a 10-day hunger strike, public opinion turned against the medical practice act. In 1922 the chiropractic licensing law was adopted by a majority of 153,751 votes in a statewide public referendum, and in 1923 Governor Friend W. Richardson pardoned all chiropractors then in jail because he believed they had been "unjustly accused."

In 1920 a similar public referendum rejected an Oklahoma medical practice act that defined chiropractic as the practice of medicine; it was followed by the legislature's adoption of a chiropractic licensing law in 1921 (Carver, 1936, pp 122–126). In 1931, 806 (13.6%) of 5,910 registered health practitioners in Los Angeles County were DOs and 1,272 (21.5%) were chiropractors. Gevitz (1988a, p 51) observed: "These figures gave the regular medical society little satisfaction." In a town of fewer than 10,000 persons in the unlicensed state of Mississippi, Schlessing (1950) found:

> Nine physicians embracing six different doctorates—a Homeopath, an old Eclectic, a Chiropractor, an Osteopath, a Naturopath, and the rest were regular Allopaths. They all met once a week at their local Kiwanis; all shared the same hospital.

The record for arrests—66 times—was held by Charles C. Lemly (1892–1970), a former pharmacist and co-owner with his brother of a chiropractic sanitarium in Waco, Texas (Dzaman, 1980, p 294). After his fellow Texan, Paul Meyers of Wichita Falls, was arrested for the tenth time, a parade with a band, many chiropractors, "patients and friends, and local celebrities" arranged in honor of his release so impressed the authorities that "he was never bothered again" (Dzaman, 1980, p 303). Carver (1936, pp 117–121) was arrested for being in contempt of the Oklahoma Senate in 1917 after publishing a newspaper article titled "Was the Oklahoma Senate Bought?"

Supportive patients often aided chiropractors to obtain licensure. The largest such group was the American Bureau of Chiropractic, organized about 1923 by Dr. William H. Werner of Brooklyn. Its initial objective was to acquire funds to pay bail bonds for chiropractors arrested for practicing medicine. On January 23, 1932, it filled Madison Square Garden in New York City with an estimated 12,000 cheering chiropractic supporters (Lombardo, 1990; Figure 21). However, licensing was achieved in New York only in 1963.

President James N. Firth of Lincoln Chiropractic College in Indianapolis described to me in a letter (April 20, 1948) how the Indiana law was administered:

> In 1927 the legislature enacted an amendment to the Medical Practice Act which placed Chiropractic and other branches of drugless healing under the jurisdiction of this act in all respects whatsoever. The amendment also provided for the licensing of all drugless practitioners who were residents of the state and in practice on January 1, 1927. The third provision placed a Chiropractor on the Medical Board of Examiners which then consisted of five medical doctors and one osteopath. The fourth clause of the amendment provided for an injunction against anyone practicing medicine without a license.
>
> Under the law an applicant for examination must be a graduate of an approved school. To the best of my knowledge the State Board has not issued minimum requirements for an approved school since 1931. At that time among other things an approved school had to be affiliated with a hospital having at least two beds for each Senior student. This is one of the many requirements which can not be met by any Chiropractic institution which is supported solely by tuitional income. It is now twenty-one years since this law

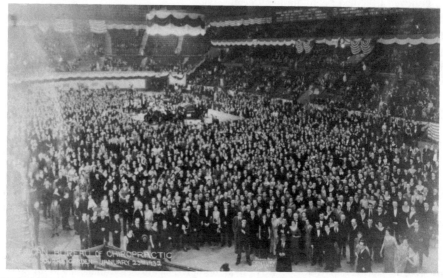

FIGURE 21.
Some of the 12,000 supporters of chiropractic at Madison Square Garden, New York City, January 23, 1932. (Courtesy of New York Chiropractic College.)

was enacted and to this date no Chiropractic School has been inspected for approval even though written applications have been filed making this request. No Chiropractic school has been approved, consequently no Chiropractors have been licensed excepting those who are licensed under the grandfather clause of the 1927 amendment.

Students entering this college are advised that the Chiropractor can not obtain a license in the State of Indiana. The law which recognizes Chiropractic is inoperative in that it does not function to examine and license Chiropractors, therefore Indiana students as a rule decide to locate in other states even before they enter school. A few do locate in the state and they are required promptly to appear in court for the purpose of being enjoined.

Only after a new chiropractic law was passed in 1955, sponsored by Walter J. Benneville, a chiropractor in the House of Representatives, were chiropractors again licensed in Indiana. Yet in addition to the Bebout, O'Neil-Ross, and other colleges, Lincoln College operated there from 1926 to 1971.

A few states had broad drugless practitioner acts under which chiropractors (e.g., Minora Paxson and Oakley Smith in Illinois) obtained licenses. In states where frontier conditions prevailed or where there was a shortage of MDs, chiropractors experienced less difficulty in obtaining acceptable licensing legislation. Dr. W.A. Budden, President of Western States Chiropractic College (WSCC), wrote me (May 12, 1948):

In the state of Oregon we are fortunate in having a very liberal law requirement of four years of nine months each, and including the use of all modalities of healing with the exception of internal medicine and major surgery. There is also, of course, a Basic Science law, which is administered in an equitable and quite fair manner, and to which, as a consequence, our objection only is having to take two examinations. . . .

In general, in the West where pioneer conditions have prevailed until very recently, legislators were inclined to be generous and were unable to see the position of special privileges obtained by medicine. This feeling continues, and has been enhanced by the growth of popular sentiment in favor of this system of healing, so that, although the effort is made sub rosa to hamper us, legislative efforts have been almost without result.

By 1927 the Universal Chiropractors Association (UCA) had defended chiropractors for practicing medicine without a license in 3,300 court cases (Turner, 1931, p 178). Geiger (1942, pp 42–43) wrote:

During the cult's first thirty years more than 15,000 prosecutions against chiropractors are said to have occurred. . . . Only about a fifth of the thousands of such actions have produced convictions. There is ample evidence, moreover, that the punishment has sometimes hurt its administrators more than the recipients. . . . Ohio, for instance, once . . . locked up 200 chiropractors at a clip. Result: so much sympathy was stirred up on the prisoners' behalf that the state promptly licensed them.

One of Ohio's last victims, Herbert A. Reaver, "paid eight fines for practicing without a license and served four jail sentences. He was warned that the next time he was arrested he would be prosecuted as a habitual criminal resulting in a stiffer penalty" ("Vision to Action," 1986). In July 1951 *Time* magazine reported that he had moved to Florida.

The kind of chiropractic licensing law obtained varied depending on whether straights or mixers predominated in the state at the time. There was often a correlation between a medically dominated state board and mixing and between a chiropractically dominated board and practicing straight chiropractic. There was also a relationship between requiring higher educational standards and a broader scope of practice. Oregon had a broad-scope law permitting chiropractors to practice obstetrics and minor surgery, set simple fractures, and sign birth and death certificates, while the neighboring state of Washington had a restrictive law permitting only adjustment of the spine by the hands only. Similarly, Maine always has been a mixer state and neighboring New Hampshire has been a straight state; indeed, according to one of my Massachusetts informants, even x-rays were forbidden there at one time because they were considered mixing. (Straights had called x-rays "the mixer's first drink.") One reason that Massachusetts chiropractors experienced so much difficulty in getting licensed was that although a majority of them were straights, there were also many mixers (mostly from New York schools) who would not enthusiastically support a restrictive law.

Chiropractors preferred separate examining boards. Still another alternative was a "basic science board" that would examine and certify candidates from all the major healing arts in the basic medical sciences, followed by an examination in each field conducted by a separate board. Wisconsin and Connecticut were the first states to install basic science boards, in 1925, followed by 21 other states and the District of Columbia. Gevitz (1988a, p 43) confirms that in Wisconsin "the major targets of the society's proposed legislation were the chiropractors." How the Wisconsin law was passed was narrated in an oral history interview by Dr. J.B. Sprague, who incidentally was also an MD (Mawhiney, 1984, p 97):

> It was in 1925 . . . that the law was passed. . . . The night before, the representative of the medical people contacted the fellows who remained in Madison. He told them, "We have a bill which will be helpful in the healing profession, and really it's something that everybody should have. It will be what we call a Basic Science Board, and the basic sciences will consist of Anatomy, Physiology, Pathology, and Diagnosis. . . . Then they can go to their own [chiropractic] board. . . . This, of course, was rank trickery, because the governor appointed professors from all of the state colleges, Marquette and the University of Wisconsin in Madison and some other colleges, and naturally these colleges, most of them, had medical departments, medical colleges, and so naturally the members were more apt to be namby-pamby with the medical profession. . . . Even though the candidates were supposed to be anonymous and known only by number, it was always known who was going where. The examinations were given from a medical standpoint. . . . Nobody passed that Board for at least ten years. . . . Therefore they could not get to the Chiropractic Board, so our Board just sat and had nothing to do. . . . These fellows went into practice anyway, and practiced without a license. . . . I don't recall that anybody was prosecuted, but some years later . . . possibly around 1943, the Naturopaths . . . were

working to try to get a bill through the Legislature. The medical profession told the chiropractors that if you will help us defeat this bill, we'll make arrangements to license your unlicensed chiropractors in the state. We will let them have examinations by the Basic Science Board, but we'll examine them on the spine only, so they'll be sure to pass. . . . Thereby they got licensed.

The Secretary of the Federation of State Medical Boards, W.L. Bierring (1948, p 111), confirmed the goal of the basic science boards:

The character of the examining questions in the different basic sciences has undergone remarkable changes, assuming more and more the type adaptable for a licensure examination, especially that of the practice of medicine. The evident original purpose of enacting basic science laws was to exclude chiropractors and other inadequately trained practitioners from being admitted to licensure.

There was an obvious predisposition to believe that chiropractors were too poorly educated to pass the basic science examinations. A pamphlet published by the International Chiropractors Association (ICA; "Basic Science a Recurring Problem," n.d.) quoted an examiner as saying: "We used to give them out [questions used in previous examinations], but the chiropractors memorized the questions and answers for future examinations. We do not believe they knew enough to answer them otherwise. Now we refuse to give them out." However, according to Lauretti et al. (1988), President W.A. Budden of WSCC "strongly supported the change in Oregon law requiring that all medical, chiropractic and other students in health fields take the same Basic Sciences examination covering Anatomy, Pathology, Physiology, Chemistry and Public Health. He felt that participation in the examination would help add credence to a field still looked on with distrust by many."

By 1980 all states had repealed their basic science laws. Their effect had been to push educational standards higher in those professions where students had difficulty passing the examination, especially osteopathy and chiropractic. Blackstone (1977, pp 409–410) states: "In the early seventies 1.5 percent of the osteopaths taking the exams did not pass while 9.3 percent of approved medical school graduates and 37.3 percent of foreign medical graduates failed." Between 1963 and 1967 a third of all medical candidates and over half of the foreign graduates had failed (Gevitz, 1988a, p 59). By 1969 chiropractic education had improved so much that four state basic science boards recognized as equivalent the certificate of the National Board of Chiropractic Examiners, established in 1963.

Section 3

An Example: The Case of Massachusetts

From a sociologic perspective, law is only one of the factors involved in maintaining an orderly society. Ethical codes, professional standards of competence, and even customs and courtesies also function as "social controls." The law also often allows loopholes and exceptions, and is not always obeyed. Hence a critical question is the extent to which the law is enforced. Massachusetts, where I began field research on chiropractors in the late 1940s, provides an excellent example. Despite the ruling by the State Supreme Court in 1915 that the practice of chiropractic is the practice of medicine, the law was not uniformly enforced. Most Massachusetts chiropractors were practicing openly when I interviewed them in the 1940s. But a significant number of chiropractors practiced just over the borders of neighboring states, and others had fled the state to avoid prosecution. Most were cautious about treating new patients, fearful of spies from the Massachusetts Medical Society or the State Attorney General.

William D. Harper (1908–1990) was then a beginning chiropractor (with a masters degree from the Massachusetts Institute of Technology), who later chose teaching as a career and served as president of Texas Chiropractic College from 1966 to 1976. He spent many hours educating me about chiropractors, noting that he habitually postponed seeing a new patient until he could check his identity insofar as possible. Some chiropractors eliminated from their offices as much of their chiropractic credentials and paraphernalia as possible to convey the fiction that they were not chiropractors. Others relied on their instincts to identify a provocateur. Most accepted only cash payment of fees, although a few were secure enough to mail written bills to the patients they trusted. A few were completely fearless because they believed they had good personal relations with police, prosecutors, judges, or politicians. Some (usually not the straights) obtained physiotherapy licenses and pretended to practice it on a suspected spy. A very few obtained local licenses as masseurs. Some would not treat the very sick, who might die under their care.

One of the first chiropractors to arrive in Boston found that the medical practice act explicitly excluded "cosmopathic healing" along with Christian Science; inasmuch as no one at the State House could tell him what a cosmopathic healer was, he decided he would be one. Compare this: according to Montenegro (1988), George Kopp of Wisconsin once said:

> [I] had determined that, if taken to court, I would say that D.C. meant Disciple of Christ. I knew that the law would not monkey with spiritual healers. . . . Dr. Kopp remembers B.J. saying that if chiropractic were to be eliminated he would declare it a religion and thereby be free from persecution.

But chiropractors in the greater Boston area who did not put their name in the classified section of the telephone directory or otherwise call attention to themselves (e.g., by gaining newspaper publicity for remarkable cures, as some did) usually were not arrested. In outlying areas chiropractors practiced more openly, often listing themselves in telephone directories. James Chaisson, a confident and prominent chiropractor, had been appointed to the Fitchburg Board of Health. In most small communities chiropractors were well integrated into the social fabric as active church participants, scout leaders, and members of civic clubs such as the Rotary or Kiwanis and of fraternal organizations; the Masonic Shrine was a particular favorite.

Practically all Massachusetts chiropractors were on good terms with at least some MDs. Most treated some MDs and referred to them patients needing medical care; and some MDs referred patients to chiropractors. One question I asked every chiropractor in the group I interviewed was what he would do if a patient collapsed or died in his office; could he count on an MD to come help him and/or sign a death certificate? (A chiropractor in Massachusetts of course could not do that.) Nearly every chiropractor was confident that he knew an MD he could call on to help out. I heard of no such an event occurring during the period of my interviewing, but it was an ever-present possibility.

When I asked John Walsh my question about medical "protection" if a patient died in his office he replied, "I guess every chiropractor in this state has an MD who will cover for him." John Murphy agreed, saying, "A chiropractor cannot practice in Massachusetts without medical connections." Several chiropractors told me they were on such good terms with MDs that they had open invitations to put patients in what I presume would have been small private hospitals, and that they occasionally did so. Another chiropractor told me that he had referred cancer patients to the famed Lahey Clinic and received back the customary reports. A prominent chiropractor who sent bills to insurance companies was said to sign his name so that the D.C. looked like M.D.

Chiropractors told me many stories about medical spies, arrests, trials, fines, and incarcerations, and that 11 chiropractors had been arrested recently; most of whem pleaded nolo contendere and were fined $100. Despite the law, juries (but not judges) almost never convicted chiropractors for merely practicing their profession. They believed that the chiropractor was trying sincerely to help the sick using an alternative to orthodox medicine. And patients were always ready to testify to the good character of the chiropractor and the benefits they had received. This was generally true across the nation. The Massachusetts situation was typical of the practice situation in those states without licensing, and especially typical of what the situation had earlier been everywhere. Even in states with licensing laws the law often was flauted, either because it too narrowly restricted the way chiropractors wanted to practice or because it was unfairly administered, especially if the licensing board consisted only of or was dominated by MDs.

Harry Runge was first arrested in 1914, along with seven other chiropractors. His four arrests resulted in fines. After one arrest he went to Vermont for a few months. In contesting his last arrest, he persuaded the attorney for the International Chiropractors Association (not the later ICA) to make an exception from its usual policy of only defending those who admitted practicing chiropractic and to argue that he was practicing physiotherapy. But after the police investigator described the treatment given, Runge was convicted of practicing medicine without a license, and fined. When he reapplied for insurance he was rejected on the grounds that he used a heat lamp and vibrator, although he claimed he used them only to prove that he was a physiotherapist. The National Chiropractic Association (NCA) also denied him insurance coverage, saying he was such a poor risk because of his four arrests. I was told that the ICA later refused to defend any Massachusetts chiropractor because of the excessive risk of arrest, in sharp contrast to the earlier period when the UCA mainly defended chiropractors arrested in unlicensed states. When I interviewed Runge in 1948 he would accept only those patients he already knew or were vouched for. Moreover, he was claiming to be a magnetic healer, a field specifically exempt from regulation under the medical practice act. Despite his many difficulties, he was still optimistic about the future of chiropractic, and asserted: "Chiropractic will not die because the principle is true. When the principle of chiropractic is properly applied the patient will get well, whether it is called chiropractic or medicine. You can blot out the name."

The *Commonwealth vs. Zimmerman* (1915) decision of the Supreme Judicial Court of Massachusetts was of great historic importance because it defined the legal status of chiropractic not only for Massachusetts but for many other states where it was often cited as a legal precedent. J.O. Zimmerman, one of Runge's classmates at the Palmer School of Chiropractic (PSC), was, like Runge, in practice in Boston by 1912. He was arrested February 20, 1914, on a complaint filed by police officer Arthur E. Keating in Boston Municipal Court, charging that he had practiced medicine from December 15, 1913, to February 20, 1914, without being lawfully authorized or duly registered by the Massachusetts Board of Registration in Medicine. On February 25 he pleaded not guilty, but was convicted and fined $100. He appealed to the Suffolk County Superior Court on April 6, and between April 28 and November 23, 1914, underwent two trials by jury, because the first jury failed to reach a verdict.

In his defense he argued that a chiropractic adjustment is not within the scope of medical treatment and that the provisions of the laws regulating the practice of medicine were unconstitutional as applied to him. Judge Dana denied his claim. By then the Boston newspapers were finding, or generating, considerable public interest in the case. The Boston *Herald* (November 21, 1914) reported the proceedings under the headline "Texas Ranger Eloquence Fails to Rope the Jury: Col. Long Came from the Plains to Defend Chiropractor in Vain." The newspaper went on to describe Attorney Colonel Sol O. Long as:

> . . . a Texas ranger and former Texas legislator and chief attorney for the Chiropractic Association. . . . Attorneys and legal luminaries crowded the courtroom all afternoon to get an idea of how the law is administered in Texas. They were not disappointed. Colonel Long brought the local color of the plains with him. He wore the typical goatee, flowing hair and drab jacket of the prairie man, and his gestures were as of all outdoors.

Despite advice to the contrary from his Massachusetts colleagues, Zimmerman appealed through his attorney to the Supreme Judicial Court, which on January 19, 1915, agreed to hear the case. Zimmerman's legal brief repeated his argument that he was not practicing medicine but chiropractic, that he was not interested in symptoms, diagnosis, or the cure of disease but merely examined and analyzed the spine for abnormalities of position and made adjustments of the vertebrae. "All evidence showed that he did not attempt a 'treatment,' but rather an 'adjustment' and there was no medical harm administered" (Edelstein, 1974, p 24). Furthermore, he was a graduate of PSC and had a reputation in the community for good moral character. Runge described it as a "clean case"; that is, there had been no injury, malfeasance, or malpractice of any kind.

More specifically, Zimmerman asked the Court, among other things, to find that Section 7 of Chapter 76 of the Revised Laws of Massachusetts of 1902, which dealt with Board examinations, was unconstitutional because it did not provide the chiropractor with the privilege of taking an examination in his own science, as was accorded the osteopath in Section 2 of Chapter 526 of the Acts of 1909, and because it required an examination in obstetrics, therapeutics, and materia medica, although these fields were unrelated to the practice of chiropractic; that Section 7 of Chapter 526 was unconstitutional because the chiropractor would have been exempt if the osteopath was exempt; that chiropractic is not the practice of medicine but "a separate, systematized, coordinated and arranged system or method . . . not a massage or manipulation of the entire body but of the spine only (Edelstein, 1974, p 27).

In making those arguments Zimmerman's attorney was clearly following the strategy urged by B.J., which in many states won separate licensing laws and examining boards for chiropractors. However, by 1915, the year in which the Zimmerman suit was finally adjudicated, only Kansas had enacted a chiropractic licensing law (in 1913), and no licenses were actually issued to chiropractors until Arkansas first did in 1915. Hence there were nearly no legal precedents for the Massachusetts courts to follow, although Indiana had ruled that a magnetic healer required a medical license because the term "practice of medicine" was generic in character (Parks vs. the State, 159 Indiana 211, 1902), and Kansas had decided that a chiropractor's actions came within the meaning of the term "practice of medicine," adding gratuitously that inasmuch as "chiropractic" was an unknown word it must have been invented as a hoax (State vs. Johnson, 84 Kansas 411, 1911).

In any event, Chief Justice Rugg's opinion for the Supreme Judicial Court of the Commonwealth of Massachusetts was clear-cut (Commonwealth vs. Zimmerman, 1915):

> Although the defendant did not prescribe medicine, and testified that he paid no attention to the patient's description of disease or symptoms, yet it is obvious that his purpose was to treat the human body in order to make natural that which he found abnormal in the narrow field of his examination. . . . It is of no consequence that the defendant abstained from the use of words "diagnosis," "treatment," or "disease" in description of what he did, and employed the terms "analysis," "palpation," and "adjustment." The acts which he did and their manifest design are to be examined rather than the words used, in order to ascertain the true nature of the defendant's conduct. A physical examination of the vertebrae, a decision whether they are in normal position or not, and strong manual pressure upon them with the end of changing the position with reference to each other of those found to be irregular, and thereby relieving pressure upon nerves, may be found to have such relation to the cure or prevention of disease or the relief of pain as to constitute the practice of medicine.

That decision governed the legal status of chiropractic in Massachusetts for a half-century. The conclusion that "reasonable classification is within the power of the Legislature," not the courts, meant that chiropractors should look to the legislature rather than to the courts to change their legal status. Although the legislative route was successful in most other states, Massachusetts, New York, Mississippi, and Louisiana resisted chiropractic legislation until the 1960s.

The *Commonwealth vs. Zimmerman* suit was the centerpiece of the campaign by the Massachusetts Medical Society to enforce the medical practice laws against the small but growing chiropractic profession, as the Boston *Herald* (January 22, 1914) noted: "For some time the state board of medicine and the state police [have] been at work gathering evidence of the practice of several chiropractors of the vicinity." The headline to that news item indicated that even before Zimmerman had been arrested another court case had been initiated: "Chiropractors Court Proceedings: President Riley of New England College Summoned into Court," and the article noted that it was "at instance of State Board of Registration in Medicine." Several months later Officer Keating cited the college in a separate complaint for granting the degree of Doctor of Chiropractic without the authority of a special act of the legislature granting the power to give degrees. Although this case did not have as far-reaching legal significance as the *Zimmerman* case, it was appealed to the Supreme Judicial Court and resulted in a major decision.

According to Runge, J. Shelby Riley arrived in Boston "about the fall of 1912" and soon opened his New England College of Chiropractic on Huntington Avenue. Ernest Carreiro, the first chiropractor my family took me to, confirmed in an interview in 1949 that Riley was operating his school in 1913 and 1914, and stated that it had about 15 faculty members (who almost certainly would have been teaching part-time), including himself in the "chair of neurology," as he put it, and two MDs. He added that the course consisted of 3 years of 6 months each and cost $350 per year. His claim that at one time the school enrolled 175 students may be doubted. Runge stated that it had "not less than twenty-five students," some of whom he described in unflattering terms as "fat old women who had practiced massage, clairvoyance, or metaphysics, and wanted to get in on this new field of chiropractic." Runge's contempt was probably not unrelated to his description of Riley as "not a Palmer man, a mixer who included everything possible under chiropractic: lamp, vibrator, medical diagnostic instruments like the stethoscope, osteopathic manipulations, and urinalysis; he was an osteopath, a lawyer, and a preacher, so we didn't know what he really was." Partial confirmation of Runge's characterization can be found on the title page of the book Riley published in 1919, *Science and Practice of Chiropractic with Allied Sciences,* which credits him as "M.D., Ph.D., M.S., D.M.T., D.O., D.P., D.C., Ph.C., Dean of the Washington School of Chiropractic." Riley used the term "chiropath" (cf. osteopath), which never gained currency. He also published *Zone Therapy Simplified* (1918), described by the naturopathic historian Cody (1985, I-17) as "an early forerunner of acupressure."

The Boston *Herald* headlined (April 2, 1914): "Fine Chiropractic College $100 for Awarding Degree." The Supreme Judicial Court agreed to hear the case on appeal. The complaint against the school was signed by seven of its own graduates, who were dissatisfied because the words "Doctor of Chiropractic" had not been put on their diplomas. But it was only after the diplomas were called in and "D.C." added that Officer Keating proceeded against the school. Since one of the student complainants was "Alfred Flower, M.D.," Edelstein (1974, p 35) suggests possible involvement by the medical society: "The list of witnesses' names on Keating's complaint suggests a possible 'plant' by the medical society. Otherwise, those who signed the complaint may simply have been the students of the New England College of Chiropractic who were dissatisfied with their degrees."

The principal evidence in the case was Dr. Flower's "certificate":

> Alfred H. Flower, M.D., having satisfactorily completed the prescribed courses of study in the New England College of Chiropractic, passed the examination and met all other requirements for graduation, has been declared a Doctor of Chiropractic. The certificate was signed by seven persons, all of whom wrote after their names the letters "D.C.," five also adding letters indicative of well recognized degrees such as B.S., M.D., D.D.S. . . . He [Flower] testified that the New England College of Chiropractic conferred that degree on him and that at the same time the degree was conferred on perhaps a dozen other persons; and that the ceremony was similar to any college or high school graduation upon a commencement day.

The Supreme Judicial Court's ruling, written by Chief Justice Rugg (Commonwealth vs. New England College of Chiropractic, 1915), held that:

> The conferring of a title made up of the word "Doctor" and a word related to the healing art may be found to be granting of a degree within the meaning of the statutes. The word "Doctor" in connection with an unusual and high sounding word could be quite as likely to impose upon the ignorant and credulous as the false use of the conventional Doctor of Medicine.

The appeal was denied, and the school was found guilty of granting a degree without the authority to do so. Furthermore, the offense was considered to be even greater because the practice of chiropractic had already been determined by the *Zimmerman* decision to be the practice of medicine, an area of greater hazard to the public than the practice of other professions for which academic degrees are awarded.

A medical source (Bowers, 1935) reported that Riley's school soon "folded its tent and silently stole away." It is likely that hostility from straight chiropractors toward Riley's mixer orientation created some of the problems for him and his school. Opposition grew in 1915 when Riley had a licensing bill introduced into the legislature. According to Runge, the Palmer men in the state banded together and opposed his bill: "They reported everything about Riley to B.J. Palmer and he told them the kind of licensing bill to get." Actually, three different bills to license chiropractors were introduced into the legislature in 1915, including one from the Massachusetts Chiropractic Association in opposition to Riley's. Runge described Riley as having "a gift of gab, making extravagant claims as to what chiropractic can do, and giving the impression of not being true-blue. He was on the wrong track chiropractically." Runge's version of Riley's disappearance was that the Massachusetts chiropractors "drove Riley out of town in about two years."

These and comments from other chiropractors testify to the depth of feeling over the straight-mixer issue in Massachusetts during the period. The division continued through the next half-century, with about two thirds of the state's chiropractors being straights and one third mixers. In the Massachusetts Chiropractic Association "you didn't rate if you weren't a Palmer man," according to John Walsh, who had attended Universal Chiropractic College in Davenport. John Murphy, an Eastern Chiropractic College graduate, said: "The Palmer men and the non-Palmer men have never gotten along well in Massachusetts."

The main effect of the division between straights and mixers in Massachusetts, as elsewhere, was to make agreement on the kind of licensing law desired nearly impossible to obtain. Even when a compromise was agreed to, there were always extreme mixers and doctrinaire straights who were so dissatisfied that they would not work enthusiastically or contribute generously to its success. The mixers, with some justification, feared that a board dominated by straights would "crack down on mixers" and function as in New Hampshire, where "if they find you are using a stethoscope they haul you before the board for diagnosing." William Cote confirmed that possibility when he told me that he and the other ICA men agreed to go along with getting a law passed in 1949, but were planning to have the board crack down later on any chiropractor who used such modalities. The mixers had different ideas. They were contemptuous of the straights' unwillingness to make proper diagnostic evaluations using standard scientific instruments and methods and of B.J.'s insistence on the "Hole-in-One (HIO)" technique. And there were always differences of opinion over how to "grandfather in" those who would be unable to pass nearly any kind of written examination and over how many recent graduates would have to pass a more stringent examination.

Predictably, mixers and straights also differed on overall strategy. The straights argued for B.J.'s idea of maximizing rather than minimizing the differences between chiropractic and medicine as a means of achieving popular, political, and legal standing. Since the courts had ruled that chiropractic is the practice of medicine, the greater the difference between one's practice and medicine the less the likelihood of being arrested for practicing medicine might be. Nevertheless, the interpretation of the law in *Commonwealth vs. Zimmerman* was so explicit that all chiropractors, no matter how they practiced, were vulnerable to arrest and prosecution for practicing medicine without a license. Walsh, who entered practice in 1916, put it this way: "It's like an axe hanging over your head, this law." Walter Swan, who began practicing in 1923, said:

> Massachusetts is unquestionably the worst state in which to practice. New York isn't so bad because there is no law against chiropractic—the way the Zimmerman Supreme Court interpretation results in Massachusetts. Consequently they practice very openly without intervention, especially in upper New York State.

Murphy, who had been in practice since 1925, said: "We in Massachusetts are martyrs to chiropractic. It's very hard not knowing whether the next person who comes into your office is OK or not." Leon Dana added: "A lot of fine chiropractors have left Massachusetts; they weren't able to stick it out." Most Massachusetts chiropractors displayed licenses from another state, often from several. But without a licensing requirement anyone, even I, as I often remarked, could have opened an office and tried to engage in chiropractic practice. The only example of uncredentialed practice I discovered was the wife of the aging and infirm Ernest Carreiro, whom he had trained to carry on his practice; she was described to me by another chiropractor as doing "a land office business."

To keep the subject in perspective, it should be kept in mind that during these years the Massachusetts requirements for medical licensure were not high. Only in 1915 was the law amended to require that applicants for medical registration possess an M.D. degree from any kind of school, even one not legally chartered ("Amendment to the Medical Registration Law," 1915). A later requirement that the degree be from a legally chartered medical school was intended to ensure that the board would no longer have applicants "who either failed to pass their examination for graduation from medical school or who [left] college under the false impression that a degree [was] of small importance in comparison with a certificate of registration." Gaucher (1992) reports discovering in his research a never disputed allegation by McNamara (1913, p 192):

> G.W. Simmons, who at the time was Secretary of the AMA and Editor of its *Journal*, had obtained his diploma from Rush Medical College after spending the whole of his time as a student away in Nebraska! What is more, he hadn't passed a single examination.

The tightening of medical licensure requirements coincided with the Medical Society's campaign against chiropractors. Since during this immediate post-Flexner period diploma mills in Chicago, Kansas City, and elsewhere were still peddling medical degrees for a fee, and others were evaluated by Flexner (1910, p 258) as "wretched," a license to practice medicine did not carry the same assurance of competence that it does today. According to two items in the Boston *American* (November 27, 1923), "Quack Led Hub Students" and "Prior's Official Probe Reaches Sensational Climax," an investigation by Dr. Charles E. Prior, head of the Massachusetts Board of Registration, found many schools where diplomas were "sold cheap, some second-hand," resulting in recall of licenses from physicians with bogus credentials.

A challenge by Massachusetts Health Commissioner Dr. C.D. Barrett to settle the question of the germ theory of disease and the efficacy of chiropractic was reported by the Boston *Herald* on March 7, 1923 ("To Fight a Duel with Germs to Prove a Point"). Chiropractor Nathan Friedman accepted Dr. Barrett's challenge to drink typhoid germs, swab their throats with diphtheria germs, and sleep with a patient with small pox. But the duel would have to wait until he got out of jail!

From 1915 to 1966 the legal status of chiropractic in Massachusetts remained unchanged despite repeated efforts to persuade the legislature to pass a licensing law. Chiropractors' risks and vulnerabilities remained much the same during that period. The numbers of chiropractors increased from approximately 35 in 1917 to 130 in the late 1940s and to about 140 in the 1950s and 1960s. And chiropractic gradually became better known and accepted by the public, if not by MDs. Chiropractors still were arrested periodically, and if convicted usually fined $100, warned, and released. Only if they persisted in practice or defied a court order to cease practice were they likely to be sent to jail, which happened less frequently.

Murphy's career is revealing. He told me that he and other students at Eastern Chiropractic Institute in New York City regularly wrote to five Massachusetts chiropractors who were serving time in jail. On graduation in 1924 he decided to settle in Massachusetts "to fight for chiropractic. . . . I was determined to dedicate my life to chiropractic." Hence it is clear that schools other than PSC instilled fighting spirit in their students. In view of the obvious difficulties he faced, it is hard to question his courage or sincerity. Although his two brothers gave up practice and left the state, he experienced little difficulty in getting established. "I never knew a lean day," he said. He said it was "like old home week" in his waiting room as patients socialized with one another. Another chiropractor told of having separate waiting rooms for men and women so they could talk more freely about their illnesses without the opposite sex present. Murphy conducted a large and successful practice in Waltham, not far from where Middlesex Medical School (then a class B medical school and later the site of Brandeis University) was still functioning. Perhaps because of his proximity to the medical school, or because he did a lot of advertising, he had been arrested four times: twice in 1927; once in 1929, when he was acquitted because his patient testified (perhaps perjuring himself) that no bill was rendered to him and no money was paid; and in 1943, on which occasion, after he had been convicted and paid his $100 fine, he appealed; then, because of his good community reputation and political contacts, he said, his case was placed "on file" (whatever that meant) and his fine was returned to him! Although his second 1927 arrest resulted in a 30-day jail sentence, the judge suspended the sentence because he knew, according to Murphy, that Murphy would appeal to a jury trial and that "juries never convict chiropractors." Of course they sometimes did. I was also told that Murphy once had to pay a fine of $375 for beating up a detective he had warned not to enter his office.

Some chiropractors, such as Leon Dana, who entered practice in 1914, never advertised. Runge, on the other hand, told how he "put on a terrific publicity campaign." He hired a feature writer from the Boston *American* to get something in the paper each week about him and chiropractic, and fed her material on cases that he or other chiropractors had successfully treated. The headline of one of her articles screamed: "Wellesley Girl Snatched from the Jaws of Death." After 5 weeks of such advertising, which he said netted him 43 new patients, a friend who worked at court advised him "like a father" to quit before he got run out of the state, telling him he was "all washed up" if he continued. Another chiropractor said, "I have nothing to fear. I am not doing anything wrong. . . . I never sent out a bill. I keep no books. Only one patient in a hundred doesn't pay."

George Smyrl, a prominent Springfield chiropractor and a former president of both the Massachusetts Chiropractic Association and the NCA, said to me: "There are two things that get chiropractors in trouble in Massachusetts: being prominent politically, as I was, and criticizing MDs. It's the Palmer men who lean toward criticizing MDs." John Murphy, who was also active politically, stated that MDs crack down on the most prominent chiropractors, hoping to scare the lesser ones off. Smyrl added that the complaints usually come from physicians whose patients have not been helped and who then went to a chiropractor and were helped. (I have often heard such stories, most recently from a Connecticut chiropractor who discovered an aortic aneurism missed by the woman's MD, who afterward berated her for going to the chiropractor!) George Kopp, interviewed in Wisconsin after 39 years of practice, was quoted as saying (Montenegro 1988, p 9): "My best cases were always those who did not get results under medical care."

A serious problem was created if a patient died under chiropractic care. Three such cases in Massachusetts are documented. The Boston *Herald* headlined (December 10, 1920) "Chiropractor held in $800 in Death of Girl" when Walter Crawford, a graduate of Riley's school, was arraigned for the death of an 18-year-old patient he had been treating. The conviction of Ernest Grandchamp was upheld in the death of Mrs. Whipple on appeal to the Supreme Judicial Court (Alfred A. Whipple, Administrator, vs. Ernest S. Grandchamp, 264 Mass. 40, 1927). And so was John G. Whitney's conviction in the 1935 death of a woman he treated for a year and a half for high blood pressure (Mildred H. Deward, Administrator, vs. John G. Whitney, 298 Mass. 41, 1937). I was told that Whitney was assessed $7,500 in damages (of which the ICA paid its maximum liability coverage, $5,000), fined for practicing medicine without a license, and left the state.

After the 1915 *Commonwealth vs. Zimmerman* decision the best alternative to improve the situation was to go to the legislature. Runge told me there had been a Legislative Committee in the MCA for 37 years, a claim that may have been exaggerated, because it would have to have been established in 1912, which is possible. Fred Sears, who entered practice in 1922 and was an officer of the ICA, told me that by 1949 he had participated in 26 legislative campaigns, that is, every year up to our interview. His statement, "We go through the motions each year," revealed his pessimism and frustration over the lack of success. Some progress had been made, however. In 1927 a bill to license chiropractors passed the Senate, but failed in the House of Representatives in a weakened version that would have made it a bad law. Even though it would have grandfathered in those already in practice, it would have required future candidates to pass the standard medical examination. That kind of law, which some other states adopted, would not have been acceptable to the profession as a whole, and especially not to B.J.

According to the *Report Submitted by the Legislative Research Council Relative to Boards of Registration for Chiropractors, Electrologists, and Sanitarians* (1956, p 10), an initiative petition for a popular referendum succeeded in getting a proposal to license chiropractors on the 1932 state ballot, where it was rejected 602,520 to 351,094, that is, 37.5% to 21.8%, with 40.7% of the ballots left blank.

Although the *Report of the Special Commission on Osteopathy, Chiropractic, Foods, Drugs, and Poisons* (1939) recommended that the legislature establish a special board of chiropractic regulation, "for it would drive out the so-called 'quacks' in the profession," the legislature did not act favorably until 1945, when the House approved a licensing bill 104 to 72 and the Senate followed by a vote of 18 to 15. Much to the dismay of the chiropractors, Governor Maurice Tobin vetoed the bill: "Chiropractic Bill Vetoed: Would Mean Double Standard, Says Tobin" (Boston *Herald*, July 14, 1945), and the House sustained his veto. There was a pervasive belief among the chiropractors that the Governor had been "paid off" to veto the bill. According to John Walsh, Governor Tobin had told several persons that he would sign the bill, then didn't:

> Tobin has [former Governor James Michael] Curley beat as a grafter. The story is that he got between $50,000 and $100,000 for vetoing the bill. Even the nurses and dentists were asked to contribute.

George Smyrl told me that some of the MDs in the Springfield area had been assessed $75 each to fight the chiropractic bill, and he assumed that all MDs in the state had. John Sloop, in practice since 1921, agreed:

> The chiropractic bill is known as a "money bill" by the politicians, not because of the money chiropractors spend on it but because the medics have to spend so much to defeat it. They often let it pass either the Senate or the House in order to raise the ante. Tobin delayed as long as possible to get more money.

I do not accept these statements as facts, but cite them to report a state of mind and rumors that were prevalent and believed by most chiropractors. There was a pervasive cynicism toward the legislative process and a belief that it mainly took money to get a bill passed. Fred Sears said categorically: "No bill gets through on its merits; money has to be passed around." Since allegations of bribery and corruption were very common when I grew up near Boston during the 1930s, it was easy for me to believe that some politicians could be bought. Murphy claimed that Governor Tobin was narrowly defeated in the next election because of opposition by chiropractors and their supporters.

Murphy, who was a member of the chiropractic delegation that visited Governor Tobin to urge him to sign the bill in 1945, told me that also in the delegation was Millard Smith, M.D., who departed by a side door so as to avoid being seen by the medical delegation waiting its turn to visit the Governor. When I later interviewed Dr. Smith he confirmed the story. Because he had investigated a variety of alternative healing systems, he was in danger of losing his medical appointments. He also told me that he had visited PSC, and considered B.J. Palmer one of the three geniuses he had met in his life. Retired after practicing radiology in Wyoming for 30 years, he wrote me (April 1990): "During this period I've enjoyed a working relationship with the Chiropractic Community. In this area they have always stayed within their professional competence and sought consultation when necessary."

In Massachusetts, despite all the setbacks there was always the hope that "next year" things would be different. The need for a licensing bill was compelling because there was no visible alternative. Hence each year new leaders came forward, money was raised, and the effort made again.

In 1949 I attended the legislative hearings and final debate in the House of Representatives on a proposed law. I had two purposes in mind: to observe the process and to demonstrate to my chiropractic respondents where I stood on the issue. I lobbied my own representative and senator in favor of the bill, which I felt should be adopted.

On March 1 the Joint Public Health Committee held a hearing at which each side was allotted 2 hours to present testimony. It was chaired by Senator Stanton, the sympathetic Mayor of Fitchburg who had appointed James Chaisson, D.C., to his city's Board of Health. Among those speaking in favor were several legislators; an elderly MD; Roger Dunham, Public Relations Counsel of the ICA; and John Nugent, Educational Director of the NCA. Opposed were Dr. John Conlin, Director of Information and Education of the Massachusetts Medical Society, the Massachusetts Commissioner of Health, the presidents of two county medical societies, the dean of a local physiotherapy school, and the counsel of the Massachusetts Osteopathic Society. The Public Health Committee reported out the bill favorably by a vote of 9 to 6. Next a hearing on it was held by the Ways and Means Committee, at which much of the same testimony was repeated, plus this comment by a sitting legislator:

> In 1945 the Governor vetoed this bill, . . . That man now feeds off this bill. If he had another chance to sign it he probably would do so. . . . I have three adjustments a week. I have asthma and I would be on the way to the cemetery if I didn't have chiropractic adjustments. Next to God I thank the chiropractors.

On April 27, after a late afternoon debate characterized by ridicule of chiropractors and levity in anticipation of an end-of-session party, the House of Representatives rejected the bill by a standing count of 96 to 38.

In 1955 Massachusetts chiropractors adopted a different tactic. Because 40 years of legislative efforts had been unsuccessful, they decided to try again to persuade the Supreme Judicial Court to reverse its 1915 *Commonwealth vs. Zimmerman* decision. A combination of two concurrent cases—an appeal from arrests made in 1954 (Commonwealth vs. Peter Antonio (and Three Companion Cases), 333 Mass. 175, 1955), and a new suit (Massachusetts Chiropractic Laymen's Association Inc. and Others vs. Attorney General and Another, 333 Mass. 179, 1955)—sought the following declaratory judgment:

1. that chiropractic is not the practice of medicine;
2. that even if it is the practice of medicine, then . . . [the laws] which forbid the practice of medicine without a license [are] unconstitutional as applied to chiropractors;
3. that . . . [the laws] do not regulate the practice of chiropractic in the Commonwealth; and
4. that even if . . . [the laws] be construed as regulating the practice of chiropractic but restricting it to registered physicians, then these sections bear no reasonable relation to the public welfare and are unconstitutional.

The chiropractors argued that since the 1915 *Zimmerman* decision 44 states had recognized chiropractic as legally separate from medicine, that the courts of other states had often ruled that the practice of chiropractic is not the practice of medicine, that federal agencies had officially recognized chiropractic and had even paid for the education of the defendant chiropractor Peter Antonio under the GI Bill, that 30 million Americans were receiving chiropractic care (thus proving public acceptance), and that more than 300 chiropractors currently were practicing in Massachusetts. Hence the Court could and should now redefine its position. But it refused to do so, and granted no declaratory relief.

However, in the following year, 1956, the Legislative Research Council in its *Report* referred to above, after thoroughly considering all aspects of the question, concluded that a board of registration should be established to "drive out the so-called 'quacks' in the profession, as it would require a high school education and four years training in a recognized chiropractic college." But it took 10 more years and the leadership of Malcolm Macdonald for it to happen. Finally, the Boston *Herald* reported (June 29, 1966): "Reluctant [Governor] Volpe Signs Bill Legalizing Chiropractic." The bill established a five-member board of registration that initially consisted of three chiropractors and two physicians, but later did not require MDs. The law required three levels of examinations, depending on whether the chiropractor had been in practice 5 years, 3 years, or less, and specified that candidates after 1969 should have successfully completed 2 years of work toward a bachelors degree. Thus Massachusetts chiropractors finally got their licensing bill.

It is difficult to say how representative Massachusetts was of all states in which chiropractors struggled for legal recognition. Al Smith vetoed the first chiropractic licensing bill to reach the Governor's desk in New York. Only after a long hard fight, and partly because Governor Nelson Rockefeller urged it, did New York pass its law in 1963. In New York City the situation had been particularly desperate, according to a Massachusetts informant:

> Since most Massachusetts chiropractors are in the smaller towns where they become integrated into the social fabric, they become known—favorably known—and the prosecutors hesitate to make arrests. In New York City a chiropractor is a little frog in a big puddle, without the backing of the people. There are about four hundred chiropractors in Greater New York. They are comparatively unknown there and prosecutions can take place with impunity. If they are arrested they aren't given a jury trial as they are upstate, but only have a choice between one judge or three judges. Outside New York City chiropractors are practically immune, as they are in Massachusetts.

There is not enough space here to detail the history of chiropractic everywhere. Several state histories have been published that the interested reader may consult, for example, Alabama (Hartmann, 1984), California ("California Chiropractic Association: The First 50 Years," 1978), Oklahoma (Gallagher, 1930), Kansas (Metz, 1965), New York (Goldschmidt S, 1970), Texas (Rhodes, 1978), Wisconsin (Mawhiney, 1984), and Utah (Walden, 1989); see also the special issue "Chiropractic in Australia and New Zealand" of *Chiropractic History* (1989, vol 1).

Chapter 7

EDUCATION, RECRUITMENT, MOTIVATION

> *The profession has attracted thousands of re-*
> *cruits—retired baseball players, work-weary*
> *plumbers, truck drivers, longshoremen, bogus den-*
> *tists, dubious preachers, cashiered school superin-*
> *tendents, . . . garage mechanics, ash men and de-*
> *cayed welter weights.*
>
> H.L. Mencken (1924)

It is arguable whether Mencken more offended chiropractors or the others he named.

Section 1

Educational Standards

There are two dimensions to the question of chiropractic educational standards: the *scope* of chiropractic practice for which students are to be prepared, and the *level of competence* needed in the basic medical sciences and in chiropractic techniques and treatment. These two dimensions are of course related. When the scope of practice is broad in the range of illnesses treated and in the techniques and methods used, the student's educational preparation needs to be broader and deeper and at a high level.

The profession has been divided from its beginning over how broad the scope of practice should be. B.J. Palmer insisted on "P, S, and U" (pure, straight, and unadulterated) chiropractic and castigated those who mixed it with any medical or physical therapies. But the division between straights and mixers is by no means simple. A bimodal separation of chiropractors on this dimension has never really existed. Rather, in a statistical sense they have presented a more "normal" distribution, with most chiropractors falling somewhere in the middle rather than at either extreme. Whatever the definition of "straight" at any given time (and it has broadened over the years), most chiropractors have relied on vertebral adjustments as their primary therapeutic modality, certainly as their specialty, even when they added to it supplementary, now called "adjunctive," therapies. These have ranged from dietary and vitamin supplements through the entire range of physiotherapeutic methods and instruments to such procedures (much condemned by straights) as high-colonic irrigation.

At one time vibrators and stethoscopes were considered mixing, as were braces and traction, but they have become acceptable to straights. Techniques that were originally naturopathic specialities (e.g., hydrotherapy, heat, cold, herbal remedies, electric modalities) were taught at the schools that offered both D.C. and N.D. degrees, and were considered mixing. Today ultrasound and various forms of electrical stimulation (e.g., microcurrent) are especially popular. Some chiropractors also use acupuncture (where state law permits) or one of its variants, such as acupressure or laser stimulation, and even homeopathic remedies. A very few combine chiropractic with biofeedback or some variety of suggestive therapy, hypnotherapy, psychologic counseling, or even Scientology (Koff, 1988) and some types of "New Age" healing. But most chiropractors have been neither extreme straights nor extreme mixers. Since many state laws now require competence in physiotherapeutic methods for a D.C. license, even most straight schools provide such training, sometimes as an elective. Thus the definition of the scope of chiropractic practice has evolved and broadened as the majority of chiropractors remain in the shifting middle on that dimension.

Some straights have told me they prefer the designation "neurospinal specialist" as an alternative to "drugless physician," which sounds too much like "naturopath." Although the term "chiropractic physician" was disparaged by D.D. Palmer (1910, p 400), his death certificate so recorded him, and it was used later in the title of the "Oregon Chiropractic Physicians Association." Twenty-four states now permit use of the title "chiropractic physician" (Williams, 1991, p 25).

Lerner (1954, p 169) reports that when D.D. began teaching in 1898 the only instructional materials were two small items: one was a small printed paper, titled "Luxation of Bones Cause Disease," with D.D.'s name at the end; the other consisted of four pages "printed to simulate the size and appearance of a large, ordinary daily newspaper" and called "The Chiropractic." His first course of instruction included anatomy, physiology, pathology, toxicology, symptomatology, and obstetrics, along with practical work in nerve tracing, palpation, and chiropractic technique. The course lasted only 3 months, later extended to 6 months, and cost $500. Dye (1939, p 66) states that by 1910 the standard was a 12-month course. In an oral history interview (Mawhiney, 1984, p 62) Wisconsin chiropractor John G. Shepherd told of attending a small college in 1913 in Wichita, Kansas, which gave both a 6- and a 12-month course. He was charged $300, for which he was permitted to sign a promissory note. He paid it off before he graduated by treating patients. "We were only supposed to charge half a dollar, but most of them gave us a dollar," he said. At the Palmer School of Chiropractic (PSC) the degree of "chiropractor" was awarded after

8 months, allowing needy students to earn enough money to complete the D.C. course. It was discontinued in 1921 when the course was lengthened to 18 months. An 18-month course was offered at Carver College in Oklahoma City by 1910, but did not become standard in the profession until 1920 (Gibbons, 1987, p 12). The first college to offer a 4-year course of 8 months each was Universal Chiropractic College in Pittsburg, in 1922, followed by Lincoln College in Indianapolis, from its inception in 1926, and Western States College in Portland by 1932. Only in 1949 did B.J. increase the PSC course from 18 months to 4 years.

The quality of early chiropractic education was no doubt inferior. According to D.D.'s grandson David Daniel Palmer "Dave" (1967, p 23), the principal text that D.D. first used was "Dr. Pierce's 'Family Medical Adviser,' a classic found those days in nearly every home throughout the nation." Chemistry and dissection were largely ignored, which was the primary reason why Howard left PSC to found the National College of Chiropractic (NCC) in 1906. The 1908 PSC catalogue boasted:

> We do not waste valuable time in observing healthy and morbid tissue under the microscope . . . nor the compounding of chemicals . . . nor the analysis of secretions and excretions.

According to Dye (1939, p 66), dissection classes were held only a few times a year, "whenever B.J. was able to obtain the corpse of some poor unidentified unfortunate at the city morgue, and were usually held at the morgue of some friendly undertaker." Chemistry was added to the curriculum only in 1913. D.D. wrote (1910, p 488):

> If I had been educated in a medical college, there would not yet have been a chiropractor. . . . I would rather take a layman to educate than one who is in ruts. . . . A mind free from a therapeutic education presents a clear field for cultivation.

Theodore Schreiber, former dean of Kansas State Chiropractic College, wrote me in a letter (April 17, 1952) that D.D. even "refused to have the initials 'D.C.' attached to his name," and that he had a photostat copy of the original correspondence to prove it. A letter to me from Dr. Edward Altman (March 27, 1953) contained this fascinating comment:

> My observation has been that the less education and the lower the intellectual, social, and cultural sensitivity of the chiropractor, the better is his adjustment (no pun intended). Also, the chances are that this man has a larger practice because he associates with a considerably less sophisticated group.

B.J.'s phrase was "Education constipates the mind." Not surprisingly, many of those who arrived with some medical training, whether allopathic, homeopathic, eclectic, or osteopathic, were turned off by B.J.'s attitude. Nevertheless, five of the first 15 PSC graduates were MDs (Gibbons, 1981a), and there were always MDs on the early PSC faculty. The first director of the school clinic was W.L. Brown, M.D. (Gibbons, 1981a). Obstetrics was regularly taught and practiced at the school, usually by MDs, and Gibbons suggests (1982, pp 27–28) that D.D. was the first chiropractic "accoucheur." Alfred B. Hender, M.D., D.C. (1874–1943) began lecturing in anatomy at PSC in 1905, and delivered Dave Palmer at home in 1906; he joined the faculty in 1910 in the chair of obstetrics, and became dean in 1912. A respected physician, he had graduated from the College of Medicine of the University of Iowa, and was chairman of the board of the Davenport School of Nursing and president of the Middletonian Medical Society of Davenport (Dzamen et al., 1980, p 28). Hundreds of babies of PSC students were delivered at the school clinic, thus enriching students' clinical training. Succeeding him as dean in 1943 was his son Herbert C. Hender, D.C. MDs on the staff of the B.J. Palmer Chiropractic Clinic, established in 1935, taught classes as well as doing medical workups on clinic patients.

Primarily as a legal strategy to defend chiropractors against the charge of practicing medicine without a license, B.J. insisted that chiropractic differs completely from medicine and is in fact its exact opposite. For B.J., mixing meant incorporating into chiropractic any medical technique (e.g., stethoscope, laboratory diagnosis), physiotherapy, or the instruments introduced at NCC in Chicago, and of course drugs or surgery. After B.J.'s death in 1961 and the employment of more and more university-trained instructors in the basic sciences, objections to the use of sophisticated diagnostic instrumentation disappeared. Even straights now routinely use computed tomography (CT) and magnetic resonance imaging (MRI) for diagnostic purposes. It is ironic that of all the specialized practitioners treating the spine, chiropractors may use and benefit most from these high-tech devices for differential diagnosis of spinal disorders. I continue to hear stories of medical misdiagnoses due to failure to order these scans when appropriate.

The second major dimension of chiropractic education is the question of quality. For reasons unknown, D.D. certified his graduates both to practice and *teach* chiropractic. There is no doubt that the vast majority of early chiropractic schools were inadequate (Brennan, 1983). Perhaps fortunately, most of the worst of them never attracted many students. Although PSC and NCC as well as other schools offered correspondence courses in the first two decades of this century (Brennan, 1983a, p 26; Rice, 1912), resident instruction soon became the mode. However, as late as 1919 the following advertisement appeared (Gibbons, 1980a, p 346):

> Be a Chiropractor. Learn at home. By the American University system of instruction, you can become a Doctor of Chiropractic by studying in spare time at home or in class at the university. You do not require special talent or advanced education.

Creel in an article titled "Making Doctors While You Wait" (1915) describes his visit to that American University, where the "dean," occupying a dingy office, offered him the complete course including osteopathy, mechanotherapy, and psychotherapy for $68.75. In 1923 an article appeared in *JAMA* with the following title: "The Menace of Chiropractic: Practically No Educational Requirements Necessary for Matriculation in Chiropractic Colleges." Students were permitted to enter at any time, and at first there was no distinction between classes because, as Dye (1939, p 225) wrote:

"No school is in position to ruthlessly wave aside any matriculation fees offered to it at any time throughout the school year." Some examining boards accepted high school equivalency if the applicant could prove that he had been able to earn a living (Dye, 1939, p 223), which probably meant they accepted anybody. NCC and other colleges permitted students without a high school diploma to earn its equivalent in evening classes during their first 6 months of study (Brennan, 1983, p 29). Geiger (1942, Feb., p 96) quotes B.J. as giving the following advice to a prospective student: "In regard to educational qualifications, do not allow this to annoy you. We hold no entrance examinations." Chiropractic critic Morris Fishbein (1925, p 82) wrote:

> When Thomas F. Duhigg of Davenport for the Pennsylvania Bureau of Medical Education and Licensure reported the results of an inspection of the schools of Davenport . . . he pointed out that in 1915 the three colleges which had developed in that capital of chiropractic were really little fit to educate anybody in anything. None had a library, a hospital, a laboratory worthy of the name, post mortems or capable teachers.

As late as 1964, fake applications instigated by the American Medical Association (AMA) Department of Investigation to seven chiropractic schools by obviously unqualified applicants received five provisional acceptances and two rejections ("Requirements for Admission to Schools of Chiropractic," 1964).

The earliest serious evaluation of PSC quality was that by George Dock, M.D. (1922, p 61), who found an

> "osteological laboratory," a small room almost filled with cases containing many remarkably fine specimens of bone lesions. One striking thing about these students is the friendliness, earnestness and conviction of all, . . . as attractive a body of students as I have ever encountered. It was not difficult to discover, however, that most of them had not bridged the stage between the grammar school and the course that in medicine leads to the doctor's degree. The farm, the barbershop and the hotel dining room or kitchen would seem to be the more natural work places for a great many. Some, however, seem to have come from the teacher's platform, and a few from normal schools or small colleges. . . . They preach a Hubbardesque philosophy in rather wearisome aphorisms. . . . (Mrs. Palmer) commands the class through her presence and personality, and is urbane but energetic in manner.

When the AMA Council on Medical Education inspected chiropractic schools in 1927 ("Schools of Chiropractic and Naturopathy in the United States," 1928), it reported that an institution such as NCC "is a disgrace, and it can best serve the public interest by going out of existence." However, it rated Los Angeles College of Chiropractic (LACC) "the best equipped chiropractic school that the inspector has seen," and the osteologic collection at PSC as "without doubt the best collection of human spines in existence." As for B.J., the inspector was more critical: "As a salesman, B.J. is a success; as an educator, he does not even exist."

The most sophisticated attempt to assess chiropractic from a neutral perspective was Louis Reed's *The Healing Cults* (1932), one of 28 volumes prepared for the prestigious Committee on the Costs of Medical Care. Reed made a serious effort to obtain accurate statistical data on chiropractic education, income, and practice characteristics, even though his overall bias and his support for the medical strategy of "containing, if not eliminating" chiropractic was transparent. He located 79 schools in 1920, 40 in 1927, but only 21 in 1932. His estimates of total enrollments were "not more than 2000" in 1927, and in 1932 "a probable attendance of 1400. Thirteen of these schools had a known aggregate attendance of 1090. The remainder probably had 300 students" (Reed, 1932, p 36). Hence the earlier proliferation of schools had been considerably reduced. Regarding quality, Reed (1932, pp 41, 47) stated:

> Although many of the chiropractic schools have lengthened their courses during the past few years and have shown improvement in other ways, it is nevertheless impossible to take them seriously as educational institutions. . . . Without exception, all the schools are business institutions run for the profit of their owners. Most of them fairly reek of commercialism. . . .

> There are probably fewer than a half dozen really qualified teachers in the twenty-one institutions. Not one conducts a clinic where the really serious ailments and diseases can be studied. Not one has laboratory facilities which by any reasonable standards could be considered adequate.

In the early decades most chiropractic schools were small, privately owned, poorly equipped, with mostly part-time faculty, and lacking what medical schools would call good "clinical teaching material." Student clinics, whether they were free or charged minimal fees, usually did not lack patients, but many of these were not seriously sick. The burden of recruiting patients often was placed on the students themselves, resulting in even more relatively healthy patients as students strived to meet their quota of adjustments required to graduate. Still today college clinics fail to attract the wide variety of sick patients needed for adequate training in pathology (Nyiendo and Haldeman, 1986). Only attendance at hospital clinics, rounds, and surgery can provide the best clinical training.

However, the earliest chiropractic colleges often were associated with infirmaries where patients requiring nursing care were admitted. D.D.'s first school was the Palmer School and Cure, which continued as an in-patient facility through 1902 when he introduced the word "chiropractic" and renamed it the Palmer Infirmary and Chiropractic Institute. Langworthy's American School of Chiropractic and Nature Cure was referred to both as a "health home" and a "sanitarium." Although these and later chiropractic hospitals were not established primarily to provide clinical instruction, the students and graduates who practiced in them clearly benefited from the experience. PSC "maintained the Palmer Infirmary for the care of bed patients during much of the period between 1913 and 1920" (Quigley, 1989b). A historical note is that from 1914 to 1924 NCC students were "admitted to all clinics and autopsies of the Cook County Hospital in Chicago, . . . the largest charity hospital in America" (Beideman, 1983, p 18). George Hariman (1970, p 10), who had been a student there, informs us that for a $5.00 fee students could "make bedside visitations to patients and witness operations in the amphitheatre. . . . The privilege terminated when some overzealous students began shouting from the balcony to the surgeon, 'Have you tried chiropractic?' "

Soon after World War I, Irving B. Hall (1884–1971) established a 20-bed chiropractic sanitarium in Wakeeney, Kansas. Henry O. Gauger operated the Wisconsin General Chiropractic Hospital in Prairie du Chien from 1928 to 1934 (Mawhiney, 1984, p 155). Throughout the 1936–1950 period Roy Bakkum conducted his 30-bed Bakkum Chiropractic Clinic and Hospital in Waukon, Iowa, which included a maternity unit and a surgery installed by local MDs for their patients. Even more successful was George E. Hariman (1893–1977), who founded the 25-bed (later expanded to 60-bed) Hariman Sanitarium and Chiropractic Hospital in 1928 in Grand Forks, North Dakota, which functioned until 1981 (Gibbons, 1983, p 53). North Dakota enacted a chiropractic hospital licensing law in 1947, followed by South Dakota, Kentucky, and Florida (Hariman, 1970, p 34). Gibbons (1976, p 22) asserts: "At one time in the period between the wars, there were as many as a hundred inpatient chiropractic facilities—hospitals, sanitariums, health homes and clinics." Robert Ramsay wrote me (May 18, 1949):

> In 1920 I opened up a 15-bed hospital for the Chiropractic profession in Minnesota. We are licensed under the regular City Licenses and rules of the Health Department. We conduct our hospital as any other hospital is conducted. In this institution we have employed medical doctors, osteopaths, or any other profession when needed and necessary. We are sticking to this principle yet. We are increasing in recognition of Chiropractic Hospitals, and our small institution here in Minnesota, the Park Avenue Clinic Hospital, is well recognized throughout the United States and Canada and doing very satisfactory work in most chronic cases. We have several very successful Clinics in Minnesota.

But the largest and best known chiropractic hospital was that established in Denver by Leo Spears (1894–1956; Figure 22). An enterprising 1921 PSC graduate, in 1933 he incorporated his Spears Free Clinic and Hospital and served food daily to several hundred needy children during the 1930s depression. In 1943 he built the first 200-bed unit of Spears Chiropractic Hospital, and in 1949 the second unit, providing a 600-bed capacity. In 1948 he began a nursing school and chiropractic internships (Smallie, 1990b, p 17). In 1950 he won his 7-year lawsuit (Spears Free Clinic and Hospital for Poor Children, Inc., vs. The State Board of Health of Colorado et al., 1950) in the Colorado Supreme Court, which mandated that he be issued a hospital license retroactive to 1943 (Dzaman, 1980, p 311; Rex, 1962; Spears, 1925). According to William S. Rehm, the first president of the Association for the History of Chiropractic, who interned at Spears Hospital in 1955–1956: "There were so many patients that they occupied beds in the halls of both the Palmer and Carver Buildings. . . . The pediatrics ward always had a waiting list" (Gibbons, 1983, p 55). An estimated 250 chiropractors interned there through 1975. The gradual decline and ultimate closing of the hospital in 1984 resulted mainly from the impact of the new system of financing health care through third-party payers that would not pay for non-

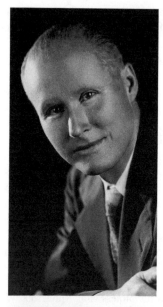

FIGURE 22.
D.D. Palmer Building, Spears Chiropractic Hospital, Denver
(*bottom*), 1943–1984, and its founder, Leo Spears (*left*).

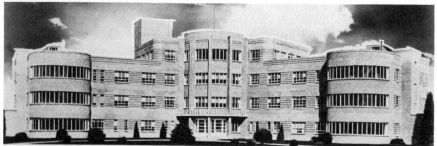

medical hospital treatment despite their increasing willingness to reimburse chiropractors for office visits.

As late as 1973 the New York State Chiropractic Association formed "a special
committee to study the concept of erecting a chiropractic hospital in New York"
(Goldschmidt A, 1973).

Relevant but less well known, especially among younger practitioners, is chiropractic management of emotionally disturbed patients and the existence of several
chiropractic mental hospitals, two of which flourished in Davenport, Iowa, for 35
years and provided internships for PSC students (Quigley, 1983). In 1922 Gerard M.
Pothoff (1889–1937) established the Chiropractic Psychopathic Sanitarium, later
known as Forest Park Sanitarium and finally as the Davenport Psychiatric Hospital,
which functioned until 1959. John Baker and Harvey Fennern established Clear View
Sanitarium as a chiropractic mental hospital in 1926 (Figure 23); it soon had 65 beds.
By 1930 it had developed a close relationship with PSC through the appointment of

Dean Alfred B. Hender, M.D., D.C., as "medical officer," and later of his son Herbert C. Hender, D.C., as "consultant." After B.J. purchased Clear View in 1951 he appointed as its director his nephew, W. Heath (Nip) Quigley (Figure 23), who had interned there. Quigley obtained a change in Iowa's law that permitted Clear View to be licensed as a "special purpose hospital" rather than a nursing home, and secured its listing in the annual publication of the American Psychiatric Hospital Association in 1955 (Quigley, 1983). However, after B.J.'s death in 1961 his son Dave promptly sold Clear View to the operator of a nursing home because of the "deplorable state" of PSC finances. Dye (1939, p 240) suggests that the term "chiro-psychiatrist" was once in vogue.

For many years the leader in the chiropractic treatment of mental health was Herman S. Schwartz (1894–1976; Figure 24) of New York, perennial president of the NCA Council on Mental Health. Author of *350 Nervous and Mental Cases under Chiropractic Care* (1950), *The Art of Relaxation* (1954), and *Home Care for the Emotionally Ill* (1957), his culminating achievement was to edit *Mental Health and Chiropractic: A Multidisciplinary Approach* (1973), which included contributions from such notables as Rene Dubos, Thomas Szasz, and Linus Pauling.

Quigley (1983, p 73) has written an epitaph to chiropractic's concern with mental health:

> With the closure of Clear View the flame of professional interest began to flicker. The flame has all but disappeared. A revival of concern and interest is doubtful but the results of the past would fully justify a serious and controlled reevaluation of chiropractic and its effect on mental illnesses, especially in light of the biologically based disorder with serious impairment of normal brain function.

The anthropologist E. Allen Morinis (1980, p 119) recommends that chiropractors return to a greater emphasis on the role of psychologic stress in illness. The ACA Council on Mental Health still claims a small but dedicated group of supporters (Ford, 1989a, 1989b).

Chiropractic hospitals and mixing both were most prevalent in California, where the conflict between straights and mixers historically was hottest. In 1933, according to Gibbons (1983, p 54), the College of Chiropractic Physicians and Surgeons in Los Angeles . . .

> offered a "Physicians and Surgeons Post Graduate Course, . . . an advanced course in medicine and surgery extending over a period of two years open to graduate chiropractors, who desire to increase their knowledge of therapeutics." . . . The course totaled 2060 hours in general medicine and surgery including 50 hours of anesthesiology and 154 hours in a course called "Clinical Chiropractic Surgery." . . . The clinical experience was . . . through an in-patient teaching arrangement with an affiliated hospital, the 1932–33 announcement detailed: "Through the facilities of the Bellevue Hospital, a 60-bed general hospital owned and operated by the Chiropractic Profession, the student receives direct instruction by the attending staff in the care of surgical and obstetrical cases, together with a wide variety of acute and chronic diseases. This is in addition to the practical work which the student secures in the College Clinic."

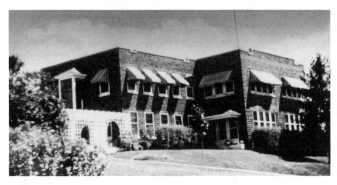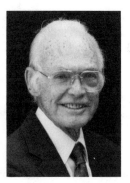

FIGURE 23.
Left, Clear View Sanitarium, Davenport, Iowa, 1926–1961 (circa 1956). (Courtesy of Patrick J. Goff.)
Right, William Heath ("Nip") Quigley, Director, 1951–1961. Quigley also was Chief Administrator of
Palmer College, 1974–1976.

The Stanford Research Institute (1960) reported that "more than a sixth of the known
hemorrhoid cases in California are healed by chiropractors." It is no wonder that
MDs became alarmed over the potential enlargement of chiropractic's scope of practice and its encroachment on medical turf! However, proposals by California medical
leaders to "solve the problem of chiropractic" by upgrading those already in practice
and cutting off further licensing, as was done there with osteopathy in 1961, met with
little favorable response from chiropractors. Even in the 1930s not many chiropractors, even mixers, wanted to practice allopathic medicine!

Obstetrics was another story. Already noted is that PSC and most other schools

FIGURE 24.
Herman S. Schwartz, Editor of *Mental Health and
Chiropractic: A Multidisciplinary Approach.*
(Courtesy of Edward M. Schwartz.)

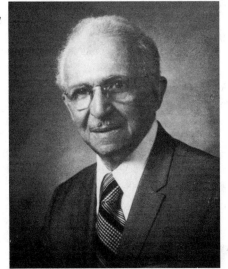

taught practical obstetrics at a time when many births were handled by midwives outside hospitals. This situation declined after 1920, but continued until the middle of the century. The 1944 announcement of Logan College in St. Louis stated that its obstetric instruction "thoroughly prepares students for practice in an ever-widening field," and the college maintained a birthing cottage on campus through 1946. Its president, Beatrice B. Hagen, recalls that Burtha Hartman, a St. Louis chiropractor, "did all of our on-campus deliveries and many of our young chiropractors of today were born under her capable guidance" (Gibbons, 1982, p 30). The 1956 announcement of Carver College in Oklahoma City offered obstetrics, as did the Los Angeles College. Gibbons (1980b, p 21) writes: "Completion of clinical work in obstetrics was a prerequisite to graduation at Carver College as well as the leading institutions such as National, Los Angeles, and Western States colleges through the early 1960s." Gibbons (1982, p 31) reports that there were 382 DC deliveries in California in 1953 and 194 in Oregon in 1981, and in California "a Society of Chiropractic Obstetricians and Gynecologists was active until the rights to OB were essentially lost in the 1960s." A 1984 Oklahoma Survey (Gemmell and Jacobson, 1989) found: "While the practice of obstetrics is a legislated part of chiropractic in this state, very few chiropractors actually practice obstetrics. One percent reported practicing often, 3 percent do so sometimes, 7 percent seldom, and 89 percent have never engaged in obstetrics."

Hence clinical experiences in both the mental health and obstetric areas hardly exist any longer. The only remaining chiropractic hospital of any significance is Kentuckiana Children's Center in Louisville, which since 1957 has furnished interdisciplinary health care to 400 multihandicapped children. If student clinical training is to be improved in the future, it will have to be in medical or osteopathic hospitals, either as part of the undergraduate curriculum or as residencies in hospitals offering chiropractic services, a new area of cooperation just commencing.

Section 2

College Accreditation

The quality of education is best monitored through an effective system of accreditation. Unlike the accrediting of academic institutions by regional associations, the accrediting of professional schools in the United States is carried out by a national agency established separately by each profession when recognized as qualified to do so by the U.S. Office of Education. The process by which a chiropractic accrediting agency finally became recognized was long and tortuous (Miller RG, 1981). It began in 1935 when the National Chiropractic Association (NCA) created a Committee on Educational Standards (renamed in 1947 the Council on Chiropractic Accreditation) with Claude O. Watkins (1902 (or 1903)–1977) as its first chairman. In 1941 John J. Nugent (1891–1970; Figure 25) was appointed NCA's first Director of Education. In

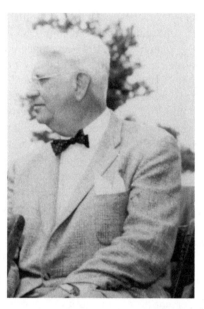

FIGURE 25.
John J. Nugent, Director of Education, National
Chiropractic Association, 1941–1961;
"Chiropractic's Abraham Flexner." (Courtesy of
National College of Chiropractic.)

the same year 12 colleges were provisionally approved under criteria established by
Nugent (1946). Gibbons (1980a pp 348–349; 1985) summarized his achievements:

> John J. Nugent was destined to change the course of chiropractic education in the next
> 27 years. Like B.J. he was persuasive and articulate, with great political instincts and
> the ability to communicate with intellectual sectors who had consigned chiropractic as
> but a distasteful cultist experience. Yet to many within the profession he appeared as
> arrogant, with a condescending air that seemed at times little more than a diatribe
> against anything and everything Palmer. Nugent had been "expelled" from PSC by B.J.
> in 1922 "for disloyalty, disrespect and insult to the President" but was reinstated by fac-
> ulty action three weeks later.

Yet John Nugent brought his classic training at the University of Dublin (he also
attended the U.S. Military Academy at West Point) into service for chiropractic, testifying before countless legislative committees, meeting with educators who believed
he had a hopeless task of elevating "trade schools" to professional status, visiting
with virtually every chiropractic school head between 1935 and 1960. He carried
with him his totally unpopular message that smaller schools must merge, all schools
must teach "4 years of 9," all institutions must become nonprofit and professionally
owned, and curriculums must be standardized, facilities strengthened, and clinical
opportunities expanded.

Nugent, one chiropractic lobbyist offered in the late 1950s, "had become the
most hated name in chiropractic." He was the Antichrist to readers of *The Fountain
Head News,* and many a mixer school owner had less reason to like him; yet 13 years
after the NCA had called its first meeting to discuss methods of raising educational
standards the results of Nugent's missionary work began to unfold. By that time, the
NCA reported:

"46 of the 51 private school owners had surrendered their equities in 19 schools, upon mutually satisfactory terms negotiated by the Director of Education. Some of these 19 schools were closed and others merged to form eight, non-profit accredited schools." . . .

Not honored in his time, he may yet gain posthumous recognition for the thankless role that he played—and which may earn him the distinction of being the Abraham Flexner of chiropractic.

The NCA-accredited schools were NCC, LACC, Western States Chiropractic College (WSCC), Northwestern College of Chiropractic (NWCC), Texas Chiropractic College (TCC), Canadian Memorial Chiropractic College (CMCC), Lincoln, and the Chiropractic Institute of New York. When I interviewed Nugent in 1949 he described himself as "the symbol of revolt against Palmer. I criticize chiropractors severely and am hated by many of them."

The International Chiropractors Association (ICA) countered by setting up its own agency, the Chiropractic Educational Commission, which accredited all of its affiliated schools with little fuss. However, Gibbons has pointed out that in 1955 only three of the NCA-approved schools (NCC, LACC, WSCC) taught physiotherapy, whereas at least three of the ICA-approved schools also offered it!

NCC and Lincoln began offering a 32-month course in the late 1920s; WSCC offered such a course in 1932, and a 36-month course in 1936 (Gatterman, 1982). The 4-year course became standard in the 1950s. Gibbons (1987, p 13) states:

B.J. fought lengthening the 18-month course until . . . virtually every jurisdiction in North America had established the standard course for licensure, . . . and in the late 1950s fought against the two year preprofessional requirement, declaring that it is "veneer and polish . . . which will weaken the profession and [cause] a large reduction in the number of chiropractors."

Although three of the strongest colleges—Carver, Lincoln, and the Chiropractic Institute of New York—were forced to close for financial reasons and merged into NCC or Logan in the 1950s and 1960s, the overall college situation gradually improved.

In 1921 a National Board of Chiropractic Examiners was established to facilitate license reciprocity between the states (Dye, 1939, p 95). It set a minimum of 18 months of instruction and the specific subjects to be examined in. Abandoned after 2 years, it was not effectively reestablished until 1963. In 1965 it held the first National Board examinations in New York City, Chicago, Davenport, and Los Angeles (Bureau of Health Professions, 1990). National Board examinations have become accepted as the uniform examining mechanism for licensure, although all states except Alabama and Illinois require separate written and/or practical examinations as well.

The 2-year preprofessional requirement for accreditation was initiated at Columbia College in Baltimore by 1953, according to William Rehm, who initially attended that school. It was made standard in 1968 by the Council for Chiropractic Education (CCE) of the new American Chiropractic Association (ACA), successor to NCA. However, several states had much earlier required 1 or 2 years of preprofessional college credit, and some undergraduate institutions began teaching 2-year "prechiroprac-tic" programs, one of the Wisconsin State Colleges in 1966 and Morehead State University in Kentucky in 1968. The Basic Science requirement helped raise academic standards; Hariman (1970, p 19) believed that they were the primary reason:

> Neither the escalation into the pre-educational college requirement nor the inclusion of physiotherapy into Chiropractic law were intentional or premeditated. They were brought about by force of necessity in the protection of Chiropractic future interests. Combatting Basic Science enactments and studying to pass Basic Science examinations necessitated pre-college studies.

The most significant achievement came in 1974 when the U.S. Office of Education recognized CCE as the official accrediting agency for chiropractic colleges. Instrumental in obtaining this approval were three college presidents, Joseph Janse of NCC, George H. Haynes (1911–1979); Figure 26) of LACC, John B. Wolfe of NWCC, and attorney-chiropractor Orval L. Hidde. CCE control of educational standards was consolidated in 1980 when the ICA accepted its designated seat on the Council, just 1 year after CCE awarded full accreditation to Palmer College of Chiropractic (PCC). These two steps toward mutual recognition and cooperation in the educational sphere reflected the decreased hostility between ICA and ACA as they discovered that they have more to gain by working together than by fighting each other.

The results have been impressive. To become fully accredited a chiropractic college must meet fairly stringent requirements regarding its governance structure, nonprofit status; duration of program, subjects taught, and preprofessional requirements for admission; qualifications of faculty; research program; and quality of laboratories and library, teaching clinics, and other facilities. At present more than three fourths of the state examining boards require applicants for licensure to have a minimum of 2 years of preprofessional college credits and to be a graduate of an accredited chiropractic college. Some states have gone farther: Maryland, North Carolina, and Florida have legislated a 4-year preprofessional requirement for licensure in the future. LACC began requiring 3 years of college credits for admission in 1991, as did Bridgeport, which opened that year.

All colleges employ university-trained recipients of M.S. or Ph.D. degrees in their basic science divisions, and their D.C. faculty also more often possess one of these degrees. Although some with advanced degrees may not be the most prestigious in their fields, and predictably some are foreign expatriates, most continue to do research and to publish in their respective fields. In 1982 the faculty-student ratio at the accredited colleges (*Annual Report of the Commission on Chiropractic Education,* 1984) was 1:12, with a range from 1:7 at Pasadena College (now Southern California College of Chiropractic, SCCC) to 1:22 at PCC-West (Peterson and Wiese, 1984, pp 27–28). More recently Gemmell (1990) found in seven Midwest and mid-South colleges that the ratio ranged from 1:8 at Cleveland Chiropractic College—Kansas City (CCC-KC) to 1:14 at PCC. Quigley told me that in the early 1970s the ratio at PCC

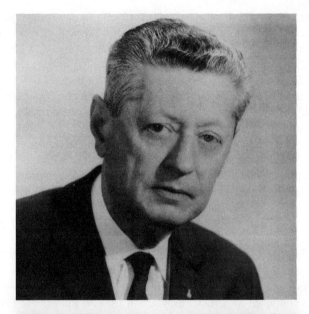

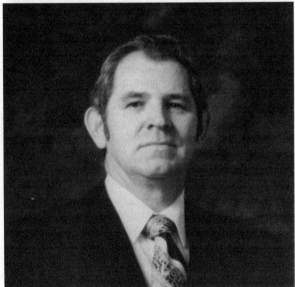

FIGURE 26.
Top, George H. Haynes, President of Los Angeles Chiropractic College, 1953–1974. (Courtesy of the Los Angeles Chiropractic College.) *Bottom,* Orval L. Hidde, President of the Council for Chiropractic Education when it won approval from the U.S. Office of Education in 1974 as chiropractic's accrediting agency.

was up to 1:70 when enrollment was 2,100 students. Libraries have been improved considerably in recent years, especially with the employment of professional librarians in all schools and the acquisition of access to electronic data bases. The three small superstraight colleges accredited not by CCE but by Straight Chiropractic Academic Standards Association (SCASA) graduate fewer than 200 DCs a year, compared with about 2,700 from the 14 CCE-accredited colleges. The Canadian, Anglo-European, and Australian (LaTrobe University) colleges are accredited in their own countries by mutual agreement with CCE.

These upgradings have won increasing respect and acceptance of chiropractic colleges in the wider academic community: 12 of the 14 CCE-accredited U.S. colleges plus Sherman College have been accredited by the regional associations of schools and colleges. Beginning with LACC and NCC in 1966, at least nine colleges now also offer B.S. degrees, usually in human biology, after completion of a combination of preprofessional and basic science credits. LACC earlier established a graduate school with a course leading to a masters degree in chiropractic, but an official of the school told me that only one such degree was awarded. In 1986 PCC received authorization from the North Central Association of Colleges and Secondary Schools to offer masters degrees in anatomy and in chiropractic science, and it enrolled the first class in its combined M.S./D.C. program in 1988. It joined with PSC-W in 1991 to become Palmer Chiropractic University (PCU). In 1990 Life College announced a new graduate program in Sports Health Science.

Texas Chiropractic College arranged for its basic science courses to be taught at San Antonio College in 1953, "apparently the first time any chiropractic school has ever had a connection with an accredited academic institution" (Stalvey, 1957, p 54). Joseph Janse told me in 1980 that NCC could become the National College of Physical Medicine of the University at Illinois Medical School anytime it wanted to, adding, "The offer is there." (I wonder if he was correct, misled, or boasting, which would have been somewhat uncharacteristic of him.) In 1974 the New York College of Chiropractic (NYCC) relocated adjacent to the New York Institute of Technology (NYIT) on Long Island, of which the New York College of Osteopathic Medicine is a component unit, and initially contracted for NYIT to teach its basic science subjects; it also integrated its library with that of NYIT. This is as close as osteopathic and chiropractic students have ever studied. Later NYCC established a joint masters program in human nutrition with the University of Bridgeport in Connecticut. In 1989 it acquired the spacious campus of the former Dwight D. Eisenhower College in Seneca Falls, New York (Figure 27), and moved there in 1991.

The first American chiropractic college to be part of an established academic institution is the University of Bridgeport College of Chiropractic, which began instruction in 1991. In Australia a chiropractic faculty is an integral part of the prestigious LaTrobe University near Melbourne; and the faculty of Sydney College of Chiropractic and Osteopathy became in 1990 the Centre for Chiropractic and Osteopathic Studies at Macquarie University in Sydney. The Anglo-European College in Bournemouth, England, has agreed to merge with Thames Polytechnic, a collegiate

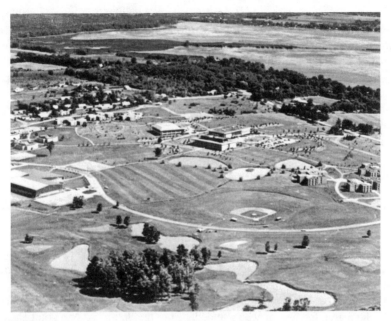

FIGURE 27.
New campus of New York Chiropractic College, Seneca Falls, 1991. (Courtesy of New York Chiropractic College.)

institution contemplating a move from London to Kent. In Toronto the Canadian Memorial Chiropractic College, though not yet successful in its attempts to become part of a University, has developed programs providing students with clinical experience in a teaching hospital.

Student preprofessional qualifications show considerable improvement, partly because of increased competition for admission. A survey (McNamee et al., 1990) of 1,296 first-and second-year students in 12 colleges worldwide (8 in the United States) found that 25% had the minimum prerequisite of 2 years of undergraduate college, 18% had 3 years, another 49% four years, and 8% had more advanced education. Eighty-three percent of the students had majored in the life sciences or a health care field. As many as 80% of candidates now enter the more selective colleges with a bachelors degree. On average, they have 3½ years of preprofessional education and a grade point average between 2.8 and 2.9 *(Chiropractic: State of the Art, 1989–1990)*. Average age at graduation is 27 years (Brennan, 1988). A survey of 534 randomly selected ACA members found that approximately 50% had earned a B.S. degree, 5% a higher degree, and 11% an associate degree, whereas 34% had no academic degree (Brennan, 1989). (It is likely that the better educated practitioners join an association.) Inasmuch as more than half of all practicing chiropractors were awarded their D.C. degree after 1977, clearly the educational level of the profession as a whole has much improved.

The proportion of women students has risen to about 25% (Gromala, 1983; Mannington et al., 1989), and more than 10% of practitioners are now women. It is noteworthy that women comprised the entire first class at NCC. A Women's Chiropractic Association was organized in 1936, with Gladys Little Ingram (1970) as its first president. In 1953 a Christian Chiropractic Association was formed, initially to provide support for two chiropractors working with lepers in Ethiopia; it currently sponsors short-term and extended stays by chiropractors in Third World countries, sometimes with and sometimes without MDs. And H.W. Evans (1978) notes that an association of Jewish chiropractors was established in 1978. Formal training of chiropractic nurses, later called chiropractic assistants (CAs) was begun in 1957 at LACC with a two-semester course, at Lincoln College in 1964 (Smallie, 1990b, pp, 21, 25), and now is common.

Although the first chiropractic patient (Harvey Lillard) was a black man, not many blacks have become chiropractors (Westbrooks, 1982). Neither D.D. nor B.J. appears to have been more prejudiced against blacks than was common in the early period, for D.D. customarily used "Mr." when referring to Lillard at a time when it was not customary to do so. And D.D. (1910, p 718) ridiculed this advertisement by an osteopath: "Clean osteopaths do not want colored or poor population." B.J. stated that the reason he did not want blacks at PSC unless they came from overseas was because he feared the loss of white students from the South. At one point Dye (1939, p 183) casually remarks: "Of course you couldn't use your portable adjusting table for both blacks and whites if you hoped to retain the white patients, . . . [and] naturally I couldn't adjust him [a black] at my office." But what was "natural" then certainly is not natural now. During the debate I attended in the Massachusetts legislature in 1949, an opponent of chiropractic ridiculed Lincoln Chiropractic College, named for the Great Emancipator, for denying admission to blacks. Nevertheless, a few blacks had become chiropractors. After World War II the Reaver School of Chiropractic in Dayton, Ohio, attracted many blacks, and the Booker T. Washington Chiropractic College in Kansas City, Missouri, obviously was designed to do so. These two colleges lasted for only 5 years or so, catering primarily to war veterans. In 1982 the American Black Chiropractic Association (ABCA) was organized to represent the approximately 1% of the profession who are black or minority, "to maintain the Harvey Lillard Scholarship fund, . . . and to recruit and support minority persons to study chiropractic" (Cartman, 1988; "Organization News," 1989). Today all colleges actively recruit black students, and many have black faculty, most often in the basic sciences. In 1990 Willard Smith, a black chiropractor, was elected president of the California Chiropractic Association.

The fact that chiropractic education has not been supported by public funds (except for veteran benefits, loans to individual students, and student stipends from Illinois and New York), and has therefore been principally dependent on student tuition, has placed severe limitations on improving quality. A federally mandated survey of the profession in 1979 (Von Kuster 1980, pp 43–44) found that tuition and fees accounted for 68.2% of the income of chiropractic colleges in 1974, but on average only 9.9% of the income of eight other types of professional schools, ranging from 4% for medicine to 36.4% for podiatry (*Costs of Education in the Health Professions*, 1974). The ACA commitment to improving education dates from shortly after it was formed in 1963, when it adopted the policy of allocating part of its membership fees to the colleges. But the college clinics do not yet attract a sufficiently diversified sick population (Nyiendo and Haldeman, 1982), and clinical training continues to be poorly integrated with the basic science subjects, as Sandoz complained (1978, p 47):

> In our schools, the criteria as to what should be taught and learned are the exigencies of the basic science examinations, instead of the requirements of actual practice. Consequently, the teaching of the basic sciences has been considerably stressed and improved, often to the detriment of the clinical sciences and chiropractic subjects, which are in complete stagnation.

More recently several of the colleges have extended their program beyond eight semesters, and some have introduced a preceptorship requirement in which students spend several months in a chiropractor's office prior to graduation. Some (e.g., Logan, TCC, LACC, CMCC) have linked up with medical schools and hospitals that offer chiropractic students clinical rotations in orthopedics, neurosurgery, or family practice. Florida has an internship requirement; a 2-year internship after graduation is mandated in Switzerland, and a 1-year requirement in some Scandinavian countries.

Two types of postgraduate chiropractic education require mention. First is continuing education. Long before other professions began requiring refresher training as a condition of relicensure chiropractors obtained state laws requiring educational credits each year or two for relicensure; 41 states now do ("Chiropractors" 1988, p 124). Beginning in 1906, B.J. encouraged PSC alumni to return to an annual Homecoming, renamed Lyceum in 1914 (Crisp, 1984). Under the "big tent" set up each year for the occasion, he worked his charisma, fostered sociability, announced new technical developments to field doctors, and softened up the market for sales of books, information tracts for patients, and practice items. Other colleges followed suit, and all still schedule annual homecomings at which credits for continuing education can be earned and enthusiasm generated for recruiting new students and donating money to the college.

The second dimension of postgraduate education is board certification by one of the ACA specialty councils: diagnostic imaging (formerly roentgenology, established in 1945), orthopedics, nutrition, sports injuries and physical fitness, neurology, occupational health, and diagnosis and internal disorders. At least 12 colleges offer full-time residencies in one or more of these areas, most commonly in diagnostic imaging, orthopedics, or sports injuries and physical fitness. Certification requirements also can be met by taking postgraduate courses one weekend a month for 3 years plus a specified amount of practical work. Other ACA councils that do not offer board certification but attract those with special interests are those for mental health, physiologic therapeutics, and technique.

However, only limited federal funds so far have been allocated to research on chiropractic. The first recipient, beginning in 1976, was Professor Chung-Ha Suh, a bioengineer at the University of Colorado whose team of researchers, including chiropractors, developed computerized models of spinal biomechanics and studied the neurophysiologic effects of spinal subluxations (Luttges and Gerren, 1980; Sharpless, 1975; Suh, 1974, 1975, 1980). The ICA alone contributed $222,598 to Suh's research between 1967 and 1979 (*ICA Newsletter,* August 1979). Research into chiropractic has been supported primarily by the profession itself and by its colleges, one of which (NCC) established a 48-bed Patient Research Center in 1981, renamed in 1983 the Janse Chiropractic Center on the occasion of Janse's retirement. NCC installed a magnetic resonance imaging machine on a contractual basis in 1990. The Consortium for Chiropractic Research was established in California in 1985 by six West Coast colleges, and has expanded to include nearly all accredited American colleges, with the goal of facilitating research. ACA's Foundation for Chiropractic Education and Research (FCER) annually awards more than a million dollars for research, mainly to chiropractic colleges. The first private donation of $1 million for research was made by Dr. William M. Harris to FCER in 1988, which awarded it to NCC for a 5-year clinical research program directed by John J. Triano. By 1990 NCC had an endowment of approximately $12 million ("National College of Chiropractic," 1989). In 1991 Harris pledged another million dollars to NWCC for its new center for clinical studies. PCC established in 1984 its Palmer Research Institute, and has an endowment of $11 million; however, it still owes the Palmer family for its physical plant, which it is paying off at the favorable rate of 4% over 40 years. Life College established a unique endowment plan based on the maturation of insurance policies over a 5-year period ("Life Chiropractic College," 1990, p 94). It also received a "Federal Grant for Disadvantaged Students" (1990) to teach the preprofessional chiropractic sciences to minority and disadvantaged students from seven southeastern states who have completed 1 year of college.

As the 1980s drew to a close, the 17 U.S. chiropractic colleges experienced increased costs and a small decrease in enrollments, which in 1991 totaled more than 10,000 students. (The average debt of graduating seniors at PCC in 1989 was $40,000.) No doubt the increased costs are due in part to the cost of better educational programs. The question of whether decreased enrollment results from decreased demand is addressed in Chapter 13, Section 4.

Section 3

Student Recruitment

Sociologists use the word "socialization" to describe the learning of any social role. Its principal components are (1) acquisition of cognitive knowledge and skills, whether taught didactically or in apprenticeship and clinical settings, and (2) internalization of the ethical norms of behavior expected in that role, which in the case of the professions are the codes of professional ethics. The role modeling provided in apprenticeships and internships should show the novice proper behavior toward patients and colleagues. Professions vary greatly in the balance between didactic and practical training. Medicine provides the longest training of any profession in clinics, internships, and residencies, whereas the legal profession offers one of the shortest, only 3 years of college with a minimum of clerkships in law offices, moot court, and such, for which it has been much criticized. Flexner (1910) properly rated as inferior those medical schools with no or poor clinical facilities.

For chiropractic students, "clinic" has always been the educational highlight. Chiropractic requires so much hands-on practice and skill in delivering adjustments that students are impatient to get to that part of their training, just as medical undergraduates are impatient to go on rounds in the hospital and assist in surgical procedures. Skill in palpation and manipulation requires much preliminary instruction, demonstration, and practice. Those who can teach these techniques well are appreciated most. As in medical schools, students resent the amount of time and effort spent on basic science courses and believe they are required to master far too many facts they will never need in practice. And like medical students they cram for exams and seek shortcuts to pass courses they consider less important.

The basic questions in this and Section 4 are: What types of people choose chiropractic as their profession? And what motivates them to become chiropractors? Since few systematic studies have been done, I must rely on skimpy data. Sociologists use the term "social selection" to refer to the process by which potential candidates for any social role enter the role. Even more important than the selection procedures of the colleges is self-selection by the candidates themselves. Unless an individual first decides that he or she wants in, college admissions criteria are irrelevant. So who become chiropractors, and why?

As noted, the antichiropractic propaganda of organized medicine always presented a distorted picture of chiropractors' motivations, denigrating them as misguided and exploited, if not exploitative and criminal. For example, Reed (1932, p 41) stated in his report to the Committee on the Costs of Medical Care that all chiropractic schools "held out to carpenters, baggage handlers, bookkeepers, pick wielders, and the like, the alluring prospect of making easy money and being a 'doctor.' " And Morris Fishbein, Editor of *JAMA,* who wrote in his famous diatribe (1925, p 98) that the chiropractor arrives "through the cellar . . . besmirched with dust and grime," quoted (1925, pp 82–84) the presumed application of an obviously "illiterate and ignorant woman," implying that she was a typical chiropractic student. However, let us not forget that many MDs then in practice had themselves graduated from schools that Flexner (1910, pp 19, 36–37) found had admitted students completely unprepared for medical studies:

> The crude boy or the jaded clerk who goes into medicine has not been moved by a significant prompting from within. He is more likely to have been caught drifting at a vacant moment by an alluring advertisement or announcement, quite commonly an exag-

geration, not infrequently an outright misrepresentation. . . . Many of the schools accept students from the grammar schools. . . . There is no protection against fraud or forgery. . . . Many of them, gotten through advertising, would make better farmers.

Turner (1931, p 37) surveyed the occupational backgrounds of PSC students:

Among the 2000 students registered in 1920 there were 102 former school teachers, 12 ministers of the gospel, 16 former school superintendents, 6 editors and 8 others from journalistic pursuits, 45 musicians, 24 pharmacists, 11 chemists, 7 dentists, 26 officers from the Army and Navy, 51 nurses, 23 manufacturers, 165 from other schools, several osteopaths, doctors of medicine and veterinary surgeons, engineers, railroad men, artists, clerks, housewives, stenographers, instructors in physical training and many from still other pursuits. The foreigners represented thirty countries, New Zealand sending thirty-four students for enrollment in 1921.

That accounts for only about 600 of the students; he does not tell us what previous occupation, if any, the others held. No doubt many were former servicemen and others came direct from school. However, folklore has it that most early chiropractors held previous occupations, sometimes to a relatively advanced age.

The 24 chiropractors whom I interviewed in Massachusetts in the late 1940s (essentially all those practicing in the Greater Boston area) held previous occupations as follows (Wardwell, 1951, p 174):

Professional	2
Chemist	
Mechanical engineer	
Managerial	4
Sales manager	
Army officer	
Sales	3
X-ray equipment	
Insurance	
Magazines	
Clerical	4
Skilled work	2
Semiskilled work	4
Unskilled work	1
Student	4
Total	24

Their average age when they began to study chiropractic was 26.3 years; only five were older than 30 years. Inasmuch as their average age was 51.5 years at interview, they had experienced on average more than 20 years of harassment by medical and legal authorities. Perhaps that is why I found so few young chiropractors there. The older ones would have entered practice in the early 1920s or before, when conditions perhaps were not so adverse. Clearly many younger chiropractors had self-selected themselves out of Massachusetts either before or after entering practice.

Patricia B. Wild (1978, pp 36, 39) studied the social background of 149 students at the then new Pasadena Chiropractic College (now SCCC) and found:

> In obvious contrast to medical students, chiropractic students are from primarily working and middle class backgrounds: 40 percent of their fathers were skilled laborers, 15 percent small business owners, 14 percent managers or executives, 19 percent professionals (which included chiropractors, medical doctors, teachers, engineers), 9 percent salesmen or clerical workers and 4 percent farmers.

> Almost half (46 percent) of the students report that close relatives other than parents are teachers, 32 percent report some relatives are engineers, 18 percent have relatives who are chiropractors, and approximately 20 percent report relatives who are lawyers, medical doctors, dentists, or nurses, so there is more of a middle-class family influence than might be readily apparent from father's occupation alone.

> For the majority of students, chiropractic is a second career. Most are older and have had substantial employment experience by the time they attend chiropractic school. Only 15 percent of the students even thought of becoming a chiropractor before the age of eighteen. A definite decision to study chiropractic was made prior to age twenty-six by only 40 percent of the students, 44 percent decided between the ages of twenty-six and thirty, and fully 22 percent made this important decision since the age of thirty. As a result, 86 percent of the students seriously considered another occupation, 25 percent of which considered medicine, 19 percent an academic career, 10–15 percent considered elementary or high school teaching, law, business, or research as possible careers.

> About half (54 percent) of the students became interested in chiropractic through the influence of friends or relatives who were practicing chiropractic, with several indicating that a healing experience had been crucial to their decision.

Ten years later McNamee et al. (1990) found that students now more often choose chiropractic at an earlier age and less often as an alternative to medicine or osteopathy. Chiropractors frequently have come from the related fields of sports, physical education, nutrition, or nursing.

Section 4

Motivation to Become a Chiropractor

Why do chiropractors choose chiropractic? My analysis of college catalogues in the 1940s revealed three main recruiting themes: *humanitarian motives, status aspiration,* and *financial ambition.* The following innocuous advertisement by Texas Chiropractic College appeared repeatedly in *The Chiropractic Home Magazine:*

Graduate into a Profession

Become a Chiropractor. Secure your

future in an uncrowded profession.

The catalogue of the Columbia Institute of Chiropractic (in Baltimore and New York City) offered this answer to the question "Who Should Study Chiropractic?":

> An individual who has a sympathetic and an inborn desire to help those who are ill; he must be ambitious, dependable, diligent and persevering. Personal experience with the value of chiropractic is important, because it will engender confidence and the knowledge that Chiropractic is the science that gets sick people well. To qualified individuals Chiropractic offers economic security, social stability and true happiness in doing something for which they are really fitted.

The following perspective was provided by a chiropractic student (Schmidt, 1948, p 14):

> What should be the mental attitude of the student of chiropractic?
>
> *First* and most important he or she must have an interest in people, and a desire to alleviate their illnesses. This interest in people may be latent and can be developed if the student has the right spirit.
>
> *Secondly* he must really want to learn, and must have the intelligence and mental ability to learn. He must be willing to give time to study, as well as time to clinical practice, in order to make himself efficient.
>
> *Thirdly* he must have the determination to finish that which he has started. He must keep in mind that he can do or have anything he wants, if he is willing to make the effort and the sacrifices necessary to obtain it.

My classification resulted in the following distribution of consciously expressed motivations in the Massachusetts respondents (Wardwell, 1951, p 180):

Motivation	Number of Chiropractors
Humanitarian motives	9
Status ambition	3
Financial gain	6
Drifted into chiropractic	4
Unclassifiable	2
Total	24

Thirteen of these chiropractors previously had wanted to become physicians, including one who had begun a dental course and was forced to abandon it. The following suggests humanitarian motivation:

> All my life my hobby has been sick people. When I was a kid, instead of playing baseball I would go visit sick people and do things to make them comfortable, favors and so on. I always wanted to be a doctor.

And so does this remarkable testimony, which rings with sincerity:

> I don't feel I should get three dollars. My people are poor people. They can afford two dollars better than three dollars. . . . Fifty percent of my work is charity work—better, "pioneer" work. I feel that I am teaching people, educating them in a new science, just as people went across the plains in covered wagons to a new world. I'm making a living, earning fair pay; but money has never interested me. My whole life has been doing good for others, analyzing their cases and helping them. . . . My flowers are my people. I see them come in sick and with their money gone. To see them building up and getting better is like changing the water on a bouquet of flowers. After twenty-five years I am more thoroughly imbued than ever before. I believe that chiropractic should be put to the Golden Rule. It should not be denied to those who want it.

Harry Runge revealed his status ambition:

> I was going with a girl who lived in the same house where Dr. Shegataro Morikubo lived (in La Crosse, Wisconsin). She insisted that chiropractic was the career for me and that I must come over and meet him. I had always wanted to be a doctor. He told me that chiropractic is a fine profession for a young man and emphasized the good I could do with my hands. He also mentioned the remunerative side but didn't emphasize it so much. He compared it with salaried occupations and the slow promotions in a bank.

> I always admired the horses and buggies of the MDs outside the hospital in my home town. They had beautiful horses and fine blankets for them. And some had rubber tires on their carriages. That was something in those days! I wanted a horse and buggy like those. Then one day I helped carry an injured man to a wagon, and went to the hospital with him. I got acquainted with an MD there and came back to see and talk with him a number of times. We talked about my being a doctor, but the course of preparation for an MD is long and hard, and what the chiropractor and the girl said made more and more sense to me.

Money clearly provided the motivation for this chiropractor:

> An osteopath friend used to tell me I should take up osteopathy, that I could make a lot of money at it. Another friend of mine did this and was very successful in California. His uncle was a chiropractor so I went to see him. I investigated both chiropractic and osteopathy. I decided on chiropractic because I felt (and still feel) that it goes farther than osteopathy. It makes more specific adjustments. . . . I was probably a damn fool to choose chiropractic from the point of view of making money; I could be licensed like the other osteopaths around here. But I'm not sorry. There are plenty of osteopaths who make no more money than I do.

And as is often true of vocational selection, some drifted into chiropractic:

> My brother went to PSC two months before I did. I can't say why I decided to become a chiropractor, but I thought I would like the work and I liked the idea of going out West to school. I probably had as little reason as anyone for taking it up. A lot of the students had been personally helped by chiropractic but I wasn't. Some of them went to PSC for treatments and while they were there they took the course too.

Finally, some didn't know:

> I really don't know. I was a kid, had to have an occupation to earn a decent living. These fellows who are philanthropic, who take up chiropractic to help the world, I don't believe that.

Dye (1939, pp 39–40) acknowledged:

> Of course, in the early days of chiropractic, it was but natural that some of the students were of the charlatan type, men and women who took up the new healing art because they felt that by becoming graduate Doctors of Chiropractic they could take advantage of the early publicity and cash in on the early returns before, as they thought, the public realized its worthlessness. In this connection, however, I am glad to state that many of these would-be-charlatans became firmly convinced of the merits of this new system and became truly worthy exponents of its practice on entering the field as graduated Doctors of Chiropractic.

Dr. Joyce Tattleman of Boston, only 4 years into practice, is a happy practitioner (Moore C, 1989, p 7):

> My patients come in excited because they'll be feeling better soon. They leave happy. I spend my day in bliss.

Two other reasons why individuals became chiropractors are well known (White and Skipper, 1971). One was being cured or vastly benefited from a serious illness that MDs had not helped. Such individuals often became the most dedicated and enthusiastic chiropractors, with the conviction and zeal to do for others what had been done for them. The other main reason for becoming a chiropractor was the stimulus of a relative or friend who, as a chiropractor role model, sometimes pressured the person to take up chiropractic. In many cases whole families became chiropractors, then often practiced together in a sanitarium, "clinic," or chain of offices. There are already some four-generation chiropractic families. The Stucky family boasts 13 chiropractors, beginning in 1950 with four brothers in the first generation and nine in the second, including three completing their studies (Mickelson, 1989, p 20); the Toftness family boasts 17 chiropractors in three generations ((Williams, 1990b); and the Lensgraf family produced 22 chiropractors in three generations. However, the tendency for chiropractic students to have family role models is decreasing. The survey by McNamee et al. (1990) of 1,296 students in 12 colleges found only 15% in that category, almost exactly the same as the 14% Radis (1981) found in a comparable survey of students at 11 osteopathic colleges.

The most systematic study of chiropractic students' characteristics and motivations was that by Wild (1978), who found . . .

> real divergences from medical students. . . . Medical students are much more apt to rank factors associated with technical and medical expertise as important for success . . . . [Chiropractic] students feel that it is most important that the chiropractor maintain an air of confidence even when he is not feeling confident.

Several measures were employed to determine if the chiropractic students entertained any characteristic personality traits, but their scores were not outstanding in either direction on the Rokeach Dogmatism Scale or on the California F-Scale. The typical response was slightly nondogmatic and slightly nonauthoritarian. The Eron Cynicism and Humanitarianism scales were also administered to the chiropractic students, and the typical score was low on the cynicism index but quite high on humanitarianism. . . . Finally, the Allport-Vernon-Lindzey scale of values was administered, and the chiropractic students' scores were found to be very similar to other college population norms.

For her doctoral dissertation Yvonne L. Brockington (1987) administered the Edwards Personal Preference Schedule to a class of 125 students at PCC, and likewise found that on most personality variables they were similar to the norms found for medical students and other college populations. Medical and chiropractic students resembled each other more than either group resembled the general population. The principal difference was that medical students scored higher on Achievement. She concluded:

> The personality trait Change was the deciding factor with the traditional students opting for medical school and the more adventurous or less scholastic students applying to a chiropractic college.

Sociologist Phylis Lan Lin (1972) identified three contingencies involved in students' decisions to become chiropractors: (1) role models or contact with "significant others" in chiropractic; (2) benefit received from chiropractic by oneself, a relative, or close friend; and (3) situational factors such as dissatisfaction with current employment and having the required educational qualifications and finances.

Peter New (1960) found that most of the 103 osteopathic students he surveyed at four of the six then existing osteopathic colleges had chosen osteopathy second, and that 69 of them had previously applied for admission to medical school. Most of them experienced ambivalence (he used the term "dilemma") about entering what they considered a second-class profession. The later (1981) Radis survey of 506 students at 11 osteopathic colleges found that 32% originally had preferred a medical school. Baer (1989a, p 1108) cites evidence that osteopathy is often still a second choice to medicine.

Ambivalence certainly is common among chiropractic students. David Sternberg studied students at Columbia College of Chiropractic (now NYCC). Modeled after the classic study of medical student socialization *Boys in White* by Howard Becker (1961), Sternberg titled his study *Boys in Plight: A Case Study of Chiropractic Students Confronting a Medically Oriented Society* (1969). He described them (1969, pp 163–164) as ambivalent toward their careers, "besieged by hostile groups and forces. . . . The image then is of a threatened self, torn between its own relatively positive and worthwhile view of the status of chiropractic student and the negative view of most of society." He found that although 55% of the 89 students he surveyed entered chiropractic college . . .

with a substantial degree of unconflicted commitment, . . . twelve percent might best be termed "aimless" or "indifferent" regarding chiropractic upon entrance, while thirty-two percent (those preferring another line of work), might be called "frustrated" or even "hostile." . . . Twenty-five percent of the twenty-nine persons who would have preferred another occupation, or eighty-six percent, wanted to be another type of health practitioner (a medical doctor, an osteopath, a veterinarian, or a pharmacist).

Sternberg (1969, p 35) concluded:

Stigma and professionalization are strange bedfellows. . . . That simultaneous "loading" should be a stable condition through time not tending toward resolution in one direction or the other, is sociologically unorthodox.

It is not surprising that many early chiropractors abandoned their profession, as R.J. Martin (1949) explained:

The professional mortality of chiropractors has always been the highest of any of the healing professions. This, no doubt, has been caused by earlier low educational standards. The chiropractor has not invested enough in the profession in either time or money to prize his position highly. As a result, when outside temptations attracted him to other lucrative fields, he did not have any strong reasons to resist the influence of these non-professional attractions. The present educational program of four years of nine months, with prospects in the not too distant future of required prechiropractic college courses, will undoubtedly have a strong compulsive effect toward keeping graduates of the future from dropping out of the profession.

Sandoz (1978, p 47) blamed chiropractors' insecurity for their "endless search for 'systems' cleverly entertained by unscrupulous parasites in our profession." He referred to the practice-building entrepreneurs.

William Bachop (1991, p 36), long-time faculty member at NCC, has provided a current but somewhat cynical categorization of chiropractic students:

At one extreme are those who come from "chiropractic families," where a parent or grandparent had been a chiropractor. Their chiropractic faith is pristine. At the other extreme are the erstwhile pre-meds who hand't been accepted to medical school and have settled for chiropractic as a substitute route to wealth, status, and being called "Doctor." They know little of chiropractic philosophy and care less. And in between these extremes are all the rest. There are nurses, fed up with being the doctor's handmaiden and the patient's maid. There are the physical therapists, no longer content to be flunkeys at the medical doctor's beck and call. One meets psychologists and pharmacists who think they somehow will be able to combine those professions with chiropractic and be better off. There are all kinds of technicians, therapists, and paraprofessionals who resent the medical doctor's smug arrogance in the hospital setting and are anxious to escape from deadend jobs. There are those repelled by the abuse of drugs and surgery who are drawn to the notion of "[w]holistic" and "natural" healing. There are many others who don't fit into neat categories.

Following is a somewhat idealized summary of chiropractors' motivations (Roberts, 1989, pp 15–16):

> Chiropractors are "people" doctors. Their enforced isolation has them relying on their hands, their heads and their hearts for the treatment of patients. . . . Chiropractors have not been able to take the attention that rightfully belongs to their patients and give it to sophisticated machines. They rely on their heads for much of their preliminary diagnostic impression, the laying on of their hands as a major portion of their treatment, and their hearts for the setting of fees.

My own analysis has led me to conclude that the principal sources of personality conflict and strain for a chiropractic student are:

First, the discrepancies between the chiropractic philosophy of disease and the standard medical texts from which the student gains his basic knowledge of physiology, biochemistry, pathology, and such, continually raise questions about the validity of chiropractic principles.

Second, clinical training, which teaches how to perform the standard techniques for diagnosing the entire range of human diseases, reveals how limited is the therapy that a chiropractor can provide. Although able to help many patients, the chiropractor learns that there are those who must be referred to physicians, those for whom it would be too risky to assume responsibility even though chiropractic treatment might help, and those for whom chiropractic might offer some palliative relief but no cure. There are surgical cases the chiropractor cannot operate on, diseases treatable by drugs he or she cannot prescribe, and patients needing hospitalization whom he or she cannot admit.

Third, the student is well aware of the continuing split within the profession between straights and mixers. Whichever type of college the student attends, he or she knows that the leaders and colleagues in the profession are not in agreement as to the proper scope of practice. The laws of some states narrowly restrict its scope, whereas other states permit a wide variety of options. The same is true of third-party payers: some reimburse for only a limited range of services, others pay for nearly anything a chiropractor does.

Consequently, the student faces critical decisions at every stage of a career: choice of college, state in which to practice, and finally, the type or scope of practice he or she will engage in and which expensive instruments and equipment to buy for that type of practice.

Finally, more students enter chiropractic today with no or minimal acquaintance with chiropractic. Many are attracted by its holistic approach to health and its emphasis on natural foods, physical exercise, healthful living, and aversion to drugs. Others find chiropractic a more available career than medicine. Still others see in chiropractic an opportunity to escape from a less interesting or less remunerative occupation. For most it is a step up the ladder of social and economic success. Certainly chiropractors have much less to apologize for now than they used to. A 1988 study published in *Jobs Rated Almanac,* based on the six criteria of salary, stress, work environment, outlook, security, and physical demands, rated chiropractic the tenth best occupation in the United States and first among the health professions. Chiropractic has indeed come a long way!

Chapter 8

MEDICAL OPPOSITION

*Sin has many tools but a lie is the handle which fits
them all.*

Oliver Wendell Holmes (1857, p 124)

Section 1

Organized Medicine's Campaign against Chiropractic

Organized medicine has a long history of opposing types of healing that might en-
croach on its "turf," whether that encroachment be piecemeal as with the "limited"
professions (e.g., dentistry, podiatry, optometry, psychology) or more comprehensive as with thomsonism, homeopathy, osteopathy, naturopathy, and chiropractic.
When medicine's fundamental tenets are challenged, as they were by osteopathy and
chiropractic, its opposition is stronger than when a speciality such as ophthalmology
or psychiatry is encroached on. In the former case, *all* MDs, especially general practitioners, may feel threatened. As osteopathy began to relax its stance against the
pharmacopeia and medical theories of disease and therapy the weight of medicine's
opposition turned more toward chiropractic. Perhaps medicine had initially felt more
threatened by osteopathy because it was closer to medical practice and because chiropractic could be dismissed as not much more than bonesetting. Although osteopaths
were accepted, "the chiropractor, by contrast, was never allowed by the medical profession to forget he was an enemy" (Inglis, 1964, p 115).

　　Although a single MD in Davenport viciously attacked D.D. Palmer and other
irregular practitioners in 1899 (Lerner, 1954, pp 202–208), it was only around 1910
that organized medicine began to notice chiropractic (Ratledge, 1971, p 66). The first
paper on it (Schaller, 1911–1912) actually was favorable in tone. However, things
changed rapidly after that (Rice, 1912; "Chiropractic," 1914), with opposition peak-
ing under the leadership of Morris Fishbein, Secretary of the American Medical Association (AMA) and Editor of *JAMA* from 1924 to 1949. Called the "Medical Mussolini" by his opponents (e.g., Bealle, 1939), he began a 50-year campaign of
vitriolic propaganda against chiropractors, using both professional and popular publications.

His main thrust was that chiropractic is an unscientific cult and that chiropractors are either bumbling incompetents or greedy quacks preying on gullible citizens. Later the phrase "rabid dogs" was used, "playful and cute but they're killers" (McAndrews G, 1982, p 22). The cures that chiropractors achieved were attributed either to psychologic suggestion or to the body's natural recuperative powers. Consequently, few MDs took the time or trouble to investigate chiropractic seriously, and those who did were condemned for doing so or were ostracized and in danger of losing their hospital privileges.

Louis Reed (1932, p 35), a generally reliable source, in his report prepared for the Committee on the Costs of Medical Care, quotes a chiropractic Jeremiah as saying in 1930:

> Eight years ago . . . officials of the American Medical Association met in secret conclave in Chicago and adopted the slogan, "Chiropractic must die." They gave themselves ten years in which to exterminate it.

Since Reed does not disavow the event, presumably it occurred. Although in 1949 the AMA "withdrew its Seal of Acceptance from Morris Fishbein, beat his head in, cut his heart out, and kicked him into the street," because "physicians who were interested in something besides their fees resented their identification with his low-comedy routine" (Mayer, 1949, p 76), it continued its antichiropractic campaign. In 1971 H. Doyl Taylor, Director of the AMA Department of Investigation and Secretary of its Committee on Quackery, submitted a memorandum to the AMA Board of Trustees (Trever, 1972, p 4):

> Since the AMA Board of Trustees decision, at its meeting on November 2–3, 1963, to establish a Committee on Quackery, your Committee has considered its prime mission to be, first, the containment of chiropractic and, ultimately, the elimination of chiropractic.

Indeed, the original name of the Committee on Quackery was the Committee on Chiropractic (McAndrews, 1982, p 24). In its first annual report to the Board (Trever, 1972, pp 4–5) the Committee outlined its strategy:

> The Committee has recommended to each state medical society that corresponding committees on quackery be formed on the local level so proper coordination of activities at the local, state and national levels may be accomplished. . . . The involvement (and indoctrination) of State Medical Society leadership, in our opinion, is vital to the success of the chiropractic program. . . . We hope and believe that, with continued aggressive AMA activity, chiropractic can and will be contained at the national level and that steps are being taken to stop or eliminate the licensure of chiropractic at the state level.

It was reported that the chairman of the AMA Committee on Quackery was paid $50,000 a year. In 1962 I attended an AMA-sponsored Congress on Medical Quackery in Connecticut where Oliver Field of its Bureau of Investigation detailed the disciplinary procedure that the AMA had adopted for use against wayward MDs who might associate with "quacks."

Four campaign goals were enumerated in a confidential memorandum summarizing discussion at a "Meeting of the Committee on Quackery, September 15, 1967" (Trever, 1972, p 123):

> Basically, the Committee's short-range objectives for containing the cult of chiropractic and any additional recognition it might achieve revolves about four points:
>
> 1. Doing everything within our power to see that chiropractic coverage under Title 18 of the Medicare Law is not obtained.
> 2. Doing everything within our power to see that recognition or listing by the U.S. Office of Education of a chiropractic accrediting agency is not achieved.
> 3. To encourage continued separation of the two national chiropractic associations.
> 4. To encourage state medical societies to take the initiative in their state legislatures in regard to legislation that might affect the practice of chiropractic.

The AMA model plan for state medical societies included enlisting the aid of outside groups (Trever, 1972, p 123):

> Other members of the scientific community and voluntary health organizations (such as the state cancer society, heart and arthritis associations) should be encouraged to adopt policy statements on this subject (chiropractic), and to implement informational programs for their members and the public. . . . The state's interprofessional association or health council should involve itself in a public education program on the subject of quackery, and it should emphasize the subject of chiropractic.

An interdepartmental Task Force on Chiropractic was established at the AMA headquarters in Chicago, designed to include (or influence) its divisions of Law, Communication, Medical Practice, Health Services, Community Health and Health Education, Physical Medicine and Rehabilitation, Health Care to the Poor, Council on Legislative Activities, and Liaison Committee to the American Bar Association. Through its liaison with the Joint Committee on Health Problems in Education, the National Education Association was persuaded to adopt the following resolution (Trever, 1972, p 5):

> That the resource units currently being developed under the sponsorship of the American Medical Association on consumer education and health be widely distributed and used in the nation's schools.

The committee also distributed "10,000 pieces of AMA propaganda" to educators and guidance counselors, and reported to the AMA Board of Trustees (Trever, 1972, p 100):

> The Committee was instrumental in blocking the inclusion of a chiropractic chapter in a Health Careers Guidebook being prepared by the United States Department of Labor for distribution to guidance counselors and others throughout the country.

In support of the Committee's goals and strategy the AMA House of Delegates in June 1970 adopted the following resolution (Trever, 1972, p 81):

That the American Medical Association encourage medical schools to include specific information in their curricula regarding the nature of the health hazard to individuals who make up the general public which is posed by quackery in general and the unscientific cult of chiropractic in particular; and . . . the AMA be encouraged to offer bibliographic materials to each medical school and to other appropriate bodies relative to the health hazard posed by quackery.

However, a sarcastic reaction came from Professor Richard Cross of Rutgers Medical School (Trever, 1972, p 83):

It seems to me that the resolution sounds more like propaganda than like education. . . . Please don't tell anybody, but I had a chiropractor come and speak to our students last spring along with an osteopath, a general practitioner, a member of a medical group, etc. . . . I think the students ended up with a fairly good understanding of both pros and cons of chiropractic . . . and may even know more about the subject than the framers of your resolution.

Finally, the Committee on Quackery acted to place copies of the booklet "Chiropractic: The Unscientific Cult" in every MD's waiting room and to "plant" articles critical of chiropractic in *Readers' Digest, Consumer Reports, Good Housekeeping,* and other widely read magazines. It also sponsored publication of Ralph Lee Smith's book *At Your Own Risk: The Case against Chiropractic* (1969). His involvement is documented in a confidential letter from the AMA dated May 13, 1971, to Dr. Stephen Barrett of Allentown, Pennsylvania, Chairman of the Board of the Lehigh Valley Committee against Health Fraud (Trever, 1972, p 46):

After talking with you on Tuesday, I had the opportunity to talk to Doyl Taylor and Bill Monaghan of our Department of Investigation. You and your Committee are to be congratulated on the magnitude and impact of your program against health fraud and particularly against chiropractics [sic] in Lehigh County.

Thank you for sending me your promotional flyer advertising "The Medicine Show," published by Consumers Union, and the book, *What Do You Know About Chiropractics* [sic] by Ralph Lee Smith. As you know, we worked very closely with Mr. Smith while he was writing this book and has since sold approximately 200,000 copies.

The AMA's opposition to the initial accreditation of the National College of Chiropractic (NCC) by the New York Board of Regents and by the Illinois Superintendent of Public Instruction is documented by Ronald Beideman (1990, pp 5–6).

Section 2

The Surgeon General's Study

In 1967 Congress required Secretary Wilbur J. Cohen of the Department of Health, Education, and Welfare (DHEW) to make a study relating to the inclusion under the supplementary insurance program (part B of Title XVIII of the Social Security Act) of services of additional types of licensed practitioners performing health services in independent practice. The Secretary shall make a report to the Congress prior to January 1, 1969.

Despite expectations that an outside agency would be engaged to make an objective, unbiased study, the decision was taken that the Surgeon General of the United States Public Health Service (USPHS) would do it in-house using outside consultants. The report, *Independent Practitioners under Medicare* (Cohen WJ, 1968), was given final approval by an Ad Hoc Consultant Group consisting of 22 representatives of major health professions and institutions, a few other professionals and businessmen, the AFL-CIO, the Congress of Senior Citizens, plus Senator Maurine Neuberger of Oregon. For each practitioner group to be studied an Expert Review Committee was established. I was honored to be invited to serve on the committee for chiropractic and naturopathy. The other members were five MDs and three PhDs, one of whom chaired the department of anatomy at the University of Texas Medical Branch at Galveston and also the Committee. Perhaps I was intended as a neutral participant, because no chiropractor or naturopath was included.

Two things particularly surprised me about the work of the Committee, which met in Washington, D.C., only twice. Although we were given masses of data and reports to review and were invited to submit our recommendations for circulation within the Committee, it was clear that the report was to be written by the USPHS staff; in fact, I discovered at our first meeting that much of it already had been drafted. My second surprise was that there was more support for chiropractic in the Committee than I had anticipated, not only from John Mennell, a practitioner of manual medicine, but also from several others. However, the number of comments favorable to chiropractic decreased over the 4 months of our work, and between our preliminary and final votes there were several vote switches.

Although the higher level Ad Hoc Consultant Group, designated to advise the Surgeon General, decided not to hear or consider material from any professional group other than those being studied, and that no outside observers would be allowed, lest they influence or inhibit discussion, Doyl Taylor, Director of the AMA Bureau of Investigation, and Joseph A. Sabatier, Chairman of the AMA Committee on Quackery, met with USPHS staff responsible for preparing the report and supplied much of the raw material and documentation used in it (Wilk, 1976, plaintiff's exhibit no. 239). There was no *formal* involvement of the AMA because, as the USPHS staff officer who was responsible for drafting the report wrote on October 2, 1968, to a member of the Committee on Quackery (Wilk, 1976, plaintiff's exhibit no. 332): "testimony by the AMA or by the medical profession is unnecessary, as *the final answer has already been determined*" (italics supplied).

William Trever published *In the Public Interest* (1972) based on documentation provided by a disaffected AMA staff member (named "Sore Throat" after "Deep Throat" of Watergate fame). In it he included photocopies of inculpating AMA correspondence and detailed how members of the Expert Review Committee were subjected to behind-the-scenes pressure orchestrated by the AMA to produce a report critical of chiropractors. A member of the Committee was recruited to keep the AMA informed of its deliberations (Wilk 1976, Plaintiff's Exhibit #337):

> As indicated in our conversation, it would be helpful if we can be kept informed as to the progress of your committee work. Any reports or proceedings received will be quickly reproduced and returned to you. Your help is very much appreciated.

At a private luncheon during the second Washington meeting Dr. Mennell told me about the pressure on him. And as far removed as I was from the medical establishment, I received two communications concerning my work on the Committee: one from my personal physician, who knew me better than to try to pressure me directly; the other a letter (dated November 18, 1968) from the Dean of the University of Connecticut Medical School, which began: "I am informed that you are a member of a Federal Government committee with respect to the role of chiropractic in Medicare and Medicaid . . ." He enclosed some AMA propaganda on chiropractic. (He did not mention naturopathy, although it was and still is licensed in Connecticut.) There is documentation that the Chairman of the Committee had earlier been contacted by an associate in his medical society: the latter reported back to the AMA in a letter dated August 23, 1968 (Wilk, 1976, Plaintiff's Exhibit #228), well before completion of the Committee's report, that the Chairman

> is most anxious to do everything he can and is completely sold on the idea that chiropractic benefits should not come under the Medicare program. In our discussion it was realized that if anywhere in your records or reviews there are authenticated evidence of injury or evidence of delay of proper treatment caused by use of a chiropractor, this would give him good ammunition.

Taking all this into consideration, it is not surprising that the final recommendation to the Congress by DHEW Secretary Cohen (1968) was that chiropractic services *not* be included in the Medicare program. The following reasons were cited:

> Chiropractic theory and practice are not based upon the body of basic knowledge related to health, disease, and health care that has been widely accepted by the scientific community. Moreover, irrespective of its theory, the scope and quality of chiropractic education do not prepare the practitioner to make an adequate diagnosis and provide appropriate treatment.

Chiropractors and their supporters were naturally disappointed by the negative recommendation to Congress. They reacted with the first-ever effective cooperation between the American Chiropractic Association (ACA) and the International Chiropractors Association (ICA) in preparing jointly "Chiropractic's White Paper on Health, Education, and Welfare Secretary's Report" (1969). As a result, in 1970 Congress was flooded with an estimated 12 million letters and telegrams urging that chiropractic be included in Medicare, and in 1972 Congress disregarded the DHEW recommendation and legislated reimbursement for chiropractors (but not for naturopaths) under the Medicare program.

I was not surprised to see AMA pressure behind the scenes, the way the Expert Review Committee functioned, and its negative recommendation to Congress. It was exactly what I had expected, inasmuch as I was already well aware of organized medicine's campaign against chiropractic and its ability to influence federal agencies. While I was flattered to be invited to serve on the Committee, my personal reaction was curiosity and absolute delight at the opportunity to observe first-hand the AMA's tactics in its effort to "contain and ultimately eliminate" chiropractic. Incredibly, when USPHS records were subpoenaed for the Wilk trial, none could be found! Fortunately for the chiropractors, I had saved every scrap of paper I had received from the Committee, which as my legal obligation I willingly shared with the attorneys for both sides. I repeatedly told the two attorneys who interviewed me for the AMA and the American College of Radiology that if I was called as a witness my testimony could not help them. I was not called.

The AMA Committee on Quackery, following its success in turning the DHEW report into a condemnation of chiropractic, widened its efforts to involve other medical and health-related groups in its antichiropractic campaign. A memorandum from the Committee to the AMA Board of Trustees dated January 4, 1971, summarized its perceived achievements (Wilk, 1976, Plaintiff's Exhibit #464):

> This, then, might be considered a progress report on developments in the past seven years. The Committee has not previously submitted such a report because it believes to make public some of its activities would have been and continues to be unwise. Thus this Report is intended only for the information of the Board of Trustees. . . .
>
> Two major occurrences in 1966 are noteworthy. First, the U.S. Supreme Court affirmed a federal district court decision holding, in effect, that a state has the right to refuse to license chiropractors unless they have the same qualifications as Doctors of Medicine. Your Committee and its staff assisted in this case. Second, as recommended by your Committee and as submitted by the Board of Trustees, the AMA House of Delegates, for the first time, adopted a specific statement of policy on chiropractic.
>
> This was the necessary tool with which your Committee has been able to broaden the base of its chiropractic campaign. With it, other health-related groups were asked and did adopt the AMA policy statement or individually-phrased versions of it. These, in turn, led to even wider acceptance of the AMA position. . . .
>
> During 1970, there have been many other developments, including the report by the HEW Task Force on Medicaid and Related Programs (opposing federal funds for chiropractic under State Medicaid programs), public statements in opposition to chiropractic inclusion under Medicare by the AFL-CIO, the Consumer Federation of America, the American Public Health Association, the Association of American Medical Colleges, the American Hospital Association and others.
>
> The hoped-for effect of this widened base of support was and is to minimize the chiropractic argument that the campaign is simply one of economics, dictated and manipulated by the AMA.

Granted a certain amount of puffery in this self-serving report, "dictation" and "manipulation" by the AMA are precisely what the Committee on Quackery was designed to do, and did. Examples of its use (and misuse) of the mass media were an article "Should Chiropractors Be Paid With Your Tax Dollars?" by Albert Q. Maisel (1971) in *Reader's Digest* and two unsigned feature articles, "Chiropractors: Healers or Quacks?" in *Consumer Reports* (1975), which its managing editor, Eileen Denver, later explained in an interview with the Hartford *Courant* (November 5, 1989) "meant attacking the entire institution of chiropractic." Shortly after submission of the Cohen report and before the Wilk (1976) antitrust suit the AMA eliminated its Bureau of Investigation and its Committee on Quackery, stating budgetary reasons.

Section 3

The Antitrust Suits

In 1975 The United States Supreme Court (Goldfarb vs. Virginia State Bar, 421 U.S. 773) established for the first time that the learned professions are not exempt from antitrust laws but constitute trade and commerce because they engage in economic competition. And in 1982 it ruled that the Federal Trade Commission (FTC) has the power to enforce these laws against medical societies (FTC vs. AMA, 455 U.S. 676). Strenuous efforts by the AMA to persuade Congress to reallocate that power to the U.S. Department of Justice (which would permit jury trials where the AMA's likelihood of success is greater) were thwarted when the chiropractors joined in a coalition with 27 other health organizations, the United Steel Workers, and the United Automobile, Aerospace, and Agricultural Implement Workers that lobbied successfully against the AMA efforts.

The AMA connivance in making the DHEW report to Congress something other than the "independent, unbiased study of chiropractic" that was asked for was both a stimulus for and convincing evidence used in the massive antitrust suit launched by five chiropractors in 1976 in the Federal District Court for Northern Illinois. (The chiropractors had been unable to persuade the FTC to move against the AMA.) The suit was lodged against the AMA, American Hospital Association, American College of Surgeons, American College of Physicians, Joint Commission on Accreditation of Hospitals, American College of Radiology, American Academy of Orthopedic Surgeons, American Osteopathic Association, American Academy of Physical Medicine and Rehabilitation, Illinois State Medical Society, Chicago Medical Society, Medical Society of Cook County, H. Doyl Taylor, Joseph A. Sabatier, M.D., H. Thomas Ballantine, M.D., and James H. Sammons, M.D. (Wilk et al. vs. AMA et al., 1976). Sammons was Executive Vice President of the AMA, and Taylor headed its Department of Investigation. Sabatier and Ballantine had been successive Chairmen of the AMA Committee on Quackery. Although both the ICA and the ACA at first opposed the suit (even though "Sore Throat" repeatedly on the telephone urged them to support it), they soon began raising the large sums needed to support it. The plaintiffs charged that

> Commencing at least as early as November, 1963, and continuing through the present, defendants and their co-conspirators have been and are engaged in a combination, conspiracy and continuing course of conduct having as its objective first the isolation and then the elimination of the profession of chiropractic through, inter alia, unreasonable restraints on the rights of the individual members of the defendant trade associations to establish and carry on inter-professional relations with members of the chiropractic profession including the plaintiffs herein and enforcement of a concerted refusal by defendants and those acting in concert therewith to deal with plaintiffs and other members of the chiropractic profession. Such conduct constitutes an unreasonable restraint on interstate trade and commerce, a concerted refusal to deal and a group boycott, all in violation of Section 1 of the Sherman Act.

Among the specific offenses charged were refusal by the AMA and other defendants to permit MDs and DOs to refer patients to chiropractors, accept referrals from chiropractors, treat patients in cooperation with chiropractors, share office space, collaborate in research, teach at chiropractic colleges, lecture at their professional programs, and publish in chiropractic journals; also collusion to deny chiropractors hospital privileges (even taking their radiographs), efforts to persuade private insurance companies to deny coverage for chiropractic services, and "the attempt to exert concerted group pressure in an improper, illegal and sham effort to obtain executive, administrative, and juridical and legislative action by the federal and state governments adverse to the chiropractic profession." Specifically the complaint alleged:

> The defendant AMA wrongfully employed its Principles of Medical Ethics . . . whereby all members of the defendant AMA were and still are prohibited from engaging in any inter-professional relations with duly licensed and qualified members of the chiropractic profession including the plaintiffs herein. . . . The approximately 1900 constituent and component societies of the defendant AMA and, on information and belief, defendant AOA (American Osteopathic Association) have and continue to regularly communicate for the purpose of establishing and maintaining a coordinated anti-chiropractic campaign and for adopting and maintaining by the defendants ACS (American College of Surgeons), JCAH (Joint Commission on Accreditation of Hospitals), ACR (American College of Radiology), AAOS (American College of Orthopedic Surgery), AAPMR (American Academy of Physical Medicine and Rehabilitation), ISMS (Illinois State Medical Society), and CMS (Chicago Medical Society) of the AMA's Principles of Medical Ethics. . . . Defendant associations have and continue to vigorously enforce compliance by their members with the aforesaid prohibitions through threats of and actual censure, suspension and other disciplinary proceedings harmful to the professional standing and pecuniary interests of such individual members of the defendant associations. The anti-chiropractic activities of the defendants have been conducted in large measure sub rosa, and the fact that manipulative techniques used by certain members of the defendant trade associations in treating patients are "identical to maneuvers used by chiropractors" has been suppressed with the purpose and intent of misleading and deceiving the public

to the competitive detriment of the chiropractic profession including the plaintiffs herein.

The JCAH was singled out especially for its role in enforcing the AMA Code of Ethics, because the JCAH Hospital Accrediting Manual explicitly stated that failure of the medical staff and governing body of a hospital "to take all reasonable steps to ensure adherence to (the AMA Principles of Medical Ethics) shall constitute grounds for non-accreditation." In addition:

> The defendant JCAH has and continues to vigorously enforce compliance by accredited hospitals and their staffs with the AMA Principles of Medical Ethics and the interpretative rules of the Judicial Council through threats of and actual censure, suspension and other disciplinary proceedings against individual staff members and through threats of loss of accreditation as to the accredited hospitals, such threats being effective to coerce hospitals and individual staff members thereof from professionally associating with Doctors of Chiropractic.

Among the remedies sought, aside from legal costs, were (1) finding the defendants guilty of violating the Sherman Act; (2) injunctions to prevent the conspirators from enforcing the Code of Medical Ethics on their members insofar as they apply to all types of interprofessional relations with chiropractors; (3) publication of the court's finding of guilt in defendant associations' journals, along with revisions of policies stating that "it is ethical to deal with chiropractors operating within the scope of their state licenses"; (4) payment of threefold damages to each of the plaintiffs by each of the defendants; and (5) payment by the defendants of $1 million a year for 10 years to establish and maintain "an inter-professional research institute controlled equally by medical doctors and Doctors of Chiropractic for promoting inter-professional research and educational programs, and for developing a common lexicon."

On July 5, 1979, the attorney general of the State of New York filed an almost identical antitrust suit in the Federal District Court for the Eastern District of New York against 13 New York medical groups and the executive vice president of the Medical Society seeking injunctive relief and civil fines up to $15 million (State of New York vs. AMA et al., 1979). It is especially noteworthy that this suit was brought not on behalf of chiropractors but by a third party (the State of New York) on behalf of its citizens. Other court suits were filed in several other states. For example, in 1977 Pennsylvania chiropractor John Slavek and the Pennsylvania Chiropractic Society, in the Federal District Court in Philadelphia, sued the AMA, JCAH, American Hospital Association, Pennsylvania Medical Society, Pennsylvania Hospital Association, Pennsylvania Society of Radiologists, Pennsylvania Association of Clinical Pathologists, and Northern Penn Hospital, to gain access to laboratory and radiologic services (*American Medical News,* November 10, 1978). All these suits created deep tensions between the AMA and its various specialty societies over what their response strategy should be, leading the *Wall Street Journal* (December 5, 1978) to quote the AMA Counsel: "We're involved in internecine warfare. Its brother against brother."

Concerned about its financial vulnerability, especially if it lost the suit, within 6 months after the Wilk suit was filed the AMA proposed modifying its Code of Ethics to state that "each individual physician may decide for himself or herself whether to accept a patient referred by a chiropractor or other limited, licensed practitioner and whether to provide a report to whomever the patient directed" (*American Medical News,* November 3, 1978). Four specialty groups (physicians, surgeons, orthopedic surgeons, and radiologists) disagreed and demanded that the AMA withdraw proposed changes to the Code and retain the old language, contending that "the proposed code change elevates chiropractic to a status equal to that of medical doctors." They argued that the Board of Trustees lacked authority to commit the AMA to a court settlement that "conflicted with established AMA policy," and petitioned the court to enjoin the AMA proposed settlement in Pennsylvania. Despite this, the AMA, the American Hospital Association, and JCAH reached a court-approved agreement on December 11, 1978, giving Pennsylvania chiropractors access to laboratory and radiologic facilities. Many chiropractors were disappointed because they believed the settlement did not go far enough toward correcting other offenses committed by the defendants, such as those alleged in the Wilk case.

The AMA House of Delegates adopted a new Code of Medical Ethics on July 22, 1980, the first major revision in 23 years. Passed by only 11 votes more than the two thirds required, it was strongly opposed by the die-hards. Its key provision was:

> A physician shall, in the provision of appropriate care, except in emergencies, be free to choose whom to serve, with whom to associate, and the environment in which to provide medical services.

Clearly the antitrust suits had stimulated the change, as Trustee William Hotchkiss indicated in the debate (*American Medical News,* August 1/8, 1980):

> The Board of Trustees has a fiduciary responsibility to protect the assets of our membership. Legal counsel tells us that we need to change the principles. . . . If we should lose these suits, the damage could bankrupt this Association.

James S. Todd, Chairman of the Ad Hoc Committee on the Principles of Medical Ethics, said in an address to the House of Delegates on July 22 (*American Medical News,* August 1/8, 1980):

> The issue remaining is how much—should we only remove the legal pinch or should we recognize the need to modernize fully in keeping with changes in the profession and changes in society as well as changes in legal requirements? . . . It is time that parliamentary maneuvering stop, and we face up to the real issues. Do we simply reach a defiant accommodation, or do we seize the opportunity to demonstrate our deep commitment to our patients by producing ethics reflecting professional and social reality?

He was indirectly acknowledging another reason too sensitive to mention explicitly, that despite the AMA success in winning the battle over the DHEW report to Congress, it had already essentially lost its war with chiropractors. Public opinion and political pressure already had influenced Congress to grant chiropractors reimbursement under Medicare. By 1974 the U.S. Office of Education had recognized the Council on Chiropractic Education (CCE) as the accrediting agency for chiropractic colleges, the last holdout state (Louisiana) had licensed chiropractors, and Congress had appropriated $2 million for a scientific study of chiropractic. Hence 1974 was a milestone year in chiropractors' progress toward legal recognition and public acceptance. The antitrust suit in 1976 merely capped the climax. The worst fears expressed as follows by the AMA Committee on Quackery in its meeting on September 15, 1967, had been justified (Trever, 1972, p 60):

> If chiropractic coverage is ever obtained under Title 18, and if a chiropractic accrediting agency for their schools is granted federal recognition by listing with the U.S. Office of Education, the program to contain the cult of chiropractic will be considerably more difficult, if not impossible.

It is no wonder that the AMA was forced to trim its sails, cut its losses, and regroup so as to be able to continue the struggle on other fronts. After 1976 it sharply curtailed its antichiropractic efforts, especially those that were overt and confrontational. When Mike Wallace presented a television program on chiropractic in 1979 he stated that he had been unable to locate a medical doctor who would present the antichiropractic side, a radical change from earlier days when the Committee on Quackery would have leapt to such an opportunity. (As substitutes he found two disaffected chiropractors.) At about the same time a freelance writer told me that only one of 65 MDs to whom she wrote around the country requesting interviews on chiropractic would permit his name to be used, presumably because of fear of being sued. Organized medicine also became more cautious, though not inactive, in opposing legislation favorable to chiropractors at federal and state levels.

The Wilk suit finally came to trial in December 1980, and lasted 2 months. The record of the case includes 3,634 pages of transcript, 1,265 exhibits, and 73 depositions (Chapman-Smith, 1989, p 144). On January 30, 1981, the jury of the Federal District Court for Northern Illinois found the medical defendants in the Wilk antitrust suit not guilty on all charges, but the decision was reversed by the Seventh Circuit Court of Appeals on September 19, 1983, and a new trial was ordered. On February 28, 1984, the chiropractors filed a Petition for Certiorari for a discretionary review by the U.S. Supreme Court of the issues at law that would govern the new trial, but it was denied.

The American Osteopathic Association and the American Academy of Physical Medicine and Rehabilitation were the first defendants to settle out of court, in 1980. While not admitting guilt, they paid $30,000 and $35,000, respectively, to the chiropractic plaintiffs as compensation for legal expenses, and agreed to stop impeding collaboration between their members and chiropractors. Although the AMA sought an injunction against these settlements, Judge Nicholas J. Bua refused to grant one. The New York suit was settled in 1981, with the AMA agreeing that

> A physician may, without fear of discipline or sanction by the AMA, refer a patient to a duly licensed chiropractor when he believes that referral may benefit the patient. A phy-

sician may also choose to accept or to decline patients sent to him by a duly licensed chiropractor.

It [the AMA] affirms that the term "limited practitioner" includes duly licensed doctors of chiropractic.

It [the AMA] affirms that the term "other health professionals" includes duly licensed doctors of chiropractic.

It is the further position of the AMA that a physician may engage in any teaching permitted by law for which he is qualified, including teaching at a chiropractic college or seminar.

Similar out-of-court settlements were arrived at with the Chicago Medical Society in 1982 and the Illinois State Medical Society in 1985 and approved by the court (Wilk et al. vs. Illinois State Medical Society, 1985). In a surprise move the Illinois Society abandoned the position held by the AMA-related organizations and agreed to . . .

full professional cooperation with chiropractors including student exchanges, hospital training programs for chiropractic students, cooperation in research and publication, and cooperating with doctors of chiropractic in hospital settings where the hospital's governing board, acting in accordance with applicable law and that hospital's standards, elects to provide privileges and services to doctors of chiropractic.

For the retrial of the original Wilk suit in June 1987 the chiropractors dropped their claim for monetary damages so as to deprive the AMA of any opportunity to argue that the case was motivated by personal greed of the plaintiff chiropractors, which the AMA had argued in the first trial. It also allowed the second trial to be decided by a judge rather than a jury. On June 12, 1987, in the middle of the retrial and to the dismay of the remaining defendants, the American Hospital Association reached an out-of-court settlement with the chiropractic plaintiffs, requiring widespread dissemination of the following revolutionary new policy (Wilk et al., 1987):

The American Hospital Association specifically disavows any unlawful effort by any private, competitive group to "contain," "eliminate" or to undermine the public's confidence in the profession of chiropractic. The Association has no objection to a hospital granting privileges to doctors of chiropractic, where consistent with law, for the purpose of: (1) administering chiropractic treatment to patients who wish to have such treatment, whether administered in conjunction with or separate from other health care treatment or services administered by medical doctors or other licensed health care providers, (2) furthering the clinical education and training of doctors of chiropractic, (3) having new diagnostic x-rays, clinical laboratory tests, and reports thereon, made for doctors of chiropractic and their patients, and/or previously taken diagnostic x-rays, clinical laboratory tests, and reports thereon made available to them, by individual pathologists or radiologists employed by or associated with such hospital, upon the request or authorization of the patient involved.

In the retrial Judge Susan Getzendanner found the AMA, American College of Radiology, American College of Surgeons, and American Academy of Orthopedic Surgeons guilty of an illegal conspiracy, and proposed an injunction preventing the first three from impeding professional association between their members and chiropractors in the future. To avoid being enjoined, the American College of Radiology settled out of court and agreed to pay $200,000 to the plaintiff chiropractors toward legal expenses, and the American College of Surgeons settled and agreed to pay $200,000 to Kentuckiana Children's Center in Louisville ("Kentuckiana Children's Center Plans Large New Facility," 1989). Evidence had been presented at the trial that Kentucky Medical Societies had urged physicians to discontinue care at the nonprofit center because it was operated by a chiropractor. Both medical colleges also agreed to inform their members that they are free to cooperate with chiropractors in hospitals and private practice.

Judge Getzendanner ordered a permanent injunction against the AMA on September 25, 1987. Denied a stay, the AMA complied with the part of the order requiring it to publish the court's judgment in *JAMA* ("Special Communication," 1988, pp 81–82), but it appealed her order to mail copies to all AMA members and employees and to have the AMA Judicial Council revise its official "opinion" regarding professional association between MDs and chiropractors. Consequently the chiropractors cross-appealed the judge's finding that JCAH was not guilty. Although the general counsel of the AMA claimed a "major victory," Executive Vice President James Sammons, in his affidavit arguing for a stay of the injunction, wrote that the adverse effects from its publication in *JAMA* "will be the same as would result from the mailing of the order" and that the damage to *JAMA's* stature "cannot be repaired by any reversal of the order" (Wolinsky, 1988). Although the AMA continued to deny it was guilty of any conspiracy (Johnson, 1988, p 83), on February 7, 1990, the Seventh Circuit Court of Appeals unanimously upheld Judge Getzendanner's finding of guilt, and later that year the U.S. Supreme Court without comment let that decision stand. Hence all defendants in the Wilk case except for JCAH were found guilty and/or settled out of court. Although the American Academy of Orthopedic Surgeons was found guilty, it was not enjoined because it was judged to have ceased its conspiratorial activity. The chiropractors' cross-appeal of Judge Getzendanner's finding that the JCAH was not guilty, alleging that it was a party to the medical conspiracy because it is dominated by the 13 MDs on its 22-member governing board, was not adjudicated even though the State of Illinois and the nurse anesthetists submitted amicus curiae briefs in support of the chiropractors' appeal.

Chiropractors charge that organized medicine continues to conspire illegally to impede professional relationships between them and MDs. In 1990 Attorney George McAndrews initiated a new suit in the United States District Court for the Northern District of Illinois, Eastern Division, seeking damages and injunctive relief for forcing the MD co-owner with a chiropractor of The Neuro-Spine Center to terminate their relationship and for suspending the MD from the staff of Central DuPage Hospital in Winfield, Illinois. The following paragraph from the complaint reveals part of the rationale for the suit (Chinnicci vs. Central DuPage Hospital Association et al., 1990, p 16).

> Providing treatment of neuromusculoskeletal ailments by combining, in close association, the services of a chiropractor with the services of a medical doctor is a comparatively advantageous and superior method of doing business in that it provides the consumer with more treatment options and convenient, more comprehensive and superior service involving more modalities of treatment than is available from any one type of provider. It also provides a less expensive form of treatment in that chiropractic services are less expensive than the services of medical doctors and tend to minimize surgery and/or the length of hospital stays.

In 1991 an out-of-court settlement gave chiropractors the right to order hospital laboratory and radiologic services, to request CT and MRI scans, and to lease or buy space in the MD-owned Mona Rea office condominium from which Chinnicci and his MD associate had been ousted.

The antitrust suits would not have been so successful without the skill and expertise of the plaintiffs' attorney, George P. McAndrews, who combines several fortunate characteristics. First, he is the son of a chiropractor, brother of Jerome F. McAndrews (former Executive Vice President of the ICA and President of Palmer College of Chiropractic), and he has a sister and nine cousins who are chiropractors. Second, he was with a large Chicago law firm that handled technical and scientific antitrust litigation for many of the *Fortune* 500 largest corporations in the United States. He was therefore both highly motivated and well qualified to represent the weak, nonaffluent chiropractors against the vastly stronger AMA and the other defendants, with their superior legal and financial resources. The case has been expensive for all parties and has required strenuous fund-raising efforts by chiropractors. In January 1990 McAndrews estimated for me that the medical associations were believed to have spent in excess of $10 million in legal expenses plus $600,000 to settle various lawsuits with chiropractors. He also told me that the chiropractors would not settle out of court because they believed that a clean-cut victory was essential after so many years of time, effort, and money, and because the AMA has the resources to make a compromise look like an AMA victory, as it did so often in the past. Although chiropractors reportedly sought a judgment close to $14 million, including lawyers' fees, the out-of-court settlement reached with the AMA in December 1991 kept the exact amount secret. Due to tax considerations attending profession-wide fund-raising for the case, the beneficiaries, except for damages, designated are chiropractic charities. Publication of Judge Getzendanner's 1987 decision in *American Medical News* (Jan 13, 1992, pp 4–6) was accompanied by George McAndrew's "opinion" requesting continuing dialogue and by the "Revised Opinion on Chiropractors" of AMA's Council on Ethical and Judicial Affairs.

The struggle continues. In 1991 the ACA appropriated $1 million to finance a lawsuit against the Health Care Financing Agency (HCFA) of DHHS for not ensuring that health maintenance organizations (HMOs) provide chiropractic services to their Medicare subscribers as Congress had required.

Section 4

Interpretation

To what extent was the AMA antichiropractic campaign successful? Probably it delayed chiropractic acceptance for many decades. Certainly it convinced most MDs, many other health providers, and educated lay persons to believe that chiropractic is "an unscientific cult." Ritual condemnation became routine in MDs' offices and in legislative forums.

The extent to which the AMA enforced its proscription against professional association with chiropractors is illustrated in the following story related by McAndrews (1982, p 21):

> The Judicial Council of the AMA actually got letters like this, "I am a member of the local Rotary Club. A chiropractor has joined, must I terminate my membership?" And the five MDs that made up the Judicial Council scurried around looking at their precedents and finally came up with a formal ruling: "You must terminate your membership only if the Rotary Club is involved in health care matters." That's how complete this boycott was.

Gevitz (1989, p 294) writes: "However, following the judicial council's 1967 ruling prohibiting consultations, it appears that no physician was stripped of AMA membership for associating with chiropractors."

In sum, chiropractors' victories came first from patient acceptance and support, second from legislative struggles that skillfully used that support, and third from victories in the courts. The courts were actually a two-way street for chiropractors. Their early arrests for practicing medicine without a license (usually instigated by individual MDs or by medical societies) caused them great difficulty but at the same time created opportunities for favorable publicity. Public demonstrations by supporters helped, as did their attorneys' arguments before usually sympathetic juries that chiropractors were being discriminated against by jealous, economically motivated MDs losing patients to chiropractors. They also argued that patients' constitutional rights to choose the type of doctor they preferred were being threatened, an argument that led to later passage of equal-access insurance legislation at state levels. Allegations of medicine's attempts to dominate the public regulation of health care for its own advantage, familiar from the history of medicine, often succeeded in convincing juries and legislators that the chiropractors' cause was just.

The AMA campaign against chiropractors actually helped them in several ways. On one hand the campaign was overkill: MDs and patients who had the slightest exposure to chiropractic recognized this. They knew the chiropractor as their doctor or as a fellow practitioner who clearly was not as ignorant or as incompetent as AMA propaganda portrayed him. Patients who received relief needed no other evidence. MDs who were aware (and many may not have been) that after 1966 more than a hundred of their colleagues became members of the North American Academy of

Manipulative Medicine, and that osteopaths also use manipulation successfully, knew that the AMA propaganda was primarily organizationally motivated. Inglis (1964, p 112) concurs:

> So vigorously did the profession pursue this campaign that it began to take on the look of a vendetta; and the public . . . began to sympathize with the chiropractors as men oppressed.

Medicine's opposition was in general stronger at federal and state levels than in local communities. Although much of it no doubt was economically motivated, a lot of it certainly came from medicine's commitment to traditional theories of cause and cure. Its slow, partial abandonment of the "magic bullet" model of disease for a more holistic paradigm emphasizing prevention, life-style, environmental factors, and nutrition also has impeded medicine's acceptance of chiropractors as professional colleagues.

Other reasons for "quack hunting" were noted by Oliver Garceau in his classic *The Political Life of the American Medical Association* (1941, p 171):

> Perhaps the active minority [of the AMA] finds that quack hunting is personally profitable. Such sporting events give evidence of conscientious attention to duty; they appeal to the professional idealism of members, hurt no member's pocketbook, and contribute to a feeling of gratitude, obligation and even dependence on the active minority.

Sociologist Everett Hughes (1945, p 356) has suggested that the most hostile MDs may be those who are not very successful in attracting patients:

> It may be that those whose positions are insecure and whose hopes for the higher goals are already fading express more violent hostility to "new people."

It also is possible that the MDs who are less ethical or more "commercialized" in their practices project onto chiropractors their own tendencies and feelings of guilt and find it rewarding to attack chiropractors for those same tendencies (see also Luce, 1978).

Susan Smith-Cunnien has written an insightful doctoral thesis (1990) in which she shows that medicine's opposition to chiropractic was strongest during periods when it was undergoing threat or transition, first in the years following the Flexner report (1910) and its sequelae, and later when the federal government was imposing Medicare, Medicaid, and quality controls on the practice of medicine and its reimbursement. She argues that the AMA campaign against chiropractors unified the medical profession, gave MDs an added sense of superiority and status, and justified their dominance over the entire health care field. She summarizes:

> In fighting chiropractic, organized medicine is serving itself and the profession: focusing on unity in the face of factionalism, demonstrating its superiority in the face of a doubting public, and reasserting its dominance in the face of bureaucratic and legislative challenges to that dominance.

A main result of the AMA campaign was to unite chiropractors against a common enemy. Harry Vedder (1930, pp 7–8) indeed bemoaned some of chiropractic's early successes:

> Legal recognition . . . was the fatal blow . . . because it robbed us of the issue upon which our militant following had been built. Further, because it robbed us of our own militant attitude toward organized medicine. . . . *we were most prosperous when we were a militant group fighting organized medicine. . . . prosperity will return when we create an issue upon which we can again unite as a militant group fighting organized medicine.*

Although one of the AMA goals always was to keep chiropractors organizationally divided, the coordinated reaction of the ICA and ACA to the Cohen report (1968) began an era of communication and cooperation between them in political and legislative activities. In 1983 they began holding their annual Legislative Conference for lobbying purposes in Washington jointly rather than separately. As sociologist Lewis Coser argued in *The Functions of Social Conflict* (1956), conflict increases group solidarity. B.J. Palmer, a skilled practical psychologist, knew that, and a few years earlier had expressed similar ideas in his *Conflicts Clarify* (1951b).

The AMA attacks created in chiropractors and their supporters a sense of righteous indignation at being persecuted (not simply prosecuted) for a cause based partly on patients' constitutional right to a doctor of their choice and partly on the well-established right of a practitioner to continue earning a livelihood in a legitimate (especially a *licensed*) occupation. Although the division between straights and mixers gave organized medicine leverage in legislative contests, chiropractors never lost sight of who their real enemy was. Even though they are not yet fully united, they have already achieved much success.

Chapter 9

CHIROPRACTIC PHILOSOPHY, SCIENCE, ART

It is only as we advance as a science that we advance in the eyes of the rest of society. . . . The "philosophical" leaders regard chiropractic as being based upon doctrine rather than upon science. Fortunately, probably less than five per cent of our membership are of like mind but many of this five per cent still occupy official positions.

C.O. Watkins (1944, pp 4, 44)

D.D. Palmer stated repeatedly that chiropractic is a philosophy, a science, and an art. By art he meant technique, which is not problematic at this point. What is problematic is chiropractic philosophy and its relation to chiropractic science. D.D. (1910, p 116; 1914, p 1) explained these terms as follows:

> Science is knowledge reduced to law and embodied in a system. Philosophy is the knowledge of phenomena as explained by, and resolved into, causes, reasons, powers and laws.

> Chiropractic is a science and an art. The philosophy of chiropractic consists of the reasons given for the principles which compose the science and the movements which have to do with the art.

His explanation of the difference between science and philosophy is not clear, certainly not in the light of modern epistemology and the philosophy of science.

The distinction between philosophy and science made in Chapter 3 is critical here. Most of what D.D. wrote was based on his own observations and on the best empirical evidence he could glean from the scientific texts he studied. They were limited by the then current state of medical science, which had not yet profited from the breakthroughs of the 20th century and the knowledge of how to conduct clinical trials. Also, 19th century scientific writings often were admixed with religious and

philosophic concepts. To what he found in books D.D. added his own empirical observations and clinical insights gained from treating patients. Eventually his experience as a magnetic healer convinced him to abandon magnetism and to experiment
with a hands-on technique that worked better. Naturally he sought an explanation for
his successes, writing (1910, p 18):

> I desired to know why one person was ailing and his associate, eating at the same table,
> working in the same shop, at the same bench, was not. *Why?* What difference was there
> in the two persons that caused one to have pneumonia, catarrh, typhoid or rheumatism,
> while his partner, similarly situated, escaped? *Why?*

Such inquisitiveness is what is required in an empirical scientist.

Section 1

Chiropractic Philosophy

A fairly complete statement of D.D.'s philosophy comes from an essay (1914, p 10)
published posthumously by his wife:

> I believe, in fact know, that the Universe consists of Intelligence and matter. This intel-
> ligence is known to the Christian world as God. As a spiritual intelligence it finds ex-
> pression through the animal and vegetable creation, man being the highest manifesta-
> tion. I believe that this Intelligence is segmented into as many parts as there are
> individual expressions of life; that spirit, whether considered as a whole or individually,
> is advancing upward and onward toward perfection; that in all animated nature this In-
> telligence is expressed through the nervous system, which is the means of communica-
> tion to and from individualized spirit; that the condition known as Tone is the tension
> and firmness, the reniuency and elasticity of tissue in a state of health, normal existence;
> that the mental and physical condition known as disease is a disordered state because of
> an unusual amount of tension above or below that of tone; that normal and abnormal
> amounts of strain or laxity are due to the position of the osseous framework, the neuro-
> skeleton, which not only serves as a protector to the nervous system, but also, as a reg-
> ulator of tension; that Universal Intelligence, the Spirit as a whole or in its segmented
> parts, is eternal in its existence; that physiological disintegration and somatic death are
> changes of the material only; that the present and future make-up of individualized spir-
> its depend upon the cumulative mental function which, like all other functions, is mod-
> ified by the structural condition of the impulsive, transmitting nervous system; that crim-
> inality is but the result of abnormal nervous tension; that our individualized, segmented
> spiritual entities carry with them into the future spiritual state that which has been men-
> tally accumulated during our physical existence; that spiritual existence, like the physi-
> cal, is progressive; that a correct understanding of these principles and practice of them
> constitute the religion of chiropractic; that the existence and personal identity of individ-
> ualized intelligences continue after the change known as death; that life in this world
> and the next is continuous — one of eternal progression.

If this is religion, it certainly is not Christian. Basically, D.D. did not consider chiropractic a religion.

Much of what D.D. and B.J. Palmer called philosophy really is scientific hypotheses, or rather a mixture of theoretical hypotheses, philosophy, and (especially in the case of B.J.) ideology. It often is difficult to tell where one ends and the other begins. Their key concept is *homeostasis,* a well-recognized phenomenon basic to all sciences dealing with living organisms. It can even be attributed, as "equilibrium," to economic or social systems, which tend to react automatically to external stimuli to restore their status quo ante whenever their equilibrium is disturbed (Pareto, 1935, pp 1435–1442). D.D. may have anticipated the principle of homeostasis as it was developed by Walter B. Cannon in *The Wisdom of the Body* (1939). Terrett (1986, p 154) argues that "D.D. Palmer's use of the word tone is interchangeable with the current use of "homeostasis."

Since innate for D.D. characterized all living organisms, including subhuman species, it is puzzling to me why he thought it necessary to invoke the peculiarly human faculty of intelligence, which he called "Innate Intelligence" or simply "Innate," to encompass the human body's capacity to heal itself, the well-known vix medicatrix naturae, or healing power of nature. It is perhaps even more amazing that chiropractors continue to use the concept, because it is well known that reduction of subluxations in animal spines benefits them too and that at least a half dozen chiropractor-veterinarians (D.C.-D.V.M.s) practice in the United States. (There is also an American Veterinary Chiropractic Association, which offers a 100-hour certification course in animal chiropractic to both DVMs and DCs, who typically collaborate in the treatment of a particular animal.) Apparently D.D. simply redefined the word "intelligence" to mean what he wanted it to mean. Douglass Gates (1987), president of the Federation of Straight Chiropractic Organizations (FSCO) and a staunch exponent of traditional straight philosophy, seems to agree:

> All matter, small or large in mass, exists because of its organization. And its organization is the result of a principle at work—an intelligence. For the most part it [intelligence] is a term coined by chiropractic (even though the concept has been recognized for thousands of years) and represents this "principle of organization" at work in living things. It is important to point out, however, that this principle is a universal principle; it applies to all matter, living or not.

A word defined so broadly is meaningless. The question remains: Why did D.D. select the words "Intelligence" and "Innate Intelligence" for such a basic concept as "organization," or more properly "homeostasis"? Various reasons have been suggested, most of them focusing on his interest in spiritualism and metaphysical healing and his experience as a magnetic healer. He discusses these topics as well as Christian Science and the theosophic movement in *The Chiropractor's Adjustor* (1910). However, he was not so conventionally religious as many have assumed. He stated (1910, p 547) explicitly: "I do not believe in a world beyond the present one."

Although some authors call D.D.'s philosophy "vitalism," Joseph Donahue

(1987, p 23) identified spiritualism and theosophy as the most important sources of his philosophy of "Innate," which Donahue (1986, pp 32–34) summarized as follows:

> Innate is an individualized portion of Universal Intelligence or God . . . It becomes bonded with a human body at birth (with the first breath) by the soul. . . . It is capable of gaining knowledge by intuition. . . . It is a superior consciousness to the educated mind in every way. . . . It runs all the "vegetative" and "vital" physiological functions of the body. . . . It activates the vital force in an organ by the way of the nervous system. . . . The "nerve vibration" carries innate's thoughts and commands. . . . Human disease is caused by a nervous interference to innate's normal perfect control of the body, particularly by vertebral subluxations.

D.D. (1910, pp 641–642) tells us that he first introduced innate intelligence, which he called his "theosophical philosophy of chiropractic," in a 1904 article titled "Innate Intelligence" and that he expanded on it in *Science of Chiropractic* (1906), which carries both B.J. and D.D. as co-authors; but he did not publish it in full until 1910. Donahue's conclusion (1986, p 35; see also 1990) is that D.D.'s linking of "the marvelous complexity and healing capabilities of the body" with "a supernatural intelligence" was

> the basis of his innate philosophy, but was a serious scientific flaw because his conclusion far outreached the available data. . . . The whole concept of innate of course rests on accepting on faith the basic premises without hope of any concrete proof. From a strictly scientific viewpoint, innate must be rejected out of hand because it fails the most fundamental requirement of science, namely testability. From the standpoint of logic, the whole concept of innate depends on the logical fallacy called word magic. Giving names and definitions to unprovable spiritual entities like innate and soul cannot guarantee their existence. Innate philosophy's impact on the profession was far greater than it should have been, considering its scientific merit.

Donahue notes that many early chiropractic teachers and schools ignored innate completely. That was especially true at National College of Chiropractic (NCC), which had early come under medical influence and taught a more scientific approach to chiropractic. Furthermore, soon after its publication D.D.'s *The Chiropractor's Adjustor* (1910) became nearly unavailable, according to Terrett (1986, p 156):

> All copies were quickly bought up and destroyed. You could not get a copy anyplace at any price. In fact, you could not find a copy for "love or money." The leaders of the profession did not want the world to know anything about the teachings of old Dr. Daniel D. Palmer. . . . The early leaders then greatly distorted their founder's science, philosophy and vision for chiropractic, as the book wasn't reprinted for half a century, some five years after B.J. Palmer's death.

The early issues of D.D.'s *The Chiropractic* and *The Chiropractor* also were unavailable, because B.J. kept them in what Lerner refers to as his "secret files."

After falling out with his father in 1906, B.J. adapted innate philosophy to his own purposes, which caused D.D. (1910, pp 639–640) to respond with characteristic bitterness and sarcasm toward his son:

> He says, "This is a pet theory of mine." Innate and Educated Intelligence were among my earliest Chiropractic conceptions. . . . That boy should long ere this have received it as such and not continue to hold it as a "pet theory." . . . There are forty articles which have been falsely copyrighted. . . . If I should authorize the circuit courts of the United States sitting in equity to enjoin the issuing, publishing or selling of any such article marked in violation of the copyright laws, the penalties would be sufficient to blow up that pseudo fountain head.

> I have been lenient, knowing that if I should deprive the thief of my property, that it would *dispossess him of nine-tenths of all the literature he has which is characteristic of the science, art or philosophy of chiropractic.*

After the acquittal of Shegataro Morikubo in 1907 in La Crosse, Wisconsin, based on the argument that chiropractic is neither the practice of medicine nor osteopathy, B.J. embraced innate philosophy with evangelistic fervor. Perhaps because chiropractic's scientific basis doesn't really differ much from that of medicine or osteopathy, although its technique of manipulation (specific vertebral thrust) differs from osteopathy's long-lever manipulation, B.J. treated the difference as primarily philosophic. Using his father's definition of philosophy as concerned with "causes" and "reasons," B.J. taught that chiropractic treats only causes, not symptoms, and that it therefore is the diametric opposite of medicine. Clearly his need for an effective legal and political strategy dictated his philosophy, rather than vice versa. Although he insisted on the opposite—that philosophy dictated his strategy—actually he espoused philosophy in order to oppose licensure by medical authorities and control of the profession by mixers. He (1958a) came very close to saying as much:

> Chiropractic differs fundamentally and absolutely from any other method of getting the sick well. If this were not true, there would be no reason for asking state legislatures for recognition as a separate and distinct science. To justify the claim for recognition, we *should* differ from any other method; and for this reason most Chiropractors scorn to use any of the methods used by others.

In a later passage (1958a) he exaggerated the difference between chiropractic and medicine:

> The dividing line is sharply drawn: anything given, applied to, or prescribed from outside-in, below-up, comes within the principle and practice of medicine. None of this does Chiropractic do! Our principle is opposite, antipodal, the reverse, for everything within the chiropractic philosophy, science and art works from above-down, inside-out. Anything and everything outside that scope is medical whether you like it or not.

D.D. had provided the basic idea (1910, p 824): "A chiropractor is not a therapeutist. . . . Chiropractors do not use remedies. Chiropractic principles are antipodal to therapeutics."

Although D.D. (1910, p 561) had equated "diagnosis" and "analysis," B.J. insisted on distinguishing between them; for example, in chiropractic terminology "diagnosis" became "analysis," "treatment" became "adjustment," "x-rays" became "spinographs." It is clear that B.J. introduced more cultistic elements into chiropractic (see Stephenson, 1927) than did D.D. B.J.'s (1920, p 11) preposterous definition of chiropractic actually was incorporated into a proposed New Jersey statute, but had to be changed when the governor refused to sign it:

> Chiropractic is a name given to the study and application of a universal philosophy of biology, theology, theosophy, health, disease, death, the science of the cause of disease and the art of permitting the restoration of the triune relationships between all attributes necessary to normal composite forms, to harmonious quantities and qualities by placing in juxtaposition the abnormal concrete positions of definite mechanical portions with each other, by hand, thus correcting all subluxations of the three hundred articulations of the human skeletal frame, more especially those of the spinal column, for the purpose of permitting the re-creation of all normal cyclic currents through nerves that were formerly not permitted to be transmitted, through impingement, but have now assumed their normal size and capacity for conduction as they emanate through intervertebral foramina—the expressions of which were formerly excessive or partially lacking—named disease.

Some exponents of traditional philosophy still expound B.J.'s original message. Fred H. Barge, who became president of the International Chiropractors Association (ICA) after the proposed ICA/ACA (American Chiropractic Association) merger was voted down in 1988, wrote (1989, p 7; 1987):

> We must produce our own paradigm for diagnosis/analysis, design our own model of patient care and referral, develop our own distinctly chiropractic councils, diplomates, and consultants. *We do not want to become part of the "medical team." We are our own separate and distinct profession.*

Some of B.J.'s followers indulged in even more egregious flights of ideologic fancy. Gordonne E. McGowan, who had taught histology at Palmer School of Chiropractic (PSC) (without a microscope, he told me!) before moving to Massachusetts, wrote the following in the October 1948 *The Chiropractor,* which well illustrates "word magic" and the invoking of religious concepts:

> In the final analysis, the condition outside causes the condition inside called disease. In this sense, the condition inside is an effect of the condition outside that has caused it; but in relation to the body alone, the condition inside is the cause of disease. This is an important distinction. There is an outside as well as an inside cause of disease, for there could be no inside cause without an outside cause. . . . Thus the term "cause" is always relative to something else which is its effect, and the effect becomes a cause of its own effects. Every effect is accordingly a cause, but there is one cause that is not an effect and that is the First Cause, Universal Intelligence, or God, according to the conclusions of Logic.

Incidentally, McGowan practiced using the intriguing GPC (God-Patient-Chiropractor) Service Principle under which the patient was not charged a fee but was invited to donate whatever he felt the treatment was worth, a plan introduced at the 1939 PSC Lyceum (Shears, 1939), which some chiropractors believed would make them less vulnerable to arrest.

Although the more scientifically oriented chiropractors adopted some of B.J.'s special terminology, they were contemptuous of his philosophy, which they regarded as cultist and a "reflex verbal trap." Clarence W. Weiant (1981), long-time dean at the Chiropractic Institute of New York and the recipient of a doctorate in anthropology in 1943 from Columbia University, wrote that B.J.'s chiropractic philosophy could be reduced to two sentences:

> (1) The entire universe is permeated by a *Universal Intelligence*. (2) *Universal Intelligence* bestows upon every human being an *Innate Intelligence* which from the moment of birth to the moment of death controls every bodily activity that is not under voluntary control.

Weiant, Janse at NCC, Budden at Western States Chiropractic College (WSCC), Haynes at Los Angeles College of Chiropractic (LACC), Wolff at Northwestern College of Chiropractic (NWCC), and other nonideologically oriented chiropractic leaders saw no need for such a chiropractic philosophy. For them chiropractic was scientifically grounded and what it needed was more scientific research. To that we now turn. (A new and experimental journal, *Philosophical Constructs for the Chiropractic Profession*, published by NCC in 1991, attempts to revive interest in the question of whether there is a "chiropractic philosophy.")

Section 2

Chiropractic Science

Sid Williams, President of Life Chiropractic College in Marietta, Georgia, and a dedicated advocate of traditional chiropractic and leader of the opposition to the proposed ACA/ICA merger in 1987–1989, wrote the following in the same volume in which Weiant belittled chiropractic philosophy (1981):

> The human organism is a self-healing self-restoring organism. . . . Subluxations of the spine and its articulations do occur, affect biomechanical, neurological and muscular changes, do decrease the ability of the body to express its self-healing, self-restoring capability; removal of subluxations offers the body an opportunity to return to its full potential. Subluxations can be located and corrected by application of forces to an articulation, are capable of producing a wide variety of symptoms and maladies, are common to all mankind, are capable of yielding organic disease; correction may be contraindicated.

No chiropractor would disagree with these propositions. To be noted is that they are stated in such form that each proposition is testable, at least in principle, by empirical laboratory, epidemiologic, or clinical research. The word "subluxation" would have to be precisely defined, and agreed on. Much debate in chiropractic is caused by the familiar semantic problem of different meanings for the same term. If operational definitions can be agreed on, and (ideally) quantified, then each of Williams' propositions could in principle be empirically proved or disproved (validated or invalidated). Systematically interrelated, such propositions then would constitute the body of chiropractic scientific theory.

Only in the past couple of decades have most chiropractic leaders, especially those in the national associations but also even many of those in the colleges, begun to appreciate what chiropractic theory and science really are and what constitutes acceptable research. Earlier the few leaders who did understand had insufficient resources to undertake serious research, although individual practitioners often made insightful clinical observations and published case studies based on them.

Like everything else, early chiropractic research was closely tied to the concerns of B.J. and PSC. By 1910 B.J. had purchased a Sheidel-Western state-of-the-art x-ray machine and set up a "spinographic" laboratory. X-rays offered the possibility of detecting spinal displacements (Canterbury and Krakos, 1986, p 26):

> B.J. called this work spinography because the chiropractic principle in practice was confined to the research of living spinal columns of sick people, both before and after adjustment.

According to Carver (1936, p 189), B.J. "received a commission from the x-ray companies for every machine sold to a graduate of his institution." Dye (1939, p 194) notes that the rate of patient recovery after its introduction increased from 30% to 40%, to 50% to 60%. Later B.J. (1919) recognized its expanded use:

> Spinography does more than read subluxations, it proves the existence, location, and degree of exostosis, ankylosis, artificial, abnormal shapes and forms, all of which may prevent the early correction to normal position of the subluxation.

Mixers felt no inhibitions regarding full diagnostic use of x-ray studies, and soon also included "detection and diagnosis of pathological processes, fractures, and anomalies that would directly relate to the patient's health and prognosis."

Although many radiologic "firsts" have been rashly claimed for chiropractic, a medical text (Monell, 1902) had already described the use of x-rays "for spinal exposures, luxations and fractures, scoliosis, congenital anomalies, ankylosis, tumors," other diseases, "upright filming of the spine," and "stereoscopic radiography" (Canterbury and Krakos, 1986, p 28). Nevertheless, chiropractors did some original research. Full-spine radiography was first reported by Thompson (1919) using four overlapping films. In 1931 Ray Richardson described the first full-length spinograph made using a single 8 × 36-inch film, and in 1933 Warren Sausser reported the first use of a 14 × 36-inch spinograph (Canterbury and Krakos, 1986, p 27). Joy M. Loban announced the first upright radiographs used for chiropractic in the April 1924

Universal Chiropractic College Bulletin, although Dintenfass (1970, p 68) writes that they were being taken by 1918 at that college; Leo J. Steinbach (1886–1960), then dean and later president of Universal College, usually is given major credit for that achievement (Steinbach, 1941, 1957). Although full-spine x-ray films have been criticized widely as being of little value and more recently as exposing patients to excessive radiation, they are still sometimes used. It is especially impressive for patients to see an x-ray film of a full upright spine with scoliosis or pelvic tilt. However, in the earliest days patients had to be persuaded to have them. Edward Maurer told me that one tactic used was to give patients a choice: either have an x-ray examination or sign a liability release covering a hundred different conditions.

A favorite story at PSC, according to Quigley (1989b), was of a man named Jensen who had traveled the length of Iowa in the early 1920s to try the new chiropractic treatment. After being examined he was sent to the x-ray department with instructions to return. When he didn't return in an hour a phone call determined that he had left the x-ray department 30 minutes earlier. He disappeared. "In two weeks the doctor received a letter from him, painfully penciled with evident effort but filled with generous praise. The gist was that Mr. Jensen was feeling wonderfully better since the doctor had sent him for that chiropractic x-ray treatment!"

Carver (1936, p 68) wrote that in the early 1920s:

> There was a strong endeavor during the organizing period of the ACA to establish in it a real research department. . . . It was fully discussed and rejected upon the outspoken declaration, particularly on the part of Dr. Loban, that with the delegates present from the various schools, Carver would always be there, and would Carverize every proposition brought forward.

The term "whiplash," now a generally accepted medical term, was introduced by chiropractor H.E. Crowe in 1928 to describe damage to the cervical spine often caused by an automobile crash (Foreman and Croft, 1988).

B.J.'s purpose in creating the B.J. Palmer Chiropractic Clinic at PSC in 1935 was to carry out research on chiropractic. Problem cases were solicited from the field and referred to B.J.'s personal attention. He employed MDs to do complete physical examinations and standard laboratory tests on all patients at admission, weekly, and at discharge. However, true randomization and statistical controls were not used (and probably not even considered!). A partial list of research reports produced by the Clinic between 1935 and 1949 follows:

Hematological Changes Under Specific Chiropractic Adjustment, 1,054 cases
Radiological Changes Under Specific Chiropractic Adjustment, 2,006 cases
Basal Metabolic Changes Under Specific Chiropractic Adjustment, 900 cases
Cardiographic Changes Under Specific Chiropractic Adjustment, 1,500 cases
Urological Changes Under Specific Chiropractic Adjustment, 2,006 cases
Electrocardiographic Changes Under Specific Chiropractic Adjustment, 1,500 cases
Audiometric Changes Under Specific Chiropractic Adjustment, 1,029 cases

B.J. also published a 744-page tome, titled *Chiropractic Clinical Controlled Research* (1951a), based on these studies, but only chiropractors were impressed. Quigley (1988) provided this candid evaluation of the much-touted clinic:

> Unfortunately, as a research facility it contributed very little. The principal reason for this failure was the total lack of qualified research personnel. The avowed goal was to prove that chiropractic adjustments reversed disease processes but the research design was fundamentally flawed. It was essentially this: each patient was examined and tested once a week. These included blood tests, EKGs, CBCs, urine tests, conturograms, etc. All these data were collected as if in a basket. In the absence of a statistician the staff could only allow the data to pile up. For example, for a patient who remained in the clinic for six months, and many did, there would be 26 sets of CBCs, 26 sets of EEGs, 26 sets of EKGs, etc. In 1951 an effort was made to extract some meaningfulness from the imposing collection. A statistically naive staff member made a well-intentioned effort but there was not one mathematically valid technique for the testing of significance applied and there were no controls. But, aside from research, the clinic enjoyed a healthy growth.

One of the earliest proponents of valid scientific research on chiropractic was Claude O. Watkins (1902 or 1903–1977) of Sidney, Montana, the first chairman of the National Chiropractic Association (NCA) Committee on Education. By the early 1940s he was criticizing NCA leaders for not adopting a program of vigorous clinical research. According to Joseph Keating (1987, pp 13–14):

> Watkins envisioned the chiropractor as a physician-scientist. . . . "Too often," he suggested, "chiropractors do not realize that chiropractic research must be done by clinicians like themselves in their own offices because the first prerequisite for clinical research is being able to observe patients under treatment, and this must be done under normal practice conditions. . . . All should be trained in clinical research," he reasoned, "as no one can tell who might discover a promising hypothesis for testing." . . .
>
> Although Nugent was often publicly vilified and disputed, Watkins' views seem rather to have been ignored. . . . In a 1967 letter to Harlin Larson, Watkins described his career-long frustration: . . . "I gave it up back in 1945 and took it up again in 1960 and now I am about to give it up again as a hopeless cause. . . . The past year I have been working with the ACA colleges and officials to point out to them the need of getting rid of cultist principles and (basing) chiropractic on scientific principles and outlining a program by which it could be done. It would be necessary for the colleges to head up such a program, and it would spread from the colleges to the field. Most of the colleges, if not all, favor the plan but do nothing about it."

Watkins published a forward-looking document, *The Basic Principles of Chiropractic Government* (1944, p 33) in which he asserted:

> Perhaps the greatest cause for chiropractic's failure to make greater scientific progress and to be accepted as a worthy science is the cult in chiropractic. . . . However, I believe it is true that there appears to be more cult than actually exists due to a natural fact. Those possessing the scientific attitude are by nature an humble people, preferring

to remain in the background; by nature, the cultist is a boisterous, articulate individual who advances himself or is advanced because he is a natural leader and politician into positions of leadership.

One can think of many examples fitting that description! Although Watkins lived to see official recognition of the Council for Chiropractic Education (CCE) as the accrediting agency for chiropractic in 1974, he died in 1977, 6 months before publication by NCC of the first issue of the *Journal of Manipulative and Physiological Therapeutics,* the first chiropractic journal to be indexed by the National Library of Medicine and regularly subscribed to by medical libraries.

J. Robinson Verner of the Chiropractic Institute of New York, drawing heavily on the Russian neurologist A.D. Speranski (1935), attempted a systematic statement of chiropractic theory in his *Science and Logic of Chiropractic* (1941), and Janse and colleagues (1947, p 7) at NCC, following Forster's (1915) lead, spelled out five principles comprising chiropractic theory:

1. A vertebra may become subluxated.
2. This subluxation tends to impingement of the structures (nerves, blood vessels, and lymphatics) passing through the vertebral foramen.
3. As a result of such impingement, the function of the corresponding segment of the spinal cord and its connecting spinal and autonomic nerves is interfered with and the conduction of the nerve impulses impaired.
4. As a result thereof, the innervation to certain parts of the organism is abnormally altered and such parts become functionally or organically diseased or predisposed to disease.
5. The adjustment of a subluxated vertebra removes the impingement of the structures passing through the intervertebral foramen, thereby restoring to diseased parts their normal innervation and rehabilitating them functionally and organically.

Joseph Janse and Fred Illi (1901–1983; Figure 28) pioneered research on spinal and pelvic biomechanics at NCC (Illi 1940; Janse et al., 1947). From 1943 through 1975 Illi continued this research at his Institute for the Study of Statics and Dynamics of the Human Body in Geneva, Switzerland. Probably the best chiropractic researcher of his time, Illi (1951, 1965, 1971) made major contributions to understanding the functioning of the sacroiliac joint as a synovial articulation essential to fully upright bipedal locomotion. And he claimed to have identified a previously undiscovered interosseous ligament essential to sacroiliac movement, "confirmed by the U. of Bordeaux and designated 'ligament d'Illi' " (Dzaman, 1980, p 128). Illi wrote (1951, pp 12–13):

> The author constructed a wooden model, the manipulation of which made him conclude
> . . . the existence of an intra-articular ligament, whose major function is that of directing and limiting sacro-iliac movement. . . . Eager to verify my hypothesis, I traveled to Chicago, the home of the National College of Chiropractic, where I had at my disposal

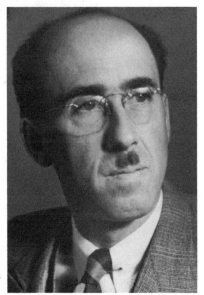

FIGURE 28.
Fred W.H. Illi, Swiss researcher noted for his
work on the sacroiliac joint.

abundant dissection material. . . . I almost abandoned the effort as being futile when I
conceived the idea of approaching the joint laterally by searching under the periosteum
of the iliac bone . . . through the succulent cancellous tissue. On the second attempt I
uncovered the ligamentous structure I had foreseen and expected. With my friend, Dr.
Janse, and some student assistants, I dissected eight more pelvises to verify and make
the discovery certain. . . . This ligament has been named "Illi's ligament." We found
some which were ruptured, others which were distorted or which showed atrophy.

James Cassidy, D.C., has questioned whether Illi actually discovered a new ligament
(McGregor and Cassidy, 1983, p 2). He wrote to me (April 5, 1990): "I am now
finishing my Ph.D. thesis on the sacroiliac joint and have dissected well over one
hundred joints. I have yet to see an "Illi's ligament." Although Freeman et al.
(1990), using dissection technique much like Illi's, found the ligament in 75% of 31
human pelves, Cassidy has written to me that he remains skeptical.

Illi (1965) based his findings on "studies over thirty-six years, in which I have
covered no less than 18,000 cases of patients examined, x-rayed, and treated," as
well as on several years of collaboration in anatomic dissection with Janse at NCC.
Baker (1985) has reviewed Illi's contributions that explained the biomechanics of the
sacroiliac joint, and "demonstrated that the sacrum acts as a 'universal joint' between
the ilia and spinal column; otherwise the irregularities of locomotion would incur
trauma to the spine." He (1985, pp 60–61) summarizes Illi's conclusions on how
"human phylogenesis" (evolution) produced adaptation to fully upright locomotion:

> In comparing the spine of a gorilla with that of a human, Illi noted that locomotion in
> the ape is accomplished in a bending position, with a rhythmical swinging of the torso.
> . . . In the full upright position, man must contend with the vertical axis of gravity

which imposes a balance of compensation heretofore inessential while man assumed the bent position. . . . Being upright necessitates torsions in one part of the spine to be compensated for elsewhere within the pelvic-spinal mechanism. When compensations are not balanced, subluxations or pathological compensations result. . . .

He further demonstrated that as the pelvis on the swing-leg side during gait assumes a motion of extension, the sacrum on that side travels posteriorly and superiorly. Meanwhile, as the pelvis on the weight-bearing side assumes a motion of flexion, the sacrum of that same side reciprocates accordingly by going anteriorly and inferiorly. Thus the sacrum, during the act of walking, is almost analogous to a ball and socket articulation, whose movements take place in definite articular crevices.

Baker concludes, at times quoting Illi (1965, pp 59–60):

His foremost concern was the neuropathological reflex. . . . Illi contended that it was not essentially the pinching of the nerve by the zygopophyses which was the cause of the irritation, but rather the swelling in and around the injured articulation. Furthermore, he was at odds with the prevalent idea of "putting a vertebra back into place" to make the patient better: "One cannot put a vertebra back in place the way one does a fracture or dislocation. What one really does is: to restore the function of a vertebra. . . . The completely performed reduction of a displacement is often followed by immediate relief [which] suddenly throws into light the intimate relationships existing between our spine and the other parts of our body."

Another American-educated European, Henri J. Gillet (1907–1989; Figure 29) of Belgium, did major clinical research, first publishing his *Belgian Notes on Fixation* in 1951, which went through 10 editions. He and his father and brother and Mar-

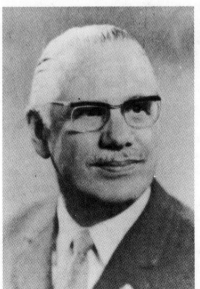

FIGURE 29.
Henri J. Gillet, Belgian researcher noted for development of motion palpation. (Courtesy of Motion Palpation Institute's Dynamic Chiropractic.)

cel Liekens (Gillet and Liekens, 1973) attempted to specify exactly what a subluxation is and in particular to discover whether it is limited to the upper cervical vertebrae, as B.J. then taught. They found not only that a "hole-in-one" adjustment appeared to correct subluxations at lower spinal levels, that is, produced generalized corrective effects on the whole spine, but that the same thing happened when they made dorsal, lumbar, or sacroiliac adjustments. In his "A Hundred Holes in One" (n.d.) he stated:

> *All* correct and effective application of *any* adjustment at *any* vertebra *always* produces, not only a change at the vertebra or area aimed at, but it also tends to produce a spontaneous correction at all other subluxations in the whole spine; this effect is generally in ratio to the degree of effective local correction. We insist: this law is true not only for the atlas, but for any other vertebra or area! . . . Later we observed that, if instead of trying to adjust all the subluxations, we started only with the tough ones, all the smaller ones tended to disappear spontaneously, with far faster results!

He is credited with introducing "motion palpation," a diagnostic technique further developed at PCC by Jerome McAndrews in 1973 and by L. John Faye (Schafer and Faye, 1989), and with emphasizing the role of "total and partial" fixations of spinal segments. Hilton S. Taylor (1961, p S-30) quotes him as saying:

> A vertebral articulation can become fixed in any of the positions it normally takes in spinal movement. Vertebrae do not "slip out of place," they are not "displaced" out of their physiological boundaries, they have not gone out of their limits of motion. When we adjust subluxations we do not "replace" vertebrae.

Dye (1939, p 165), B.J.'s apologist, appears to have agreed:

> After all, the misalignment of a vertebra termed as a subluxation is of so minute a degree that its correction to normal position would be practically impossible of determination by a mere digital palpation.

In recent years more research has been done. The colleges have attracted teachers better qualified and motivated to do research, especially those teaching the basic sciences. Furthermore, the demands to put chiropractic on a scientific footing have increased. From its inception in 1963 the ACA allocated a portion of its membership fees to education and research. In 1967 it established the Foundation for Chiropractic Education and Research (FCER) as successor to both NCA's Chiropractic Research Foundation (established in 1944) and NCA's Foundation for Accredited Chiropractic Education (established in 1958). Most FCER money at first went to strengthen education in order to prepare the colleges for accreditation. Later, because one of the criteria for accreditation is that colleges train and subsidize researchers, more money has been allocated to research. Twenty percent of FCER donation income is provided by the ACA.

There is no question that a major stimulus to chiropractic research was the landmark interdisciplinary conference on spinal manipulative therapy (SMT) sponsored by the National Institute of Neurological and Communicative Disorders and Stroke (NINCDS) in 1975 in Bethesda, Maryland. Its organizer and chairman, Murray

Goldstein, D.O., Associate Director of the Institute, edited the 310-page report of its proceedings, *The Research Status of Spinal Manipulative Therapy* (Goldstein, 1975). Political pressure from chiropractors had persuaded the Senate Appropriations Labor-HEW Subcommittee to recommend in its 1974 report to the Senate: "This would be an opportune time for an 'independent, unbiased' study of the fundamentals of the chiropractic profession. Such studies should be high among the priorities of the NINCDS." Congress authorized up to $2 million of the 1974 DHEW appropriation for that purpose. For the first time in history leading scientists and clinicians assembled for 3 days to discuss SMT. Goldstein's switching the focus of the conference from "chiropractic" to "spinal manipulative therapy" was a stroke of genius because it more accurately delineated the common ground shared by the participants rather than highlighting their differences. George Silver (1980, p 349) sarcastically suggested that it could have been "for safety's sake." Only in the program for the first evening were the differences between medical, osteopathic, and chiropractic theories presented and discussed. I was honored to be invited as the discussant for that session. In doing so I could not resist the opportunity to suggest (Wardwell, 1975, p 53), following usage of the abbreviation "OMT" (osteopathic manipulative technique, derived from initials of the Department of Osteopathic Techniques at Still's Kirksville College) that the abbreviation "SMT" could designate "spinal manipulative therapy," a usage that seems to have gained general acceptance. My remark that physical therapists should perhaps also have been invited to participate in the conference provoked no comment.

The remaining 2 days of the conference focused on the scientific principles of neuroanatomy, pathology, spinal biomechanics, radiologic diagnosis, and SMT. Among the 58 participants and 40 presenters were such leading scientists and practitioners of SMT as the medical physicians James Cyriax, John McM. Mennell, Augustus A. White, Robert Maigne (France), Alf Nachemson (Sweden), Akio Sato (Japan), and Sir Sydney Sunderland (Australia); osteopaths J.S. Denslow, Philip Greenman, William L. Johnston, and George Northup; chiropractors David C. Drum, Ronald Gitelman, Scott Haldeman, Joseph W. Howe, Joseph Janse, Martin E. Jenness, and Andries M. Kleynhans (Australia); and basic scientists Chung-Ha Suh, Irvin M. Korr, and Seth Sharpless. As expected, fundamental differences emerged, but there was substantial agreement on many points. Goldstein (1975, p 6) cautiously concluded:

> There was a plea for precise definition of terms (e.g., subluxation; clinical improvement) so that communication could be even more meaningful in the future. It was also suggested that precision of terminology would provide a basis for focused investigations, comparisons of results, and cooperative efforts among investigators. . . . The efficacy of spinal manipulative therapy is based on a body of clinical experience in the "hands" of specialized clinicians. Chiropractors, osteopathic physicians, medical manipulative specialists and their patients all claim manipulation provides relief from pain, particularly back pain, and sometimes cure, and may be dangerous, particularly if used by non-physicians. The available data do not clarify either view. However, most participants in the Workshop felt that manipulative therapy was of clinical value in the treat-

ment of back pain, a difference of opinion focusing on the issues of indications, contraindications and the precise scientific basis for the results obtained. No evidence was presented to substantiate the usefulness of manipulative therapy at this time in the treatment of visceral disorders.

In reality, William D. Miller's (1975) paper dealt with the treatment of visceral disorders by SMT. At a later date Goldstein (1978) reflected on the workshop:

> What did the Workshop accomplish? It did several things. First, it provided the Congress and specifically the Senate Subcommittee with the information it had requested: an analysis of the status at that time of the research basic to the clinical use of manipulative therapy. Second, it demonstrated that scientists from several disciplines and clinicians from several professions are able to communicate meaningfully on a research subject of mutual interest, even when the scientific and clinical aspects of that subject are as controversial as is this one. But perhaps of most far reaching importance, the Workshop documented that although there are a number of meaningful basic and clinical research questions about manipulative therapy and vertebral biomechanics that are amenable to investigation, there was relatively little quantitative data either in support or in opposition to the several clinical hypotheses. . . . I suspect the NINCDS Workshop cleared the air by demonstrating that there are precise scientific issues relevant to manipulative therapy that deserve research attention.

My opinion is that, as impressive as were the substantive conclusions of the conference regarding SMT, most striking was that the conference took place at all. It was the first public recognition that a scientific basis for chiropractic exists that merits discussion by distinguished experts in the field. It was also an illustration of how political pressure (in this case lobbying Congress) can influence scientific behavior. The symbolism of the meeting could hardly be exaggerated. Despite the reported remark by a medical skeptic, "I hope this meeting stamps out chiropractic," the face-to-face discussion among the three groups established the basis for a later series of interdisciplinary conferences on the spine, with sponsorship alternating between chiropractors, osteopaths, and the interdisciplinary American Back Society, established in 1982 under the leadership of Aubrey A. Schwartz, M.D. (Anderson R, 1989). Stemming from these conferences have come publications edited by Buerger and Greenman (1985), Buerger and Tobis (1977), Greenman (1984), Haldeman (1980; 1992a), Korr (1978a), and Mazzarelli (1982). My remark that physical therapists perhaps should have been invited to the conference may not have been misplaced after all, for they now participate regularly in meetings of the North American Academy of Manipulative Medicine and of the American Back Society. It is especially significant that the American Back Society and the new World Federation of Chiropractic met jointly in Toronto in 1991.

What has interdisciplinary research produced? In a carefully controlled study that Cassidy and Kirkaldi-Willis (1990) described as the only trial of manipulation for lumbar disk herniation, Nwuga (1982) randomly assigned 51 Nigerian women with prolapsed intervertebral disk to a conventional regimen of heat, exercise, and postural education or to lumbar rotation by a physical therapist, and found manipulation therapy superior. However, when Haldeman (1983, pp 67, 63) surveyed studies of SMT, he found that "the poorest response to manipulation in these studies was in patients with documented disc herniation," and that "the effectiveness of manipulation is greatest in patients who have acute pain and no leg or neurologic deficits." (Note that he did not say that there was *no* response to manipulation in the patients with disk herniation.) Deyo (1983) surveyed 59 trials of conservative therapy for low back pain, 14 of which involved spinal manipulation, and concluded that the two best (Farrell and Twomey, 1982; Hoehler et al., 1981) "suggested immediate benefit of manipulation but no long-term benefits."

Brunarski (1984) summarized 50 clinical trials of spinal manipulation, 14 of which made specific reference to chiropractic. With more than 8,300 subjects involved, he classified 19 of the trials as "descriptive in design," 12 as "case control studies," and 15 as "randomized control trials," and summarized:

> Overall it would seem that there is sufficient evidence to suggest that spinal manipulative therapy may be more effective than standard medical care in the management of painful neuromusculoskeletal conditions, most notably that of low back pain.

His conclusions were:

1. Manual therapy was superior to placebos.
2. There was greater mobility following manipulation.
3. The duration of treatment was shorter for the manipulated groups.
4. There was improved lateral flexion and rotation after manipulation.

Not included in the Brunarski study was the 1985 research report by W.H. Kirkaldi-Willis, M.D., and J.D. Cassidy, D.C., "Spinal Manipulation in the Treatment of Low-Back Pain" (1985; see also Cassidy and Kirkaldi-Willis, 1988), which presented impressive findings regarding chiropractic's efficacy. One of the first publications in a medical journal to recognize a chiropractor as a joint author and research collaborator, it summarizes the results of chiropractic-medical collaboration in the Low-Back Pain Clinic at the University of Saskatchewan Hospital in Saskatoon. (It is significant that this occurred in Canada and was published in a Canadian journal not read by many MDs in the United States.) Their conclusions were:

> We recently completed a prospective observational study of spinal manipulation in 283 patients with chronic low back and leg pain. . . . Our patient population was taken from a specialized university back pain clinic reserved for patients who have not responded to previous conservative or operative treatment. All of the patients in this study were totally disabled (grade 4 disability) at the onset of treatment. . . . They were given a two or three week regimen of daily spinal manipulations by an experienced chiropractor. The results of this treatment were assessed one month later and at three month intervals thereafter.

> No patients were made worse by manipulation, yet many experienced an increase in pain during the first week of treatment. Patients undergoing manipulative treatment must therefore be reassured that the initial discomfort is only temporary. In our experience, anything less than two weeks of daily manipulation is inadequate for chronic back pain

patients. . . . Almost 25% of our patients had undergone previous surgical treatment for their back pain. . . .

Manipulation requires much practice to acquire the necessary skills and competence. It is a fulltime vocation: few medical practitioners have the time or inclination to master it. Most doctors, whether family physicians or surgeons, will wish to refer their patients to a practitioner of manipulative therapy with whom they can cooperate, whose work they know and whom they can trust.

The 2- to 3-week regimen of daily SMT by a chiropractor produced improvement with "no restrictions for work or other activities" in 79% of 54 patients with posterior joint syndrome, in 93% of 69 patients with sacroiliac joint syndrome, in 88% of 48 patients with both syndromes, and in 36% to 50% of the 112 patients with more serious disorders. Yet as late as 1987 the Quebec Task Force on Spinal Disorders (Spitzer et al., 1987) concluded: "There is no properly controlled chiropractic study on this subject [spinal manipulation]."

Contrasting two modes of treatment for low back pain, Waddell (1987) comments:

Rest is the commonest treatment prescribed after analgesics but is based on a doubtful rationale, and there is little evidence of any lasting benefit. There is, however, little doubt about the harmful effects, especially of prolonged bed rest.

Kirkaldy-Willis and Cassidy agree. They survey research on low back pain in a paper titled "Health Through Activity" (1989) and document that chiropractors' mode of treatment keeping patients ambulatory and at work if possible is superior to bed rest:

1. This brief review demonstrates clearly the deleterious effects of prolonged bed rest and other forms of immobilization of the spine in treating low back pain.

2. Muscle atrophy, joint stiffness, and impairment of the circulation together with fibrosis around small nerve endings are all things that result from immobilization and lead to a very marked degree of disability. The physical changes in the structure of the back may be difficult to reverse. . . .

3. The most important practical conclusions are that bed rest, even when essential, should be of very short duration; activity should be encouraged from a very early stage. It should be increased in tempo as quickly as possible and those forms of treatment that are active in nature are clearly the most desirable.

4. These desirable methods of treatment include: (1) Back School, (2) Manipulation, (3) Physical Therapy, and (4) Local Anesthetic Injections. Each and all of these modalities should be so structured as to put the greatest possible emphasis on the patient taking the responsibility for his/her own healing—and become his/her own back doctor.

5. In educating the patient (back school) the physician or the therapist should emphasize: (a) function is more important than structure; (b) restoration of function is more important than relief of pain (the latter often follows the former).

Howard Vernon (1991, pp 380–381) offers a broader interpretation of why the "chiropractic healing encounter" works so well and often. He uses the "illness behavior model" to distinguish between *disease* and *illness,* the latter defined as "the subjective experience of the disease by the person in his/her environment." He cites Waddell's statistics that "while physical severity accounts for 40% of the disability in low back pain, psychological distress and illness behavior account for a further 31%." And like Waddell, he argues for the importance of moving "from rest to recovery," the key elements of which are emphasis on ambulatory care, rational explanation to patients in order to reduce distress, and emphasis on recovery of full function rather than on rest and symptomatic relief. Vernon (1991, p 379) therefore defines chiropractic as "a primary-contact practitioner-based system of conservative care for patients with low back pain disorders, which emphasizes an interventional, but participatory, multi-model approach to functional recovery and restoration in an ambulatory setting. Inherent principles of care involve thorough diagnosis, individualized treatment which is built around manual techniques, evaluation based on achievement of functional objectives, and a keen interest in after-care and prevention." (The more specifically psychologic dimensions of chiropractic care are developed further in Chapter 10.)

Thus far I have discussed chiropractic theory in general and presented some examples of research on SMT, but I have not discussed specific chiropractic theories. I shall now try to remedy that. Scott Haldeman (1978, p 63), a chiropractor with a doctorate in neurophysiology as well as a medical degree, published a table titled "A Few of the Proposed Mechanisms of Action of Manipulative Therapy with One Author Who Has Supported Each Theory":

1. Restore vertebrae to normal position	Galen (c. 200)
2. Straighten the spine	Pare (1562)
3. Relieve interference with blood flow	Still (1899)
4. Relieve nerve compression	Palmer (1910)
5. Relieve irritation of sympathetic chain	Kunert (1965)
6. Mobilize fixated vertebral units	Gillet (1951)
7. Shift a fragment of intervertebral disc	Cyriax (1975)
8. Mobilize posterior joints	Mennell (1960)
9. Remove interference with cerebro-spinal fluid circulation	DeJarnette (1967)
10. Stretch contracted muscles causing relaxation	Perl (1975)
11. Correct abnormal somatovisceral reflexes	Homewood (1962)
12. Remove "irritable" spinal lesions	Korr (1976)
13. Stretching and tearing of adhesions around the nerve root	Chrisman et al. (1964)
14. Reduce distortion of the annulae	Farfan (1973)

Using references such as these, Robert A. Leach in *The Chiropractic Theories: A Synopsis of Chiropractic Research* (1986) summarized interrelated hypothetical propositions comprising chiropractic theory that are susceptible to empiric proof or disproof. I am well aware of my limitations as a social scientist to evaluate these propositions, but I can note that his text is nearly unique in the field and is widely used in chiropractic education. After a few preliminary remarks, I present the propositions that seem most important. Leach (1986, p 17) accepts the definition of "subluxation" proposed in the NINCDS conference (Goldstein, 1975, p 4): "An alteration of the normal dynamics, anatomical or physiological relationships of contiguous articular structures." And from the same conference he cites (1986, p 18) the ACA definition (Schafer, 1973) used by Haldeman (1975, p 217): "A manipulable spinal lesion . . . [has] the following characteristics: vertebral malposition, abnormal vertebral motion, lack of joint play, palpable soft tissue changes, and muscle contraction or imbalance."

Leach (1986, pp 5–6, 18) lists 18 "categories of spinal and paraspinal subluxations," asserting:

> The axiom common to all chiropractic theories presented herein is that an intervertebral subluxation somehow alters the normal neurophysiological balance found in a healthy individual. There follow four important secondary hypotheses which propose that in some cases this intervertebral subluxation may cause (a) somatic afferent bombardment of the dorsal horn cells within the spinal cord, (b) spinal cord compression, (c) spinal nerve root compression, or (d) vertebrobasilar arterial insufficiency in humans. . . . The principal quarternary hypothesis is that spinal nerve root compression, axoplasmic aberration, or aberrant somatoautonomic reflexes may contribute to neurodystrophic phenomena.

He gives credit to both osteopathic and chiropractic researchers (Leach, 1981, p S-20):

> Perhaps the most clinically important of the chiropractic tenets are the Somatoautonomic Reflex (SAR) and the Spinal Fixation (SF) hypotheses (Haldeman, 1978; Korr, 1974). These hypotheses are based upon the concept of vertebral motor unit fixation, with subsequent afferent bombardment to dorsal horn cells and disturbance of autonomic function. Based upon the work of Schmorl and Junghanns (1971), Hviid (1955), Homewood (1962), Denslow (1944), Korr (1978b), and others, these hypotheses can be divided into four chronological events:
>
> 1. Spinal Fixation—vertebra in normal or abnormal position but is fixed within its normal range of motion.
> 2. Soft Tissue Insult—kinesthetic receptors and paraspinal musculature involved.
> 3. Nociceptive, Aberrant Output—somatic afferent bombardment of dorsal horn cells.
> 4. Facilitation—segmental facilitation affects normal somatic as well as autonomic reflex traffic.

Concerning the hypothesis relating to spinal nerve root compression hypothesis, Leach (1986, p 70) cautiously states:

Subluxation pathophysiology includes various stages of degenerative and regenerative processes that impair the function of the involved nerve roots, as well as clinical signs and symptoms of intermittent claudication, leg weakness, sensory changes, limitation of mobility of the involved joint, paravertebral muscle spasm, scoliosis, and depressed or absent reflexes in the area of cutaneous innervation. The conclusion is reached that although there is a definite possibility that nerve root compression or irritation may be caused by intervertebral subluxations, especially in the cervical and the lumbar spine, it has not been proven that this relationship is a common clinical entity.

Regarding the hypothesis concerning cord compression, a condition even rarer than nerve root compression, he (1986, pp 83–84) states:

Severe subluxations have been demonstrated as a cause of spinal cord compression. . . . Possible effects of cord compression include headache, numbness, tingling, paresthesias, quadriplegia, transient paraplegia, practically any combination of neurologic findings, and even death.

Regarding the spinal fixation hypothesis he (1986, p 105) states:

SF is likely to create some degree of interruption of normal neural transmission within the CNS, although the phenomena of neuronal pools, descending inhibition, anti-dromic discharge, etc., make it difficult at best to predict the effect of any given SF on CNS function.

Regarding the vertebrobasilar arterial insufficiency hypothesis he (1986, p 119) states:

It is hypothesized that chiropractors may be inadvertently correcting this condition in many individuals, by correcting subluxations.

Regarding the axoplasmic aberration hypothesis, Leach (1986, p 129) writes that it

is valid in that when spinal nerves or roots are compressed or irritated by intervertebral subluxation, AXT [axoplasmic transport] may certainly be altered with significant consequences.

Regarding the somatoautonomic reflex hypothesis, he (1986, p 150) states:

It appears from medical and osteopathic clinical research that such reflexes can set into motion a wide variety of abnormal pathological and functional processes, including such conditions as asthma, bronchitis, acute pulmonary atelectasis, muscular atrophy and degeneration, gastrointestinal complaints, coronary arteriospasm associated with ischemic heart disease, and pain actually referred to any portion of the body. . . . The SAR hypothesis may be the most logical justification for the use of chiropractic adjustment for conditions other than pain syndromes.

And regarding the neurodystrophic hypothesis "that neural dysfunction is stressful to the visceral and other body structures, and that this 'lowered tissue resistance' can modify the non-specific and specific immune responses, and alter the trophic function of the involved nerves," he (1986, p 185) states:

> There is overwhelming evidence to support the chiropractic *neurodystrophic hypothesis,* but there is scant evidence to directly link the vertebral lesion with immunological competence in human clinical studies.

Finally, Leach notes (1981, p S-22) Haldeman's (1978, pp 53–75) "four criteria that must be established through research before a neurobiologic mechanism of manipulative therapy can be properly evaluated":

1. A specific manipulative procedure must be demonstrated to have consistent clinical results under controlled conditions in the treatment of a specific pathological process.
2. The specific manipulative procedure must be demonstrated to have a specific effect on the musculoskeletal system to which it is applied.
3. The musculoskeletal effect caused by the manipulation must be shown to have a specific influence on the nervous system.
4. This influence on the nervous system must be demonstrated to have some beneficial effect on the abnormal function of an organ, tissue pathology or symptom complex under study.

Stated so simply and clearly, these criteria seem obvious. Osteopath Philip E. Greenman has argued (cited by Gunby 1983, p 3149): "Efficacy of manipulative therapy can be explained in various terms—temporal, functional, or analgesic, for example—and we have to agree on what we are trying to measure."

Scientific support for SMT can be found in medical and osteopathic sources, some of which have been cited. Osteopathic researcher Irvin M. Korr (1978a, p xv) defined manipulative therapy as follows:

> Manipulative therapy involves the application of accurately determined and specifically directed manual forces to the body. Its objective is to improve mobility in areas that are restricted, whether the restrictions are within joints, in connective tissues or in skeletal muscles. The consequences may be the improvement of posture and locomotion, the relief of pain and discomfort, the improvement of function elsewhere in the body and enhancement of the sense of well-being.

Specifically he noted (1981, p 451):

> Evidence for the trophic function of nerves includes examples of the atrophy of denervation in organs, of the way nerves influence morphogenesis, genic expression, and regeneration, and of nerve-to-muscle transmission. Research supports the view that the trophic influence of nerves on target organs depends largely on delivery of specific neuronal proteins by means of axonal transport and junctional transfer. There is also retrograde transport from nerve endings to cell bodies. Factors such as nerve or root deformation and hyperactivity of peripheral neurons may adversely affect trophic influences, resulting in aberrations of structure, functions and metabolism, and, ultimately, somatic dysfunction. The effectiveness of manipulative therapy is probably due largely to its amelioration of trophic factors.

Terrett and Vernon (1984; Vernon et al. 1986) suggest that the production of β-endorphins by SMT may explain why it helps relieve back pain. J.K. Patterson (1988) in the medical publication *The Practitioner* expands on this hypothesis:

> Every manipulation provides a massive mechanoceptive input to the spinal cord, concentrated mainly at the segmental level of its application. . . . Such mechanoceptive input results in endorphin release at the basal nucleus, which (dependent also upon many other factors) may partially or totally inhibit the transmission of nociceptive input through the "gate," so blocking pain perception. Prolongation of this effect is related to the local absence of any enzyme capable of destroying this particular endorphin in situ, and to the poor blood supply in this part of the spinal cord.

A survey and critique of relevant theory and research is presented in *Musculoskeletal Manipulation: Evaluation of the Scientific Evidence* by Tobis and Hoehler (1986; see also Curtis, 1988; Evans DP, and Hawthorne, 1985; Greenman, 1989), who show why it is nearly impossible to design a properly controlled and blinded study of the effectiveness of manipulation. However, Hoehler et al. (1981) earlier argued that "soft-tissue massage is an adequate control for the placebo effect of manipulative therapy" because it permits blinding of patients and evaluators if not of manipulators.

Much of the documentation for two early compilations of research by Weiant (1945; Weiant and Goldschmidt, 1958) came from researchers in Germany, where Manuel Medizin has been practiced by regular MDs, Naturaerzte, and Heilpraktikers (Biedermann, 1959). A Czech MD who strongly advocates manual medicine, Karel Lewit (1985, p 7), writes:

> The most important pioneer of manual manipulation, however, was [James] Mennell (1952), an outspoken protagonist of osteopathic techniques which he also taught mainly to physiotherapists. It is in a way paradoxical that his famous disciple Cyriax, whose *Orthopedic Medicine* (1975) is the classical textbook for clinical assessment of motor function, did not follow his predecessor in developing these techniques further.

Nevertheless, Cyriax has devoted much of his life to teaching SMT to MDs and physical therapists. The son and grandson of well-known medical manipulators, he is amusingly correct when he complains (cited in Terrett, 1986, p 151): "I have become known as that odd and scarcely respectable phenomenon: a doctor who manipulates and, worse still, teaches those techniques."

Lewit noted that the International Federation of Manual Medicine, formed in 1965, has 21 national associations affiliated with it. In 1966 the North American Academy of Manipulative Medicine (NAAMM), a small and not particularly prestigious group in American medicine, was founded. Among its leaders have been James Mennell's son John McM. Mennell, J.F. Bourdillon, and more recently Scott Haldeman. The NAAMM permitted the first presentation by osteopaths at its 1974 meeting in Vancouver, British Columbia, which I was invited to attend. At my suggestion the NAAMM also invited chiropractor Scott Haldeman, already a Ph.D. in neurology and at that time a medical student at the University of British Columbia. After receiving his M.D. degree in 1982, he was elected president of NAAMM (now the name changed to the North American Academy of Musculoskeletal Medicine), which now includes DOs in addition to MDs, and dentists and physical therapists as associate members. The American Back Society includes all of these plus DCs, which helps promote interdisciplinary interest and cooperation in research on SMT. The North American Spine Society includes at least four chiropractors as members, a requirement for which is 4 years of post-professional education ("North American Spine Society Gives Chiropractic Adjustments Top Rating," 1991).

In an editorial in the *Journal of Manual Medicine* Dvorak (1989) wrote:

> A recent survey by the Swiss Medical Association showed that 14 percent of all MDs went through the educational program given by the association, 24 percent of the MDs in the canton of Berne are performing their own treatments regularly, and 56 percent are referring patients to other MDs or chiropractors for manual treatment. Of the 700 members of the SAMM (Swiss Association for Manual Medicine), 97 percent are Board Certified physicians, mainly in the fields of rheumatology, general practice, neurology, etc.

A Danish chiropractor reported in 1983: "In Denmark there are 300 physiotherapists who manipulate, 600 MDs who manipulate and 160 chiropractors are respected members of the health care team and are considered to be specialists" (Brennan, 1983c). In Germany "more than 2000 regular physicians belong to the Medical Research and Work Group for Chiropractic" (Baer, 1991). Sandoz (1978), a Swiss chiropractor with an excellent understanding of the European situation, decried the iatrogenesis caused by inadequately trained MDs trying to practice manual medicine (Kleynhans, 1980, pp 361–363).

While chiropractors always feared that MDs would take up SMT and practice it under another name, U.S. MDs have mostly ignored "manual medicine." In 1960 John Mennell wrote:

> The public soon came to realize that they would find greater relief more quickly and more economically from osteopathic and chiropractic treatment of their backs than they would from orthodox medical treatment.

Mennell (1989, pp 231–232) reports that little attention still is paid to the musculoskeletal system in medical education and to the important concepts of "joint play," "joint dysfunction," and "joint manipulation," to which he contributed so much:

> I am sure we were exposed to orthopedics sometime in our clinical training. . . . Did anyone ever come to our anatomy and physiology laboratory sessions to correlate what we were learning with clinical problems of the musculoskeletal system? Maybe it does not matter very much whether they did or not, as one cannot study movement in a cadaver as movement is singular to life. Now, some medical schools, though not chiropractic schools, are even giving up having students dissect the extremities in their anatomy courses; it was always an unusual student who ever dissected the back. And to compound our problems, the simple science of mechanics has always been cloaked in the guise of something new and complicated, called kinesiology. We easily forget the simple things which are the basis of movement.

Then suddenly we find ourselves in practice faced by patients most (80%) of whom complain to us of some pain related to some part of the musculoskeletal system. Eighty percent may sound high, yet remember that visceral and systemic diseases very frequently manifest themselves initially as musculoskeletal pain. . . .

The word "manipulation" is used in medicine (when it is used at all) to mean anything from the gentlest examining maneuver, using well-defined techniques relating to the treatment of dislocations and fractures, to the greatest assaults perpetrated on the human frame of a conscious or, worse, an unconscious patient in the name of therapy. Even then, when used fairly appropriately to describe a therapeutic modality in the treatment of musculoskeletal pain, its dangers are acclaimed while its potential for good is whispered and even explained away by the suggestion that whatever might have been relieved was probably a psychosomatic phenomenon anyway. . . .

Loss of a functional movement is a symptom of something, not a cause. To understand that "something" we must return to mechanics. Everything that moves has built into it "play" between the moving parts. If the play is lost, the function of that thing is impaired or lost. . . . There are play movements in every synovial joint in the body, and these can be clearly demonstrated. They are specific to each joint but common to every joint of the same kind. The muscles cannot produce them; they can only be produced by an outside force. I named these movements "joint play" movements. Virtually all of them are less than ⅛ of an inch in range within a joint.

When these joint play movements are impaired or lost, the function of the joint in which they should be present is impaired or lost. The impairment of function in the human joint is associated with pain. . . . I call this diagnosis "joint dysfunction."

It is logical to look for a mechanical means of restoring what is lost to normal. This is "joint manipulation." With normal mechanics having been restored, it is reasonable and predictable that the symptoms will be relieved and normal function restored. . . .

Surely this brings the rather nebulous concepts of manipulation into the realm of orthodox medical and chiropractic thinking.

In a paper presented in June 1990 Mennell clarified further some of these points:

Mechanical pathology is a new concept to most practitioners of the healing arts. So far as we know, there are no changes at the cellular level in mechanics and it seems unlikely that there are because relief of symptoms on restoring normal mechanics is immediate. . . . All impairments in the musculoskeletal system are associated with symptoms of pain and loss of movement to some degree or another. . . . We have not yet adequately settled the question as to whether we treat pain or loss of movement by our mechanical treatment which we call manipulation. . . . Any reference to any topographical area in therapy is absolutely contraindicated. SMT is meaningless. One never manipulates a wrist, a foot, a knee, an ankle, a shoulder, an elbow, a hand, a hip or the spine: one manipulates a joint or each joint in any given topographical area after detecting loss of joint play in it (them) by using manipulative examining techniques designed to demonstrate normal play.

He credits Lewit with making the fundamental point that the sole consequence of loss of joint play is motion change, not structural change.

Although Haldeman (1983) concluded that the only syndromes for which there is any evidence of efficacy are somatic disorders, there is evidence of benefit in some O-type (organic) conditions (e.g., Bourdillon, 1987, p 5; Klougart et al., 1989; Kunert, 1965; Miller WD, 1975; Wiles, 1990). Australian chiropractor Lines (1989, p 2) remarks:

> How many among us cannot cite cases of asthma, dysmenorrhea, hay fever, constipation, eneuresis, among others, which appear to have responded well to chiropractic treatment?

Another chiropractor remarked: "The fun begins when a woman being treated for low back pain suddenly finds that her dysmenorrhea has cleared up." A report in an optometric journal of blindness following neck injury being cured by SMT (Gilman and Bergstrand, 1990) produced a flurry of letters by chiropractors citing similar cases from their practices (*DC* 1990 8(18):26–27). As Sid Williams (1991, p 4) concisely put it: "Chiropractic care has a narrow scope of practice with broad body implications."

A broader conception of the subluxation is reflected in the currently more popular term "vertebral subluxation complex" (VSC), which according to Swiss researcher R.W. Sandoz (1989; Dishman 1988), "takes into account the complexities of this clinical entity characterized by the variable interplay of articular, neurological, muscular, psychological and, to some extent, even visceral phenomena." As Morinis (1980, p 117) so well put it: "Subluxation is not a tangible entity but a concept in the process of being changed and revised at all times."

Some studies have suggested that although SMT often provides more rapid relief from pain, its long-range benefits may not be significantly greater than those of alternative therapies (Tobis et al., 1981; Deyo, 1983; Weber H, 1983; Gunby, 1983; Curtis, 1988; MacDonald R and Bell, 1990) and have concluded that chiropractic is therefore without great merit. However, Hadler et al. (1987) point out: "In view of the extraordinary presence of low-back pain and its pervasive impact in so many social spheres, the ability to abrogate an episode of backache, even by a few days, has major ramifications." In 1991 the total costs of back pain in the United States, including lost wages, was estimated at $40 billion ("High Cost of Back Pain," 1991). The following statement from a literature survey prepared for the National Center for Health Statistics (MacDonald MJ, 1988, p 7) therefore is pertinent:

> Overemphasis on the self-limiting nature of many of the presenting conditions, however, tends to obscure the fact that in reported clinical cases, clinical trials and retrospective studies of thousands of cases, chiropractic treatment has resulted in faster (sometimes immediate) relief and quicker return to work (or restored functioning). Moreover, as shown in the paragraphs which follow, it has done so at a cost lower than typically encountered in orthodox medicine.

An especially well designed 3-year randomized comparison in England of chiropractic and hospital outpatient treatment of low back pain of mechanical origin in 741 patients (Meade et al., 1990) concluded that chiropractic treatment

> was more effective than hospital outpatient management, mainly for patients with chronic or severe back pain. . . . Chiropractic almost certainly confers worthwhile, long term benefit in comparison with hospital outpatient management. *The benefit is seen mainly in those with chronic or severe pain. Introducing chiropractic into NHS* [National Health Service] *should be considered* [italics supplied].

This study is all the more remarkable because 72% of the hospital outpatients received manipulation by physical therapists using Maitland (1964) technique and 12% by Cyriax (1975) technique, clearly demonstrating that chiropractors' technique is superior, according to an editorial in *Lancet,* "Chiropractors and Low Back Pain" (July 28, 1990), which noted that it took 15 years after the Cochran Commission recommendation for the Medical Research Council to authorize the clinical trial. The editorial concluded that although more studies are needed to confirm the results and to "dissect the causes, . . . chiropractic treatment should be taken seriously by conventional medicine, which means both doctors and physiotherapists. Physiotherapists need to . . . take on board the skills that chiropractors have developed so successfully." However, a Dutch medical team (Assendelft et al., 1991) severely criticized the British study on methodologic grounds. It is ironic that chiropractic, a U.S. contribution, has met with so much less prejudice in other countries.

In an article in *Medical Economics,* "How Being a Chiropractor Makes Me a Better MD," Haldeman (1982, pp 132–133) wrote:

> I find no conflict or incompatibility. . . . Chiropractors throughout the world see almost a million patients every day. They fill a void that exists because the whole concept of laying on of hands—manual medicine—as a method of treating musculoskeletal problems has been almost totally ignored by the medical profession, particularly in North America. . . . I believe manipulation has a definite place in health care.

Examples of MD/DC cooperation are *The Back Power Program* (Imrie and Barbuto, 1988), based on a 10-year collaboration in a Toronto back care center serving 70 local industries and 30,000 workers; and *Conservative Care of Low Back Pain* (White AH, and Anderson, 1991). In sports medicine chiropractors collaborate with MDs as part of official medical teams serving athletes at olympics and other international sports events (Schafer, 1982). The Commonwealth of Independent States named chiropractor Stephen J. Press chief of its medical delegation to the 1992 Olympic Winter Games in France ("DC to Direct Medical Services for Soviet Olympic Team," 1991). Even hostile medical groups such as The National Council Against Health Fraud ("Position Paper on Chiropractic," 1985; Barrett, 1980) concede that manipulation can achieve some remarkable cures (citing Duke and Spreadbury, 1981; Farrell and Twomey, 1982; Kane et al., 1974) and "urge educators to work with reformist chiropractic organizations to incorporate chiropractic education into accredited universities." Medical manipulator Bourdillon (1987, p 9) states that chiropractors "should be regarded as a challenge to the [medical] profession to develop adequate theories that will explain their successes and improve methods of achieving this success."

Studies of the reliability of vertebral "analysis" of the locations of the VSC have not been especially encouraging (Keating, 1989b; Nansel et al., 1989), although such studies usually have been limited to "normal" students rather than patients with significant lesions (Robert A. Leach, personal communication, 1990). Some chiropractors, like many MDs, have even questioned whether a subluxation really exists (e.g., Brantingham, 1988). And Harry Rosenfield (1986), long-time attorney for the ACA, created a storm of resentment when he suggested that the term be dropped for political reasons because it evokes cultist images. Others would prefer the phrase "spinal adjustive treatment" rather than SMT so as to preserve traditional chiropractic terminology. Charles A. Lantz (1990) has written a strong defense of the "subluxation."

Sometimes there is residual pain after SMT, as a recent publication (Moore, 1989, p 103) designed for popular and patient consumption states: "Following manipulation 40 percent of patients are said to suffer with diffuse pain which comes on fairly soon after treatment and lasts from six to eight hours. The reaction results from release of strong adhesions around the joints and usually occurs after the first treatment; it is not so common after subsequent treatments." It also is more likely to occur in the case of a long-standing problem.

Contraindications to SMT have been noted. Kleynhans (1980), Tobis and Hoehler (1986, pp 23–26), and Terrett (1988) treat them at length, and the literature also contains some reports of serious injury (Dan and Saccasan, 1983; Gallinaro and Cartesegna, 1983; Livingston, 1971; Wilcher 1989a). James Cyriax (Schiotz and Cyriax, 1975, pp 106–121) follows his chapter on "Errors in Manipulation" with a chapter titled "Perils of not Manipulating"! Chiropractors claim that the risks have been exaggerated by critics and that problems occur far less frequently than the iatrogenesis of medication errors, side effects and toxic interactions, infections endemic to hospitals, and surgical deaths. In support of their arguments they point to the relatively low cost of their malpractice insurance compared with that of medical general practitioners and specialists, despite chiropractor Peter J. Modde's (1979) prediction that chiropractors would soon suffer many malpractice suits. In one of the documents submitted in the antitrust trial (Wilk, 1976, Plaintiff's Exhibit No. 439) an official of Blue Shield wrote: "Doyl Taylor . . . urged that we stay clear of attempts to show [chiropractors'] civil malpractice suits. With the relative weight in numbers against physicians he felt we'd be playing with dynamite." He was right. In a *Medical Economics* article Holoweiko (1987) reported that one of every 23 DCs was sued in 1986, compared with one of every five MDs and DOs, and the results of the suits were that for chiropractors (who paid an average insurance premium of $1,393) 45% of the suits were closed without payment, with an average cost of those resolved of $28,162, whereas for MDs and DOs (whose median insurance premium was $8,346) 57% of the suits were closed without payment but the average cost of resolution of the others was $80,741. Concern over malpractice prompted James D. Harrison, ICA

General Counsel since 1948, to publish *Chiropractic Practice Liability* (1990) and Louis K. Campbell and colleagues to publish *Risk Management in Chiropractic: Developing Malpractice Prevention Strategies* (1990).

In recent years the greatest concern has been whether a rotary cervical manipulation could cause a cerebrovascular accident (stroke) by compressing the vertebral artery of an especially susceptible person (Daneshend et al., 1984; Jaskoviac, 1980; Krueger and Okazaki, 1980; Schellhas et al., 1980; Simmons et al., 1982). The likelihood of stroke has been estimated roughly as one in 1 million adjustments, varying perhaps from one in 400,000 to one in 6 million adjustments (Sullivan, 1989, p 12). A medical source (Dvorak and Orelli, 1985) has estimated the risk at one in 20 million, and contrasted it with the estimated risk of death of one in 700 that the Food and Drug Administration accepted when it reapproved (after banning) injection of the drug chimopapain for treating herniated spinal disks (Fager, 1984, p 326). The Midwest Research Institute report to the National Center for Health Statistics (MacDonald MJ, 1988, p 6) concluded: "The number of such complications each year is so low that a percentage calculation is meaningless." Chiropractors are well alerted to this risk and know how to cope with it (George et al., 1981).

Regarding the allegation that chiropractors overuse x-ray studies, the Midwest Research Institute (MacDonald MJ, 1988, p 5), using 1980 data from the National Center for Health Statistics, reported that "chiropractors take x-rays for approximately 6 percent of patient visits, a slightly lower frequency than the 7.3 percent for medical doctors." Since chiropractic patients usually have more repeat visits, there may be more x-ray films per patient. However, because the conditions that chiropractors treat often involve potentially serious spinal disease they often require use of x-rays, computed tomography (CT), and magnetic resonance imaging (MRI) for differential diagnoses in order to distinguish cases requiring referral and those where SMT is contraindicated, both to practice "defensive medicine" and to better serve their patients.

One of the best lay explanations of chiropractic can be found in "Chiropractic: All That It's Cracked Up to Be?," in Judylaine Fine's *Conquering Back Pain* (1987).

Section 3

Chiropractic Art (Technique)

A. Earl Homewood (1988) wrote: "The *Art of Application* makes for success of the method, not the brand of technique." Clarence Weiant (in Weiant and Goldschmidt, 1958, p 117) cites a German physician:

> I see in chiropractic no science, but an excellent method of treatment, a handiwork, as the name implies. And I must state that I prefer a well understood handiwork to a badly understood science.

Leach (1986, p 15) defines a chiropractic adjustment thus:

> Chiropractic manipulation is called *adjustment* and involves the utilization of short-lever, specific, high-velocity, controlled forceful thrusts by hand or instrument which are directed at specific articulations. Although the actual techniques of chiropractic adjustment differ fundamentally from those of any other form of manipulation, the most significant difference lies in the theories behind its application.

It should be apparent that there is a fairly general consensus that SMT works. How it works, why it works, for what conditions it works, for whom (patient or chiropractor) it works, and which of the many techniques of SMT work best for which kinds of conditions all need to be studied in carefully controlled basic and clinical research. Some chiropractors still accept the simple conclusion that "chiropractic works," and want no explanation beyond that of traditional chiropractic philosophy. Some have concerned themselves only with technical matters, such as whether patients should lie prone, supine, side posture, kneeling, or sitting, and with "new moves." Chiropractors always have believed it important to differentiate a chiropractic *adjustment* from osteopathic *long-lever manipulation*. Instead of multiple osteopathic movements chiropractors insist on the importance of a quick, forceful thrust on a specific vertebral joint chosen by skillful palpation, x-ray analysis, or deduced from the patient's symptoms using "nerve tracing" expertise. In the earliest days, according to Dye (1939, pp 162–163), chiropractors often had little interest in the patient's self-report or medical records: "The history of symptoms from the patient was never considered a reliable factor. . . . Very little reliance was placed, as well, on any medical diagnosis the patient may have previously had."

Dye (1939, p 163) summarized the evolution of adjusting technique taught by B.J., from the "meric system" through "majors and minors" and "toggle recoil" to what he called "scientific chiropractic." The earliest adjustments were performed with the patient face down on a padded bench, sometimes with bags of sand on the chiropractor's shoulders to provide more force. Bloody noses were common (Dye, 1939, p 157) until special adjusting tables were designed with an opening for the nose. The Palmer Hi-Lo table, introduced about 1911, at first used compressed air to lower the table from a vertical to a horizontal position and back; later the air was replaced by springs, and finally by an electric motor (Dye, 1939, p 180). By 1910 "hot boxes" (a term introduced by D.D., referring to the inflammation caused by a subluxation) were being located by palpation along the spine (anticipating the neurocalometer), and adjustments were made, depending on the patient's symptoms, at the "heart place" (second or third dorsals), the "kidney place" (tenth to twelfth vertebrae), and so on (Dye, 1939, p 168). Dye (1939, p 117) stated that the Palmer Recoil Adjustment began in "1909–1910 and is still the basic fundamental of the present Palmer Torque-Toggle-Recoil in use in Hole-in-One." He explained (1939, p 266):

> The application of the adjusting move consists in a quick, spontaneous thrust with the hand upon the bony process of the misaligned vertebra. The effect of this thrust is not alone to move the vertebra back toward its proper position. The spontaneity of the thrust also serves to restore to a balanced tonicity the ligaments on either side of the vertebra,

and thus permit it, automatically, as it were, to return to its proper position. The imme- diate effect of the thrust on the vertebra is, therefore, a momentary relaxation of the contracted ligaments on one side. This permits the ligaments on the other side, which have been stretched beyond the limit of their elasticity, to return to their normal condi- tion. A slow continuous pressure will not accomplish this. On the contrary, it will ag- gravate the contraction of the ligaments.

Other improvements in adjusting technique came from other schools. For example, Logan basic technique emphasized the importance of the proper relationship of the sacrum to the pelvis as the basis of good posture, or alternatively of compensatory distortions. B.J. made his own contribution in this area, according to Dye (1939, p 158), when he performed the first coccygeal adjustment in the men's room of the PSC clinic (Smallie, 1990b, p 5, cites 1905 as the proper date).

What does chiropractic therapy consist of today? The report of the Midwest Re- search Institute (MacDonald MJ, 1988, p 5) offers the following explanations:

> Chiropractic Adjustment refers to the correction of a subluxated, hypomobile, or fixated vertebral or pelvic segment(s) by making a specific, predetermined adjustment. Most common among these adjustments is spinal manipulation therapy (SMT).

> Physiotherapeutic measures refer to a variety of therapies used adjunctively to the more traditional chiropractic adjustment. Procedures such as diathermy, ultra-sound, acuther- apy and hydrotherapy are often used to assist healing and strengthening in injuries of the extremities to enhance the effects of corrective treatments during recuperation. . . . Di- etary advice and nutritional supplementation, as well as professional counsel, are used as adjunctive therapies and not generally as independent treatment modalities. Advice may be given in areas such as attitudes affecting health, personal hygiene, posture, and rest to enhance the effects of the chiropractic adjustment.

Other adjuncts also are used, including exercises, traction, and orthopedic bracing. Additional chiropractic techniques were listed by Janse (1975, p 29):

> Soft tissue procedures have been developed, such as triggerpoint, pressure point and re- flex techniques for physiological input and perhaps utilizing a mechanism such as dis- persal of triggerpoints (Nimmo, 1957), reciprocal inhibition of muscles (Goodheart, 1970) or a gate control mechanism. Manipulation of the extremities has been practiced since the earliest beginnings of chiropractic.

Also often used is a simple instrument called an "activator," which has a spring-acti- vated plunger adjustable to produce a controlled force over a selected vertebra. The second National Institutes of Health grant for chiropractic research was awarded to Arlan Fuhr, D.C., in 1985 for the development of activator technique (Osterbauer and Fuhr, 1990). Tobis and Hoehler (1986, p 17) conclude:

> There are wide differences among the techniques of various manipulators. In practice, however, it would appear that all methods are empirical and there is a wide overlap of maneuvers employed by all. Perhaps the greatest difference in technique resides in the intensity of the force applied. Thus they extend from the gentle to the very powerful thrust.

P.W. Kfoury (1977) edited a catalogue of chiropractic techniques, and the ACA Council on Technic (1986) proposed consensus "Guidelines for Technic Evaluation." According to William Meeker (1990), more than 200 different brand name chiropractic techniques have been described. In 1989 a new journal, titled *Chiropractic Technique,* began publication.

The recent "NCC Announces Profile Practice of Chiropractic" (1989) outlines "the concepts and scope of practice of a graduate of National College":

> The National College of Chiropractic holds that the practice of the chiropractic physician embraces the whole person with emphasis upon conservative health care which facilitates the inherent potential of the human organism to develop and maintain a state of self-regulation and to invoke self-healing processes with minimal therapeutic risk at reasonable cost.
>
> Chiropractic practice embodies:

- Recognition of a diversity of factors which impact upon human physiology, among which are biomechanical dysfunction, genetics, trauma, hygiene, microorganisms, nutritional status, exercise, motion, posture, environment, stress, emotion and human relationships.
- Primary care of patients based upon diagnostic evaluation, including patient history, physical examination, clinical laboratory data, diagnostic imaging, and other special diagnostic measures, as well as those procedures which are unique to the chiropractic evaluation of human spinal and structural balance and integrity.
- The application of a diversity of spinal and other adjustments and manipulations for the treatment, correction, and prevention of neurologic, skeletal or soft-tissue dysfunction and the production of beneficial neurologic effects.
- The use of other conservative means including, but not limited to, nutritional counseling, physiologic therapeutics, meridian therapy/acupuncture, trigger point therapy, lifestyle counseling, emotional support and stress management.
- The chiropractic doctor is a primary-care, first-contact physician who practices within the legal scope of licensure, emphasizes the importance of the doctor/patient relationship, recognizes the need for other kinds of treatment when indicated, and who, therefore, interacts fully with other members of the health care delivery team, always in the best interest of the patient.

That is a comprehensive statement of current chiropractic practice from a broad-scope perspective.

Chapter 10

PSYCHOLOGIC DIMENSIONS OF CHIROPRACTOR-PATIENT RELATIONSHIP

The secret of the care of the patient is in caring for the patient.

Francis Weld Peabody (1927)

The art of medicine is not the same as medical science. It comprises the doctor's "bedside manner" and "clinical skill." It is the core of the doctor-patient relationship. Here I exclude the substantive therapeutic effects of biochemical or physiologic procedures, for example, drugs, vaccines, surgery, bracing, and manipulation.

With chiropractic it is especially difficult to separate physiologic from psychologic effects. Inasmuch as 90% or more of chiropractic patients receive spinal manipulative therapy (SMT), there is more bodily contact than when an MD writes a prescription after examining some bodily part, or even when he or she uses a suturing needle or scalpel, and especially when the patient is anesthetized. Hence the chiropractor-patient relationship, as many writers have observed, usually is more intimate, warmer, and therefore more meaningful to the patient. The impersonality of medical practice was described many years ago in a quotation attributed to the distinguished Harvard MD physiologist turned sociologist, L.J. Henderson (1935; 1936, p 2):

> The patient is sometimes, I think I may safely say often, a mere *case* which (not who) passes through the doctor's office, his past, present and future unknown, except within the meager abstractions of etiology, diagnosis, and prognosis, and his personality and relations with other persons not even thought of.

Henderson, whom Talcott Parsons invariably referred to as "the late, great L.J. Henderson," also is known for the following often quoted observation (cited by Gregg 1956, p 13): "I think it was about the year 1910 or 1912 when it became possible to say of the United States that a random patient with a random disease consulting a doctor chosen at random stood better than a fifty-fifty chance of benefitting from the encounter."

Sir William Osler insisted that it is as important to know the patient who has the disease as to know the disease that affects the patient. Because the chiropractic patient usually lies prone or supine, all the symbolic significance of regression to child-like dependence on a parental surrogate is available to the patient, and indeed to the doctor, if either of them has a psychologic need, usually unconscious, to indulge any relevant gratifications.

In this chapter I discuss various psychologic dimensions of the chiropractor-patient relationship, exclusive of the motivations to become a chiropractor, which were covered in Chapter 7. First I treat the psychologic dimensions of *any* doctor-patient relationship.

Section 1

Doctor-Patient Relationship

The social structure of the doctor-patient relationship and conceptualization of the sick role from a societal rather than from the patient's point of view first were clearly delineated by my mentor at Harvard University, Talcott Parsons (1951, pp 428–479). Unlike social relationships where equality between two persons is "insti-tutionalized" (i.e., supported by cultural norms), for example, husband-wife today, brother-brother, friend-friend, work associates, or fellow citizens, the doctor-patient relationship is fundamentally unequal because the doctor possesses a monopoly of the professional knowledge and skill that the patient needs. Because of expertise, the doctor has authority to direct the care of the dependent patient seeking help. (Even the etymology of the word "patient" suggests not only "suffering" but also "depen-dency.") The doctor *diagnoses* the problem, *orders* the patient to bed, *prescribes* therapies. He or she *decides* whether the patient is really sick, only imagines he is, or is malingering. Only a doctor can legitimate a sick status. If the doctor concludes there is nothing wrong with the patient, there is no legitimate illness: the patient is *not really sick.*

The inherent authority in the doctor-patient relationship gives chiropractors leverage in the health care market. Chiropractors have always accepted patients that medicine could not cure or help, as well as those rejected by MDs because they could not find a medical diagnosis or problem. Partly because chiropractors often forswore diagnosis in favor of palpating the spine for subluxated vertebrae, they welcomed patients rejected by MDs. They legitimated illness not only in the patient's eyes but in the eyes of society as well. Hence they fulfilled an important social and psychologic function for such patients.

When patients suffer, their illnesses become confounded with their personality needs, as Joseph (1942, p 2) said so well:

> When a person cries for help and response, let me say, shamelessly, because less re-
> strained by inhibition—or even if he does not express it outwardly, but is able to cover

this cry with a dignified silence, being nevertheless keenly aware of his inward cry—when such a person does not get a total response, but only a partial one, total therapy has not been achieved. The sore throat may be cured, the streptococci in the blood stream may be destroyed, but what is left is a series of usually subconscious feelings of frustration, shame, vague dissatisfaction and again insecurity, which show themselves as hate, criticism, aggression, or what the physician from his point of view calls "ingratitude."

The doctor-patient relationship provides the patient with a cluster of what psychologists call "secondary gains." Besides having his possibly doubtful sick status legitimated, the patient is relieved, at least temporarily, of whatever responsibilities he previously enjoyed, or didn't. He need not go to work or school or attend to normal, perhaps burdensome duties. He can relax, let others take over, and in an ironic sense "enjoy" being sick. If confined to bed he can regress to infantile dependence on the caregivers who "nurse" him. This maternal symbolism is especially meaningful for some patients: he is fed, washed, dressed, rubbed, and "babied." What could be more gratifying?

Jerome D. Frank, in *Persuasion and Healing* (1961), listed physicians, osteopaths, chiropractors, naturopaths, clergymen, marriage counselors, and others among those conducting psychotherapy, and argued that the characteristics of psychotherapy are common "also to methods of primitive healing, religious conversion, and even so-called brainwashing" and that "the administration of an inert medicine by a doctor to a patient is also a form of psychotherapy." What all of these have in common is the professional-client relationship and, of course, suggestion.

An important additional benefit of chiropractic treatment that has psychologic implications that may hasten recovery is that their patients usually are encouraged to remain ambulatory. They not only walk into the chiropractor's office, they usually walk out as well. (Sometimes they walk out even when wheeled or carried in.) After receiving SMT they sometimes are instructed to rest for a short time on a couch in an adjacent room, but not for long. Bed rest seldom is urged on patients. In Chapter 9 evidence was presented confirming that patients kept ambulatory recover faster than those prescribed bed rest for many spinal conditions; indeed, bed rest now is often contraindicated (Kirkaldi-Willis and Cassidy, 1989; Waddell, 1987).

It is impossible to separate completely the psychologic from the physiologic effects of *any* therapeutic procedure. Mind and body are intertwined irretrievably in ways no one has ever understood fully. L. Eugene Emerson (1929, p 40) cited Plato:

> It is not only the body which, by a sound constitution, strengthens the soul, but the well-regulated soul, by its authoritative power, maintains the body in perfect health.

The "$64,000 question" is: How do mind and body interact? Through cartesian parallelism, some process involving electrical or neural (D.D. Palmer would have said "mental") impulses, or what? That question is beyond the scope of this book and my competence.

It is apparent that both mental and somatic sensations are present whenever emotions, dreams, fear, or pain are experienced. In psychosomatic illnesses the causal chain usually is presumed to go from the psyche to the soma. But the causal chain can go in the opposite, somatopsychic, direction; somatic injury *always* produces psychic manifestations. The most common psychologic reaction to serious illness, beyond the pain and damage, is depression. Usually there is also anxiety over whether one will recover completely, or die, as well as about what might happen to one's job and family. Even if no psychologic factor (e.g., stress, tension, accident proneness) was involved in the cause of the illness, the somatic injury soon acquires a psychologic overlay. Hence, whether an illness is primarily somatic or psychosomatic, the therapist must take into account the psychologic factors that derive simply from being sick, from occupying what sociologists call the "sick role."

To summarize, the doctor must understand the special significance of the unequal social relationship with patients, an understanding that he or she probably did not acquire through didactic instruction but through apprenticeship (internship) and role modeling. Because the doctor commands the technical knowledge and skill that the patient lacks, he or she can choose to be authoritarian and "play God" to the patient (the topic of many jokes); in different ethnic or subcultural groups playing that role could make the therapy more successful or less successful. But even if the doctor chooses to play a more "collegial" role with the patient (most needed in long-term rehabilitation from chronic disability), he or she remains a prestige figure, a counsellor, the leader of a team effort, and a most "significant other" for the patient and family. As such, the doctor's manner and actions can convey the suggestion of healing and therapeutic benefit to the patient and are an important component of the "placebo effect" of treatment. Whether it is the chiropractor's adjustment, the physician's injection, or the surgeon's knife, the power of suggestion is unavoidable. A good bedside manner conveys a sense of optimism and reassurance that all will be well, that the medicine will work, or that the spinal adjustment will eliminate the cause of the illness. That is why it has been said: "The doctor is his own best medicine," which someone called "iatroplacebogenesis."

Section 2

Suggestion

The power of suggestion accounts for most of the therapeutic benefits derivable from placebos, bedside manner, impressive treatments (whether due to the pain they cause, their cost, the prestige of the practitioner, or the distance and effort required to obtain them), hypnosis, faith healing, magic, quackery, much of folk healing and primitive medicine, and also much of modern medicine. I am not implying that there is anything wrong with either intended or unintended suggestion. A therapist would be foolish not to use whatever will facilitate cure or relief from symptoms. Turner (1931, p 83) quotes Sir William Osler as saying in *Modern Medicine* (1907):

> Most drugs have no curative effect whatever on the diseases for which they are admin-
> istered. . . . We do not now feel under obligation to give any drugs at all, except where
> the patient's attitude, or the attitude of his family, makes it expedient, in order to create
> in him the buoyant expectancy which is the real curative agent.

Later Osler (1910, p 1472) objected to the "orgy of drugging," which he named
"polypharmacy." Medical practice has not changed much: the conventional wisdom
today is that more than 99% of all MD visits involve a drug prescription.

Nortin Hadler, M.D., professor at the University of North Carolina School of
Public Health, phrased it well at the International Conference on Spinal Manipulation
sponsored by the Foundation for Chiropractic Education and Research (FCER) in
1989 in Washington, D.C.: "A goodly proportion of the therapeutic value is in the
eyebrows of the healer." Voltaire is cited as cynically saying: "The role of the doctor
is to amuse the patient until nature effects a cure or does not" (Norbeck, 1989).

Suggestion is a problem only when it is a substitute for, detracts from, post-
pones, or counteracts valid therapy. A pilgrimage to Lourdes, with its moving cere-
monies, processions, chanting, and piles of discarded crutches and braces, is not
likely to cure cancer, although it has benefitted hundreds of the faithful (Cranston,
1955). Similarly, ingestion of laetrile is not likely to cure cancer, although palliation
of symptoms may be experienced. Oral Roberts heals bodies before vast audiences
only when his imperious command ("Heal, God!") convinces hopeful devotees that
he can do so (Jacobs, 1962). The eulogy for a particularly successful chiropractor
given the Lee-Homewood award (Willis JR, 1989) emphasized particularly his "faith,
enthusiasm, and religious fervor." Rose (1968, p 134) makes the profound observation that the value of "suggestibility . . . as a therapeutic agent seems to depend as
much on the healer's faith in his methods as on that of the patient." Also striking is
this testimony by a surgeon (Goddard, 1899, p 460):

> I have opened up the abdomen in two cases when I did not know what was the matter,
> and don't now, but the patients both got completely well.

The chief difference between faith healers and quacks is that faith healers credit *supernatural* powers, whereas quacks ascribe their success to *natural* forces such as
electrical impulses, potions, or diets. Although some quacks are thoroughly disrepu-
table, as are some scientifically trained doctors, they may come to believe in the cu-
rative powers of their remedies because they clearly produce cures.

Hypnosis involves suggestion. An aural stimulus (the hypnotist) and sometimes
also a visual one (e.g., a glass ball) can concentrate attention and help exclude other
sensations, internal or external. Two other bodily senses may be employed: tactile
(e.g., holding hands, swaying, marching) or olfactory (e.g., incense). Suggestion
also can be conveyed by powerful stimuli such as commanding personalities in elaborate settings, religious symbols and representations, or impressive electronic devices, for example, Abrams' (1910, 1914) radionics machines. A visiting priest (a
man not unappreciative of the suggestive value of settings) described the B.J. Palmer
Chiropractic Clinic thus (Hilary, 1948):

Everything about this Clinic is arranged for the purpose of bringing about the greatest amount of soothing relaxation . . . the rest rooms, the subdued lighting, the silence, the carpeted floors, the signs to speak softly: all most conducive to complete relaxation. This inspires confidence in the patient thru the realization that the greatest personal interest is centered on him and so predisposes him to yield to the action of the powers of nature to restore health. . . . Add to this all the interest-catching displays in the Museums and Lecture Hall, and ingenious mechanical inventions in the physical therapy room, the soft, soothing oriental color appointments, the faint fragrance of exotic incense to lull the senses and hypnotize the mind away from self, and you have a psychotherapeutic setting unequalled anywhere.

My family chiropractor, Paul Bemis of Everett, Massachusetts, told of his cure at the hands of a chiropractor:

In France in the First World War I got hit by shrapnel, which caused me to lose a testicle. Then I got hit again in my lung. Then I got gassed and shell-shocked, and lost my voice for 368 days. The doctors told me I would get quick TB when the gas got to the injured lung. I was in a number of hospitals but they couldn't help my voice. They even tried diving me in an airplane to make me cry out. The MDs said nothing could help me. When I got back home my mother's sister took me to a local chiropractor. He examined me, took an x-ray, and said: "Boy, I'm going to make you talk." He adjusted the fifth cervical and I could talk immediately.

Since he had escaped combat after being shell-shocked (called "battle fatigue" in World War II) and had told me that his initial attitude toward chiropractic was optimistic, it is probable that his voice loss was a hysterical manifestation and that his recovery was due solely to suggestion.

Regarding the use of suggestion in chiropractic, D.D. (1910, pp 75, 92) reproduced a letter he had received from Willard Carver advocating it, then explained why he rejected suggestion. Here is how he quotes Carver:

There are a large number of ills which affect the human body that have nothing whatever to do, per se, with the body structure and exist where there are no luxations. . . . Suggestive Therapeutics is the natural father of Chiropractic and is all the sufficient extraneous aid that it needs. . . . It can be but a short time till you include a scientific suggestion as a necessary companion to the adjustments. I know that you will do this, because as the discoverer of Chiropractic you have demonstrated your intelligence and freedom from dogmas. You will see that Suggestion and adjustments are the all powerful and inseparable twins. . . . It is impossible for the Chiropractor to practice without using suggestion. . . . You cannot possibly adjust a subluxated joint without leaving some impression on the life-mind.

Although D.D. (1910, p 359) had listed "autosuggestion," along with "traumatism" and "poison," as the "determining cause of disease," he devoted 20 pages to refuting Carver, continually repeating that a chiropractic adjustment is all that is needed to cure all mental and physical diseases; for example (1910, pp 81, 97):

You seem to think that Chiropractic and Suggestion are "inseparable twins." Such a coalition would be incongruous. It would be the uniting of two opposites; two adverse methods which are antagonistic; two contradictories; two propositions which are diametrically opposed to each other in thot [sic] and action. . . .

Chiropractors have no more need of suggestion when replacing a luxated bone than a lady has when adjusting her hat or collar. Suggestion and policy are business tactics, cunning devices used to sell goods to the unwary.

But D.D. did admit (1910, p 93) that a patient's autosuggestion of improvement could follow upon an adjustment. Carver continued to insist that D.D. used suggestion in his adjusting without knowing it (Gaucher-Peslherbe, 1992), which is probably true.

It is relevant that many of the reported cures and improvements attributed to suggestion are musculoskeletal disabilities, such as the ability to walk, and conditions such as arthritis that vary in intensity from time to time for reasons not well understood. These are the kinds of conditions that chiropractors, as well as faith healers, frequently and successfully treat. In an Australian study Parker and Tupling (1976, p 375) concluded:

It may be that chiropractors have successfully combined a physiologically effective therapy with an elaborate healing ritual in such a way that they can help more people by spinal manipulation than would respond to a doctor or physical therapist performing the same manipulation without the trimmings. . . . There may be both physically and psychologically effective therapies involved in chiropractic healing.

Section 3

Psychological Implications of the Chiropractor-Patient Relationship

Setting aside the strictly physiologic effects of SMT, what more can be said about chiropractic's psychologic benefits beyond the reassuring support provided by any therapist, its placebo effects, the symbolism of "laying on of hands," the soothing effects of massage, and legitimation of the sick status of someone who has been told there is nothing wrong? Medical critics, in their zeal to deny any physiologic benefits to SMT, preferred to believe and usually claimed that it was the psychologic benefits that caused patients to prefer chiropractors to MDs. While they also commented on chiropractors' more informal behavior and solicitous concern for patients' welfare, they reasoned that recovery was due to suggestion, the laying on of hands and the relaxing manual treatment that could temporarily relieve symptoms. Because "backache is one of the human crossroads where body and mind meet" (cited by Weiant, 1947), let us examine the specific psychologic benefits of chiropractic treatments. An MD who has produced the best analysis of the chiropractor-patient relationship states that chiropractors have the "therapeutic core qualities" (Coulehan, 1991) that are also needed for success in psychotherapy: "acceptance and positive regard for the patient, . . . empathy and genuineness" (Coulehan, 1985, p 371). Chiropractors also have what Osler (1910) called "the faith that heals" (by which he clearly meant "faith in himself"), which unquestionably derives from the conviction that chiropractic works. Coulehan adds (1985, p 362): "It seems likely, however, that some reproducible benefit of spinal adjusting is in fact a necessary condition for the overall integration and maintenance of the chiropractic profession itself even though not for a successful individual case."

In sociologic terms, there may be less social distance between the chiropractor and the patient. This was especially true in the past, when chiropractors more often shared a working-class background with their patients. Chiropractors spoke the same language as their clientele and were not so likely to "put on airs," as some patients complained that MDs did. They took more time to listen to what their patients wanted to say, and patiently explained to them the *cause* of their illness and how their treatment would help. Using a real or imitation spine, chiropractors demonstrated how vertebrae could be twisted out of place and impinge on nerves as they leave the spinal cord. They showed patients x-ray films of their or someone else's spine, often displaying a curvature or pelvic tilt. They told patients much more than they ever heard from an MD. And in making these explanations they demonstrated respect for patients' intelligence while satisfying their curiosity about chiropractic. As a result, chiropractors' relationships with patients tend to be less formal, less authoritarian, more intimate and personal, more patient oriented and less disease oriented. A detailed model for the process of becoming a patient of a nonmedical practitioner has been presented by Semmes (1990).

Many patients went to a chiropractor as a last resort. Often they were not only desperate for help but had been racked emotionally by a series of failed medical treatments and by being rejected by MDs unable to cure them. Confused, ambivalent about their previous therapy, seeking counsel and effective treatment, what they needed often was what the chiropractor could offer, something new and different, without distasteful medicines, injections, or surgery. The patient is invited to lie prone on the adjusting table. The chiropractor's sensitive fingers palpate the patient's neck and spine. Various maneuvers and tests are performed to assess the patient's problem. Since the chiropractor usually also offers advice regarding changes in living habits, posture, exercise, sleep, and diet, the patient is involved in a participatory relationship that works to keep him or her ambulatory and active and encourages the patient to take responsibility for his or her own well-being. Sulzer (1965) highlights this point:

> The patient is given technical explanations centering around the role of stress, of postural defects and of psychosomatic factors, and he may also be offered psychological encouragement on a non-technical supportive basis, in keeping with his level of sophistication. . . . Some manipulation and massage may be used to reduce tension and aid the patient in establishing and maintaining good body tonus, posture, and affective state. This direct treatment may be supplemented with a course of exercises, diet and mental

health practices which he is to follow at home. . . . It is likely that the homework assignments tend to maintain the relationship between the patient and the D.C. between office visits, and also give the patient a greater sense of participation in the treatment and a feeling of more responsibility for his own recovery.

Wild (1978, pp 41–42) concurs:

> The chiropractic doctor assumes the burden of health resides with the patient, and it is within the patient that the motivation and ability for health accrue. . . . Cooperation, therefore, on the part of an active patient is part and parcel of chiropractic treatment. Therefore, the most aggravating patient is an apathetic patient, one who is not willing to practice for health maintenance. Chiropractic treatment, as differentiated from other modes of therapy, places the burden of health primarily on the patient, and the burden of motivating the patient primarily on the healer.

She quotes two students' remarks concerning the patient who is "pessimistic, apathetic, or uncooperative":

> If he were able and willing to want to get well, I would keep him as long as he showed effort to improve (even with occasional lapses into apathy). If it became obvious that the patient did not really want to confront being well, or never made any reaches, I would refer him to other kinds of therapy, but I would drop him.

> I would ask him if he wanted to be well, if he was willing to do as I recommend. If not, then there is nothing more I can do to assist his recovery. I would let him know that unless he changed, he was wasting his money being my patient.

Doing so could help exclude some of the less suggestible patients. The archetypal contrast with the MD therefore is that, rather than telling a patient to stay home from work or school, to go to bed and rest, and to take medicine, the chiropractor is more likely to recommend changes in living and eating habits that require active control and participation by the patient in his or her own recovery process, plus invitations to return, that should assist in generating a more positive attitude toward cure. Vernon (1991, p 383) concludes that in the "chiropractic healing encounter" a form of transference reaction occurs which allays distress and focuses the short-term recovery on positive concrete goals."

Cherkin et al. (1988, 1989; see also Coulehan, 1985, pp 372–373) comment on the greater confidence and comfort demonstrated by chiropractors compared with MDs in managing back pain, and attribute much of chiropractors' success to that fact. Brian Inglis (1964, pp 117–118) observes that: "Some practitioners realize that the success of their treatment depends on the establishment of *rapport* with the patient; they freely admit that they achieve their best results when their hands take over, as it were, and manipulate without conscious direction: and a few find that this only happens when *rapport* has been established." Turner (1931, p 50) insightfully emphasized another point:

> Chiropractic . . . does not recognize disease in the prevailing sense of an invading en-

emy but as a disturbed condition. The Chiropractor's patient consequently comes to understand that there is no invisible monster lodged in his vitals for the purpose of destroying him, but that there is simply a mal-condition. He feels less apprehension and therefore is minded to help competent nature exert its cure as nerve pressure is relieved—by opening up the pathway so that vital energy may be restored to every cell in the body. The Chiropractor merely sets about to right the body so that it will function. Primarily concerned with subluxations he explains his task to the patient and does not permit mystery to enshroud his case.

An MD once said to me that if he had been a layman he would have been thoroughly convinced by chiropractic's simple logical explanation. Louis Reed (1932, p 55) agreed:

> It is evident that in any case the treatment has a large amount of suggestion. The patient is told, with evangelistic fervor, that his troubles are due to just one thing, a subluxated vertebra; the chiropractor sets about to "adjust" that vertebra; using, perhaps, great force and causing the bone to "crack." He assures the patient that the nerve is no longer impinged, and that his troubles are over. The patient is quite likely to believe him and, if there is nothing seriously wrong, to be "cured" by his belief.

Reed's observation contains merit. However, regarding the "crack," a different interpretation was introduced as evidence in the Wilk (1976) antitrust trial by Irvin Hendryson, an orthopedic surgeon and trustee of the American Medical Association (AMA), who testified regarding his successful use of chiropractic manipulation (Wilk, 1976, Plaintiff's Exhibit 241):

> In the presence of an objective "pop" or "snap," it was felt by the patient and also by the manipulator that the total end result seemed to be better and more impressive than if no objective "pop" were noted. I have no real explanation for this except for the fact that there may be some psychosomatic factor involved; there conceivably could be unlocking of ligamentous structures in the facet region which permitted this audible sound; or, quite possibly, there may well have been some pathology present that we were not able to evaluate in view of our limited means which was of significance.

An additional explanation is provided by R.C. Schafer (1991a): "Most authorities feel that breaking the joint seal permits an increase in mobility (particularly that not under voluntary control) from 15–20 minutes, allowing the segment to normalize its position and functional relations as much as possible, if post-adjustment rest is allowed."

Nortin Hadler (1988, p 5) explained the origin of the term *"ruptured disk"*:

> Between the two world wars, backache evolved from a highly prevalent predicament to a highly prevalent illness—and a nemesis for the military, for industrial medicine, and for medicine at large, due to coincident developments in medical theory and in social legislation. Between 1910 and 1939, each of the states enacted a separate Workers' Compensation Statute. However, in 1934, Mixter and Bare, surgeons on the staff of the Massachusetts General Hospital, described a syndrome of persistent backache and, in half their patients, cauda equina syndrome resulting from herniation of the nucleus pul-

posis. This clinical observation was a landmark. However, in writing about their observations, they labeled the condition a "ruptured" disk, even in the title of their paper, to connote their pathophysiological hypothesis. This concept of "rupture" found ready ears in the Workers' Compensation establishment attempting to define the limits of "personal injury." . . . Predicament gave way to illness and then to injury, and a surgical remedy was offered as primary therapy. This dramatic revolution was a fait accompli within a decade of the introduction of the pathophysiologic hypothesis inherent in the label "rupture." . . . For chronic low back pain, recourse to surgery should be exceptional indeed. . . . However, the message has not reached all primary physicians and certainly not the public at large. . . . People with the predicament of backache often choose to be patients because of anxiety resulting from the concept as much as from discomfort itself.

Reed Phillips (1981, p S-124) surveyed 871 chiropractic patients randomly selected from the files of 30 Utah DCs in the Wasatch Front area. He reported that in addition to the usual approximately 75% with neck or back pain, "a number of conditions that could be related to stress are found to occur in a rather high frequency, i.e., tension headaches, nervousness, shoulder pain, asthma, indigestion, constipation, and colitis." Some of these conditions could have been of psychosomatic origin and therefore potentially helped by suggestion.

The back carries special symbolic value for many persons. A study conducted in World War II hospitals by Sargent (1946, pp 427–430) revealed that only 4% of the cases of backache had an organic base alone; some were due to hysterical conversion symptoms, others to "functional backache caused by muscular tension and fatigue." A soldier, knowing that a coward is considered "spineless" and "lacking backbone," may discover that his back won't carry his weight (and his fear). During World War II, I noticed that the most popular complaint about things in general was: "Oh! My aching back!" A woman whose husband is "a pain in the neck" may develop one. Freud had said, after all, that the ego is first of all a body ego. John E. Sarno (1984, p 15) insists that regional back pain is not due to any mechanical cause but to what he calls "tension myositis syndrome" (or TMS). He even decries what he calls the "ape-myth": that human back problems derive mainly from imperfect adaptation to upright posture. Rather, he cites Russell Baker's *New York Times* article (August 16, 1981, p 14) "Where Have All the Ulcers Gone?," and suggests that the decrease in ulcers is related to the fact that "neck, shoulder and back pain have become so common in recent years." Gilchrist (1976, p 101) found that "patients with a history of low-back pain were more likely to have had a diagnosis of 'anxiety,' " though not of "depression."

A *Time* magazine article ("That Aching Back!," July 14, 1980) quoted Charles Wahl's characterization of the "backache personality" as "hard driving but lacking in self-confidence, . . . likely to repress anger and avoid conflicts," and John Basmagian's quip: "Back pain is just a tension headache that has slipped down the back." Kirkaldi-Willis and Cassidy (1988, pp 6–7) note that "psychological problems are more frequently associated with low back pain [citing Sarno, 1984], and that depression, anxiety, hypochondriasis, and hysteria are related to unfavorable outcomes for both chemonuclolysis and operative treatment for lumbar disc disease." However,

Australian investigators (LeBoeuf et al., 1989) found 41 chronic low back pain sufferers to lie within normal limits on the Middlesex Hospital Questionnaire measuring
"six aspects of milder psychological dysfunction." As is well known, the boundary
between normal and abnormal personality functioning is permeable.

Quigley (1973, pp xix–xx) tells us why chiropractors originally began treating
mental illness:

> Early in the history of the chiropractic movement, every type of patient and disease was
> brought to chiropractors for cure. This variety also included the range of mental disor-
> ders. Although no controls existed and no standard measurement was employed, except
> the rule of thumb, "social recovery," chiropractors reported successes with a variety of
> mental disorders. Eventually in the early twenties, chiropractic mental hospitals (sanito-
> riums) were built for the care of the violent and disturbed patients. The results from one
> such sanitorium in Davenport, Iowa, were so impressive to a Judge in a nearby State,
> that he consistently refused to commit a patient to the State mental hospital unless the
> patient had at least three months care in the chiropractic sanatorium first.

Reflecting on his extensive clinical experience with mental patients Quigley (1973,
pp 115–116) added:

> When I first joined the staff of Clear View Sanitarium in 1940, I held strongly to the
> view that mental disorders were of emotional origin. I frequently saw agitated schizo-
> phrenics, dangerous to themselves and others, arrive at Clear View in straight jackets,
> completely out of contact with the world of reality. They were not responsive to words,
> care, or any type of ministration. However, after chiropractic adjustments a dramatic
> change occurred, in which the patient began to orient himself by asking questions as to
> who we were, where he was, what had happened to him. Soon he was released from
> restraints, had freedom of the ward and was eventually released from the Sanitarium. At
> first I felt this represented those persons who will make spontaneous recovery with or
> without care. When this type of experience was observed in patients who had been un-
> der psychiatric hospitalization for years, the change was difficult to reconcile with a psy-
> chological rationale alone. For the most part, the major recovery occurred before one
> could perform any significant therapy. Certainly, the patient did not have an opportunity
> to develop "insight," but it was clearly evident that he was perceiving the world from a
> much different and healthier frame of reference.

Herman Schwartz, former president of the National Chiropractic Association
(NCA) Council on Mental Health and editor of *Mental Health and Chiropractic,* insisted (1973, p 163; see also Regardie, 1948) that "the results chiropractic obtains
(with mental patients) are primarily due to the neuromuscular structural changes that
the adjustment produces, and that the psychology inherent in chiropractic is only a
contributory factor." Yet he (1973, pp 164–166) wrote:

> From the moment the chiropractor places his calm, relaxed hands upon the patient's
> neck or shoulders, he senses that he has the attitude of a doctor who cares. Every human
> being has an inborn need for kindness and empathy, especially when ill. . . . The adult,
> when in mental distress, no less than the infant, needs kind and concerned attention. .
> . . When he finds himself under the care of a humane and competent D.C. who really

cares for him, that situation alone may tend to raise his self-esteem and become a force toward his recovery. . . . When the doctor allows his relaxed hand to rest upon the patient's upper thoracic region for a few moments, it induces relaxation in an important area of the respiratory muscles with the result that the nervous patient's tense, alert, attentive, and restricted breathing is usually eased. Furthermore, this primary contact conveys to the patient much more than words: a friendly protective, empathic, as well as comforting attitude. . . . It is interesting to speculate that the chiropractic adjustment, in essence, may evoke what may be considered to be the primary and basic biological reflex of life, the stretch (myotactic) reflex. The patient starts to become more active and alert. . . . The dynamic chiropractic thrust can be considered as a specifically planned stretch of the constricted holding elements of the articulation.

MD manipulator Bourdillon (1973, p 115) agrees:

Among those sent for examination because of back complaints the neurotic without back pain is a comparative rarity. It is much more common to find that even in a patient who appears to be seriously neurotic, there is physical evidence of back trouble requiring treatment. In some of these cases the neurosis is due to the back trouble and will respond dramatically to its treatment. Unfortunately in others the neurosis acts as a tiresome complicating factor which makes treatment considerably more difficult.

For psychoanalysts the back can be associated with fixation at the anal level of personality development, which could explain why certain patients are attracted to those few chiropractors who emphasize cleansing the body of poisons and waste products through high colonic irrigation. However, psychosomatic conditions must be treated carefully. Jurgen Ruesch (1946, p 68) discovered in his pioneering research on rehabilitation that the medical treatment of psychosomatic conditions can be iatrogenic:

In 13 percent of the cases the doctors were definitely the cause for fixation of psychogenic symptoms since they had treated these originally psychogenic symptoms as physical disease.

While a chiropractor might do the same thing, he or she would be more likely than an MD to emphasize that it is the innate healing powers of the body that will cure the condition. That should create in the patient's mind a more wholesome attitude toward recovery.

Georg Groddeck, named the Father of Psychosomatic Medicine by Carl Grossman (1965, p 13), discussed the psychologic benefits of massage in his *Exploring the Unconscious* (1933, pp 47–50). Calling himself the "Wild Analyst," he developed, independently of Freud, parallel psychoanalytic theories at his Sanitarium Groddeck in Baden Baden, Germany, where, as chiropractors will appreciate, he obtained remarkable cures by avoiding most drugs and relying on diets, exercises, and baths. He wrote:

Massage, in whatever way it is carried out, must have some psychical influence upon the unaccustomed organism and . . . is an important though incalculable weapon for psychotherapy. . . . Massage can be of service both in diagnosis and in treatment. . . .

The patient's changing expressions reveal hidden secrets of his soul that in no other way could come to the knowledge of his doctor. Unconscious impulses and deeply buried traits of character betray themselves in his involuntary movements, so that a massage treatment can hardly ever be given without enriching the doctor's diagnostic knowledge of his patient.

In the course of time human life brings about certain functional disturbances and anatomical changes which have little importance to the healthy man, but which retard the recovery of the sick, and nearly all of these can and should be put right at the cost of some trouble and care in massage. In the first place their removal at once releases energy though for present purposes nothing need be said on this point: at the moment we are chiefly concerned with psychotherapeutic influences. The mere discovery of these almost universal injuries has an invaluable effect upon the patient's conscious and unconscious will to be healed, and hence upon the strengthening of the mysterious forces which make for health, the eternally insoluble X of medicine.

Sulzer goes further in a paper titled "Chiropractic Healing as Psychotherapy" (1965):

It also seems likely that the physical contact with the practitioner acts to increase the personal element in the relationship. . . . In the relaxation therapies physical contact and subsequent relaxation may be unconsciously related to feelings the infant enjoyed when stroked and patted by an affectionate mother. Thus, aside from its possible beneficial effects on the neuromuscular apparatus and the autonomic system, the physiotherapeutic approach may tend to evoke feelings of infantile comfort and security and, by association, imbue the practitioner-patient relationship with affectionate feelings which were originally directed toward the mother. These feelings, however vague, would tend to weaken the patient's reticence to talk over highly personal problems with the practitioner, and would thus tend to increase openness. Assuming that improved body tonus, release of tension, "talking it out," and openness are all conducive to therapeutic change, the occasions for interaction and increase in these factors afforded by chiropractic treatment may account for much of its apparent effectiveness.

It may be useful to have some patients under the simultaneous care of orthodox "talking" psychotherapists and D.C.'s or other somatic therapists.

The psychoanalyst Wilhelm Reich, whose unorthodox psychotherapeutic practices got him sent to jail, offered the most thought-provoking theory concerning the relationship between psychic and muscular tensions, that is, between mind and body, in *The Function of the Orgasm* (1948, pp 201, 210–211, 235–236):

Around 1929 I began to grasp the fact that the original pathogenic conflict of mental disease (the conflict between striving for pleasure and moral frustration) is structurally anchored in a physiological way in the muscular disturbance. *The psychic conflict between sexuality and morality works in the biological depths of the organism as a conflict between pleasurable excitation and muscular spasm.*

I found that, whenever I dissolved a muscular inhibition or tension, one of the three basic biological excitations made its appearance: *anxiety, anger, or sexual* excitation.

True, I had been able to bring this about before, by way of dissolving purely character-ological inhibition and attitudes. The differences lay in the fact that now the break-through of biological energy was more complete, more forceful, more thoroughly experienced, and it occurred more rapidly. Also, it was accompanied in many patients by a spontaneous dissolution of the characterological inhibitions. . . . The character armor now showed itself to be *functionally identical* with muscular hypertension, the muscular armor. The concept of "functional identity" which I had to introduce means nothing but the fact that muscular and character attitudes serve the same function in the psychic apparatus; they can influence and replace each other. Basically, they cannot be separated; in their function they are identical. . . .

Again and again it is striking to find how the dissolution of a muscular rigidity not only liberates vegetative energy, but, in addition, also brings back into memory the very infantile situation in which the repression had taken effect. We can say: *Every muscular rigidity contains the history and the meaning of its origin. A certain psychic structure is at the same time a certain biophysical structure.*

In great many cases psychic inhibitions give way only to a direct loosening of the muscular tensions. . . . *The rigidity of the musculature is the somatic side of the process of repression, and the basis for its continued existence.* It is never a matter of individual muscles that become spastic, but of muscle *groups forming a functional unit from a vegetative point of view.*

A comparison of Reich's technique with chiropractic was made by David Elkind (1971, p 68):

His [Reich's] character analysis became a "vegetotherapy," which was a manipulative therapy aimed at eliminating the "armor" of stiffness in all parts of the body. The procedure involved not only massage but also breathing exercises of various sorts. The aim was to free the person to be himself. It was a kind of chiropractic self-realization therapy.

Reich's student, psychoanalyst Alexander Lowen (1958, pp 83–92), using what he called "bioenergetics," specified how muscular tension and personality characteristics are related to each other:

Reich introduced the concept of physical energy as a counterpart to Freud's concept of a mental energy. . . . But one can go much further than Reich. There is no neurotic problem which does not manifest itself in every aspect of the individual's function. This follows logically from the gestalt concept of the organism as a unity. . . . Most important, however, is the physical appearance at rest and in movement. No words are so clear as the language of body expression once one has learned to read it. . . .

Despite the subtleties and nuances of body expression there are many body signs which are clear and unchanging. . . . The severe contraction of the nuchal muscles at the base of the skull is the root, I believe, of the tension headaches that plague so many people. . . . It is surprising how quickly such headaches can disappear if one loosens these tensions. . . .

One reads little about the backbone in analytic therapy. As an important structural element in the body, a weakness in the backbone must be reflected in a serious personality disturbance. The individual with a sway back cannot have the ego strength of a person whose back is straight. On the other hand backbone rigidity while adding strength to support decreases flexibility. In addition, such individuals frequently develop lower back pain. I have treated many patients with this complaint. In each case reduction of the tension in the lumbosacral muscles, mobilization of the pelvis, analysis of the repressed conflict and a resolution of the problem of the inhibited drive results in the complete disappearance of the pain and disability. The rigidity of the backbone is not only evident in the loss of flexibility in movement, it can be palpated in the tension of the lumbar muscles. . . .

We shall now continue our analysis of the body in a segmental way starting from the shoulders down. The position and motility of the shoulders are as significant to the ego functions as the legs and pelvis are to the sexual functions. Several attitudes are easily discerned. Retracted shoulders represent repressed anger, a holding back of the impulse to strike; raised shoulders are related to fear; square shoulders express the manly attitude of shouldering one's responsibilities; bowed shoulders convey the sense of burden, the weight of a heavy hand. . . . There is an antithesis between the upper and lower halves of the body. . . . The relative underdevelopment of the lower half indicates that the functions of energy discharge are severely restricted while the discharge of energy in movement and sex is greatly reduced.

Chiropractor Clyde W. Ford (1989a, pp 2, 14, 17–18; 1989b) reports still stranger reactions to treatment (see also Ashley Montagu, 1984):

I began to pay attention to the many ways that people responded to touch. In most people touch induced a variety of bodily changes — decreased pain, increased muscular relaxation, decreased stress and tension. These were expected clinical findings. But my patients also reported other occurrences when touched: a feeling of leaving their body; vivid mental imagery; changes in their perception of time; or spontaneous insights into the emotional, psychological, or spiritual issues underlying their physical pain or illness. . . .

Robert Assagioli called his therapy (of healing through the mind) *psychosynthesis;* I coined the term *somatosynthesis* to describe my work. . . .

A basic assumption of somatosynthesis: that one can find a larger, non-physical framework within which to understand and treat physical signs and symptoms. . . .

Touch has the power to recall events recorded by the body. Early life events fall into this category and therefore are often accessible through touch. Touch, after all, is the main sense that programs our brain from the earliest stages of pregnancy until several years after birth. Before we have well-developed mental structures, we experience the world through our bodies, and this occurs because we touch. Later on, touch can recall those early events.

It may be relevant that Whitcher and Fisher (1979) found that females reacted far more positively to touch than did males in a hospital setting.

I am not aware of attempts to refute the insightful and suggestive theories of Groddeck, Reich, Lowen, and Ford, which are difficult to test in any case. They may help to explain why *any* doctor's ministrations involving hands-on bodily contact (chiropractors in particular) can be both therapeutic and psychotherapeutic. It is not my purpose to insist on any particular theory but to outline a range of possibilities. For it is doubtful whether future investigations, even though properly controlled, will ever sort out the many confounding interrelated variables in psychosomatic or somatopsychic illness or therapy. I remind the reader that I have explicitly excluded from the present discussion the physiological benefits of SMT reviewed in Chapter 9.

Chapter 11

ACCEPTANCE OF CHIROPRACTIC

*The exact contrary of what is generally believed is
often the truth.*

De La Bruyere, 1700

I distinguish several dimensions of chiropractic's acceptance: (1) by patients, demonstrated by chiropractic's growth in numbers (see Chapter 5, Section 3), (2) by legislative action (see Chapter 6), (3) by the public, as revealed in opinion surveys, the popular press, literary productions, and such, and (4) by the medical profession and the scientific community generally. Points 3 and 4 are discussed in this chapter.

Section 1

Acceptance by the Public

H. W. Evans (1978) cites two early examples of public support of chiropractic: in 1929 the National Red Cross approved a resolution authorizing its nurses to serve patients under the care of licensed chiropractors and osteopaths, and in 1945 the annual convention of the American Legion adopted "a resolution to the Veterans Administration requesting payment for treatment of service-connected disability by a licensed chiropractor." Again in 1989 "the Legion adopted a resolution officially endorsing chiropractic as a medical option for its members" (Gibson, 1989). Symbolically important was the decision to change the classification of chiropractors from "semiprofessional" to "professional" in the *United States Dictionary of Occupations*. In 1951 President Truman signed the Universal Military Training and Service Act, which deferred chiropractors and chiropractic students from the military draft ("Vision to Action," 1986). In the same year Mutual of Omaha became the first major insurance company to advertise coverage of chiropractors' fees in their health insurance policies. Even before that the states had begun mandating the availability of chiropractors in Workers Compensation cases. At chiropractors' urging, in 1955 President Eisenhower proclaimed May 1–7 Correct Posture Week (Smallie, 1990b, p 20).

The anthropologist Thomas McCorkle (1961) proposed an explanation of why chiropractic at first seemed to be a primarily rural phenomenon. Disregarding the fact that chiropractic (and osteopathy) originated in the rural Midwest and quickly spread to the sparsely settled Far West, he argued that chiropractic's "congruence with rural Midwestern culture" was what had caused its "continued high rate of acceptance." Specifically he wrote that chiropractic

> offers a "common sense," single-cause theory that is capable of effective presentation by mechanical analogy. The system also upholds the sanctity of the human body and makes use of the healing power of the laying on of hands, two things calculated to appeal to people exposed to regular Christian teaching.

He overstates his case. Desire for a simple explanation and dislike of surgery and inoculations characterized not only the farm folk of Iowa, where he did his field work, but city folk as well. Chiropractic spread rapidly over the entire country. The explanation of why it was more popular in rural areas is far simpler. It began in the Midwest when most eyes turned still farther west for lifelong opportunities. In some rural areas (e.g., Maine) MDs were so scarce that chiropractors filled a demand for delivering babies, setting fractures, performing minor surgical procedures, and in some places at times even dispensing (probably illegally) controlled drugs. In the earliest days such states needed whatever practitioners they could get, and did little regulating of health care. Even after chiropractors became licensed, the perennial shortage of MDs in rural areas offered them greater economic opportunity. Since many chiropractors came from rural areas, they often returned there willingly (just as rural recruits to Huey Long's new medical school in Baton Rouge filled the need for more MDs in Louisiana). Not needing hospital privileges or a heavy investment in equipment, chiropractors could with relative ease open a practice and attract a following, at least in comparison with what they and MDs require today.

A comparable theory by Steven C. Martin, M.D. (1989) to explain chiropractic's early success is no more convincing than McCorkle's. Martin asserts that chiropractors' appeal was based on

> the traditional value of a simpler, pastoral life [with] orthodox science as the servant to religion [and] careful observation of God's universe, using inductive reasoning to produce scientific knowledge and laws. . . . By emphasizing drugs and surgery as therapies, physicians were seen as rejecting the healing power of nature and thus implicitly rejecting the beneficence and wisdom of God Himself.

He also argues that midwestern populism favored chiropractic over powerful eastern medical monopolies. Like the doctrinaire Marxist interpretations (e.g., Baer, 1984, 1989b; Willis E, 1983), which tend to see chiropractic as a kind of proletarian revolt against bourgeois medical domination, Martin's argument fails to explain chiropractic's success in competing with medical orthodoxy. The simplest explanation, in addition to the geographic one, is that most chiropractic patients previously had been treated by MDs without success and that they tried chiropractic hesitatingly at first and stayed with it only if they were helped. (I discussed the nature of the benefits chiropractic patients received in Chapters 9 and 10.) Enough patients felt helped by chiropractic for it to survive and prosper.

The ratio of chiropractors to population (Table 2) continues to be highest in the West and in the Plains states, where in 1989 it was 27 per 100,000 and 25 per 100,000, respectively, compared with a national ratio of 19 per 100,000. New England and the South had the lowest ratios, at 14 per 100,000 and 12 per 100,000, respectively. Ratios in the urbanized states of New York, New Jersey, and Pennsylvania were slightly higher than the national average, at 20 per 100,000. The state with the highest ratio was Oregon, at 34 per 100,000, followed by Iowa, Minnesota, and Arizona, at 29 per 100,000; California, at 28 per 100,000; and Missouri, at 27 per 100,000. The national ratio of chiropractors to population is projected to be 20 per 100,000 in the year 2000, 21 per 100,000 in 2010, and 23 per 100,000 in 2020 (*Seventh Report to the President and Congress on the Status of Health Personnel in the United States,* 1990).

Table 2 also permits comparisons of DC/MD ratios in the various states and regions of the United States. The range extends from 1:5 in Iowa and Oregon to 1:30 in Virginia, 1:51 in Maryland, and 1:69 in the District of Columbia. The ratio in the plains states is 1:7, and in the West is 1:8; the national ratio is 1:11. The disparity in these ratios suggests there should be ample career opportunities for chiropractors in those states where the ratios currently are low.

In 1954 the International Chiropractors Association (ICA) commissioned a comprehensive survey of problems facing straight chiropractic. Its four-volume report, (Saunder Associates, 1954), was not widely circulated, presumably because it displeased B.J. Palmer. A quota-type sampling procedure of the entire United States resulted in 658 face-to-face detailed interviews. It found that 39 of every hundred families (20,420,000 Americans) had received chiropractic care at some time, with higher use by lower income, educational, and occupational groups. Growth potential was indicated by the younger ages at which patients were first visiting chiropractors, by their 70% favorable attitudes, and by recognition that chiropractors, though less prestigious overall than MDs, have greater skill in their particular area. Even at that early date (1954), 70% favored chiropractic inclusion in prepaid health plans and in veterans' hospitals. Inasmuch as most respondents associated chiropractors with physical manipulation rather than with the provision of dietary supplements and physiotherapy, the study concluded:

> The public conception of chiropractic corresponds more nearly to ICA thinking. However, there is a marked trend among patients toward NCA philosophy. . . . People who think in NCA terms, i.e., "physiotherapy," "vitamins, diet, etc.," "blood tests," etc., are basically more favorable to chiropractic than ICA conceptual groups. . . . To some people a doctor is simply not a doctor unless he "gives pills."

Parker and Tupling (1974) published the following "study of 84 patients under chiropractic care for the first time" in the *Medical Journal of Australia:*

> Eighty-two percent had received and failed to respond to previous medical treatment,

TABLE 2.

Number of Resident Chiropractors, and Ratios of Chiropractors to Population and to MDs, by State: 1989

Region/Subregion/State	Number of Resident DCs*	DCs/100,000 Population†	DC/MD Ratio†
National total	44,904	19	1:11
Northeast	9,442	18	1:14
New England	1,860	14	1:19
Connecticut	423‡	13	1:21
Maine	168	14	1:12
Massachusetts	835‡	14	1:22
New Hampshire	193	18	1:10
Rhode Island	149	15	1:15
Vermont	92	17	1:14
Middle Atlantic	7,582	20	1:13
New Jersey	1,915‡	25	1:9
New York	3,630	20	1:15
Pennsylvania	2,037	17	1:13
South	10,712	12	1:14
South Atlantic	6,121	14	1:13
Delaware	57	9	1:21
District of Columbia	52‡	8	1:69
Florida	2,908‡	23	1:8
Georgia	1,325‡	21	1:7
Maryland	274	6	1:51
North Carolina	578	9	1:19
South Carolina	421	12	1:12
Virginia	379	6	1:30
West Virginia	127	7	1:25
East South Central	1,548	10	1:15
Alabama	398	10	1:15
Kentucky	469	13	1:12
Mississippi	218	8	1:15
Tennessee	463	9	1:19
West South Central	3,043	11	1:14
Arkansas	302	12	1:11
Louisiana	441	10	1:18
Oklahoma	546	17	1:8
Texas	1,754‡	10	1:16
North Central	11,169	19	1:10
East North Central	6,687	16	1:11
Illinois	2,029	18	1:12
Indiana	614	11	1:13
Michigan	1,844‡	20	1:9
Ohio	1,132	10	1:18
Wisconsin	1,068	22	1:8
West North Central	4,482	25	1:7
Iowa	809	29	1:5
Kansas	546‡	22	1:7
Minnesota	1,250	29	1:7

Missouri	1,397	27	1:7
Nebraska	197	12	1:13
North Dakota	121	18	1:9
South Dakota	162	23	1:6
West	13,581	27	1:8
Mountain	3,043	23	1:7
Arizona	1,003	29	1:6
Colorado	830‡	25	1:8
Idaho	175	18	1:7
Montana	174	22	1:7
Nevada	200	19	1:8
New Mexico	276	18	1:9
Utah	296‡	18	1:10
Wyoming	89	19	1:7
Pacific	10,538	28	1:8
Alaska	112	22	1:6
California	8,012	28	1:8
Hawaii	284	26	1:8
Oregon	943‡	34	1:5
Washington	1,187	26	1:8

*Figures for resident chiropractors were obtained from the *1990 Official Directory of the Federation of Chiropractic Licensing Boards*.
†Figures for state populations and for "active physicians" (excepting osteopaths, federal physicians, and dentists, as of Dec 31, 1986) were obtained from the *Statistical Abstract of the U.S. Bureau of the Census: 1989*, ed 109. Washington, DC, US Government Printing Office.
‡Figures for resident chiropractors in these states were interpolated between those estimated by the ACA and those published in Tamulaitis C: *ICA Review* 1989; 45:29–52.

nearly sixty percent gave a desire for pain relief as their sole reason for attendance, and two-thirds affirmed that they visited the chiropractor as a last resort. At a ten week follow-up, all but eleven percent reported some improvement and seventy-four percent were sufficiently satisfied with their treatment to affirm that they would return to a chiropractor if their condition recurred.

In 1978 the National Center for Health Statistics published a study, "Utilization of Selected Medical Practitioners: United States, 1974," using interview data from the National Health Survey, which for the first time broke down chiropractic usage by age, race, income, work status, and residence (Table 3). It exploded several myths. First, chiropractic is not a primarily rural phenomenon. In the 12 months preceding the interview only 500,000 of the 7.5 million Americans who had used chiropractic services were farmers; hence clearly the vast majority of chiropractic users were not farmers even though farmers' rate of utilization was nearly double that for the country as a whole. The second myth destroyed was that chiropractors treat primarily the aged; persons aged 25 to 64 years see chiropractors the most. The third myth was that chiropractic is used mainly by the poor and uneducated. On the contrary, the study showed that middle-income persons use chiropractic most, and that whites do so far more than nonwhites. The proportion of male and female patients was approximately the same, although most later studies have found that more fe-

TABLE 3.

Persons Receiving Chiropractic Services in the United States, 1974*

	Number of Persons Receiving Service (thousands)			Persons Receiving Services as Percent of Total Population		
	Male	Female	Total	Male	Female	Total
All persons†	3,811	3,715	7,527	3.8	3.5	3.6
Age						
Under 6 years	69	61	130	0.7	0.6	0.7
6-16 years	336	197	533	1.5	0.9	1.2
17-24 years	478	488	966	3.4	3.2	3.3
25-44 years	1,229	1,206	2,345	5.0	4.6	4.8
45-64 years	1,326	1,325	2,650	6.5	5.9	6.2
65 years and over	374	438	812	4.4	3.6	3.9
Color						
White	3,680	3,572	7,252	4.2	3.8	4.0
All other	132	143	275	1.1	1.0	1.0
Family income						
Less than $2,000	52	156	208	2.0	3.3	2.8
$2,000-$3,999	192	314	506	3.0	3.2	3.1
$4,000-$6,999	504	559	1,064	3.7	3.6	3.7
$7,000-$9,999	494	592	1,086	3.7	4.3	4.0
$10,000-$14,999	1,111	1,005	2,115	4.2	4.0	4.1
$15,000 or more	1,303	927	2,229	4.1	3.0	3.5
Usual activity status‡						
Going to school	486	352	837	1.8	1.3	1.6
Working	2,669	1,389	4,058	5.3	4.8	5.1
Keeping house	—	1,856	1,856	—	4.7	4.7
Retired	482	15	497	5.6	2.0	5.3
Other	105	43	148	3.3	2.1	2.8
Geographic region						
Northeast	837	808	1,645	3.6	3.1	3.3
North Central	1,156	1,198	2,353	4.3	4.2	4.2
South	818	839	1,657	2.6	2.5	2.5
West	1,001	870	1,871	5.5	4.5	5.0
Place of residence						
SMSA§	2,189	2,078	4,266	3.2	2.8	3.0
Central city	794	737	1,531	2.7	2.2	2.4
Outside central city	1,394	1,341	2,735	3.6	3.2	3.4
Outside SMSA	1,623	1,638	3,260	5.1	5.0	5.1
Nonfarm	1,340	1,419	2,760	4.8	4.9	4.9
Farm	282	218	500	7.2	6.0	6.6

*From Utilization of selected medical practitioners: United States, 1974. Vital and Health Statistics of the National Center for Health Statistics, No. 24, 1978.
†Includes unknown income.
‡Excludes children under 6 years of age.
§Standard metropolitan statistical area.

males than males go to chiropractors. Hassenger et al. (1975) reported that between 1965 and 1973 in a 20-county rural area of Missouri the number of chiropractors increased from 39 to 43, whereas the number of MDs, osteopaths, and dentists decreased; all four groups tended to move from smaller places to those with 25,000 or greater population.

A 1977 survey of 14,000 households by the National Center for Health Services Research and Health Care found that almost a fourth of the American population had used a nonphysician in that year (Berk, 1985). After nurses, chiropractors were used most frequently, with $606 million (15.7% of the total) spent on them. The percentage of respondents earning more than $12,000 a year who used chiropractors was nearly twice that of those earning less (19.9% vs. 10.3%). Only 10.6% of those with less than a high school education used a chiropractor, compared with 21.7% with a high school education, 17.3% with 1 to 3 years of college, and 11.5% with 4 years of college. Hence the stereotypical view that it is mainly the poor and uneducated who use chiropractors is no longer true, if it ever was.

Deyo and Tsui-Wu (1987) analyzed data from the Second National Health and Nutrition Examination Survey based on interviews between 1976 and 1980 with 10,404 United States adults older than 25 years. Fifty-nine percent of those with low back pain had consulted a general practitioner, 37% an orthopedist, 31% a chiropractor, and 14% an osteopath, with some going to more than one of these. Geographic distribution of those using a chiropractor was 45% in the West, 38% in the Midwest, and 30% in the South and Northeast. For blacks it was 14%, for whites 39%. It was 37% for those with a high school or college education, whereas for those with an elementary school education it was 33%, caused partly, no doubt, by the larger number of nonusing blacks with less education. Although chiropractic is still more popular in the West, it is clearly no longer mainly rural nor used mainly by those less well educated or in lower occupational or income categories. Based on an analysis of 1979 Canadian data, Ian Coulter (1989, p 21; see also Kelner et al., 1980) similarly reported that "the factors of education, occupation, and income do not have a great impact on the utilization of the chiropractor."

The Harris polling agency prepared *The Nuprin Pain Report* (1985) based on a representative nationwide sample of 1,254 Americans older than 18 years, plus two groups assumed to be under stress: 102 account executives in New York–based advertising agencies and 63 floor traders from the New York Stock Exchange. While headaches were the most common type of pain suffered (73% had at least one in the previous year), more than half also had had backache (56%), muscle pain (53%), or joint pain (51%). Those groups under stress suffered more frequent and more different types of pains. The most troublesome type of pain was backache, and of those with backache 41% had visited a chiropractor. Of the total, 18% had visited a chiropractor, varying from 10% to 27% with increasing age and from 24% in the West to 17% in the rest of the country. Use by occupation varied from 21% in the professional and managerial group to 13% in sales and service, but was only 5% for the advertising executives.

The first public opinion survey I found of *attitudes* toward chiropractic was re-ported in *The New York State Chiropractic Journal* (1948, pp 17–18). Although few technical details were published, 507 residents of New York City, Westchester, and Long Island "from widely diversified sections of the population" responded to a ques-tionnaire:

> Nearly half (47%) of the people in the greater New York area were ignorant of chiro-practic. Many said they had "heard the name" but "could not place it. . . . Of the 507 interviewed, 51 (approximately 10%) reported they had gone to a chiropractor for treat-ment. Of these, 41 reported the results as "good," six as "fair," and four as "poor."

More recent data are available from opinion surveys conducted by university or commercial research organizations. A 1976 interview survey of a probability sample of 544 adults in Pinellas County in Florida reported that 39% of the respondents or a member of their household had been treated by a chiropractor, 10% within the past 12 months (Harding, 1977). In Wisconsin a 1978 telephone survey of a probability sample of 1,000 respondents found 12.5% of them had used the services of a chiro-practor in the preceding 2 years, and that 35.8% had done so at some time in their lives (Duffy, 1978). A 1979 telephone survey of 500 residents of Holland, Michigan, found that 42.8% of the respondents or a member of their family had received chiro-practic services at some time (Silver BC, 1979).

Statewide surveys provide more reliable data. The Gallup Organization (1982) conducted telephone interviews with 1,035 randomly selected New York State resi-dents. More than 90% had heard of chiropractors, and 88% said they knew what chi-ropractors do, nearly all of whom answered correctly when asked what they do. Twenty eight percent of the respondents had been examined or treated by a chiroprac-tor at some time, 10% in the past year. Usage did not vary by education or income. When asked about chiropractic's effectiveness, 72% of recent users rated it very ef-fective, 22% somewhat effective, and 6% rated it ineffective. Asked whether they would go again to a chiropractor for the same problem, 92% of recent users and 72% of all users stated that they definitely or probably would. When nonusers were asked whether they would go to a chiropractor if they had a problem chiropractors treat, 41% said they definitely or probably would. Despite these favorable attitudes, the public still is not well informed about chiropractors. Only 63% knew that chiroprac-tors do not prescribe drugs; 20% said they do, and 17% said they didn't know.

In California, where nearly one fifth of all United States chiropractors practice, a telephone survey of 400 households (Communications Consulting Group, 1983) found that 99% knew what chiropractic is and that at least one member in roughly half the households had been to a chiropractor; half of these had first seen an MD, and 10% had been referred to a chiropractor by an MD. Of the total interviewed 79% had a favorable image of chiropractors, compared with 88% for MDs. Negative im-ages of chiropractors were held by 14%, compared with 7.6% for MDs. Although fewer persons with some college education or more used chiropractors than did those with a high school education or less, they still held a 3:1 favorable image of chiro-practors.

A North Carolina survey (Brigman, 1983) of 786 respondents interviewed in person and by telephone found that 36% had received chiropractic care within the past 3 years, 66.8% of them considered the treatments successful, and an additional 21.9% considered them moderately successful, for a total of 88.7%. Another North Carolina study (Rosenfield, 1987) of 585 randomly chosen adults found that 7.2% had used chiropractic services within the previous 12 months. Average income was the same for users and nonusers. Sixty-four percent were male. Based on several additional questions asked, the author concluded: "The chiropractic patient—perhaps more politically liberal, affluent, and well-read than the nonpatient—may be more concerned with preventive medicine and health maintenance."

A stratified random sample survey ("Attitudes Toward Health Care in Oklahoma," 1984) of 400 households in the state where D.D. Palmer and Willard Carver established early chiropractic schools found that 58% of the respondents or a member of their household had been to a chiropractor. Sixty-eight percent of these were female. (Perhaps mixers attract more females, straights more males.) Seventy-nine percent were very or somewhat satisfied with the treatment. There was almost no variation in use by education, occupation, or income, perhaps partly because the percentage of users was more than half the population. An unusual aspect of this survey was that it contrasted the responses of the public with what chiropractors expected those responses would be. Although there was agreement on many items, the chiropractors' stereotypes of patient attitudes were not always correct. They thought that more respondents would say they have no real knowledge of chiropractic than actually did (36% vs. 14%), that fewer would say that chiropractic is an acceptable part of health care and fills a void (61% vs. 86%), that more respondents wanted treatment of headache than did (15% vs. 5%), that more came for a routine visit ("check-up") than did (7% vs. 1%), that fewer were recommended to them by MDs or other practitioners (4% vs. 14%), that more came because of failure of other treatment (18% vs. 10%), and that more came as a result of advertising (7% vs. 1%).

A Pennsylvania State University study (Hearne and Smalley, 1985), based on telephone interviews with 971 randomly selected residents of the state, found that 31% had visited a chiropractor, 11% within the past year. The chiropractic patients were older, less well educated, and less often white-collar workers than were patients of MDs, but not so much so as in their 1981 survey. A surprising finding was that more chiropractic patients (67%) than MD patients (54%) were very satisfied with their last visit, and that 68% of the chiropractic patients said their last treatment was very effective, compared with 57% of the MD patients. Asked if chiropractic services should be covered by health insurance, 73% of the total sample agreed, as did 60% when asked if chiropractors should be able to treat patients in hospitals. Misperceptions also were found: 15% thought that chiropractors prescribe drugs and medications, and 20% thought they are members of the American Medical Association (AMA)!

A University of South Dakota telephone survey (Lewis, 1985) of 416 respondents discovered that 36.5% had a "personal chiropractor," and approximately one fourth of the respondents had visited a chiropractor in the previous year. Some member of 62.5% of the households had used a chiropractor at some time in the past. Seventy percent thought that chiropractors should be permitted to admit patients to hospitals, and 67% thought that chiropractors should be able to prescribe "pain relievers and muscle relaxers."

An Ohio study (Tuchfarber, 1989) based on 820 randomly selected adults found that 43% lived in a household where at least one member had visited a chiropractor (46% of whites but only 17% of blacks) and that 78% of those who had done so would go again. Bimodal distributions by education, occupation, and income were inconsistent: those at the middle level of education (i.e., high school graduates) and occupation (i.e., skilled and semiskilled) used chiropractors somewhat more, whereas those at middle income levels used chiropractors somewhat less. Only 13% of those who had not visited a chiropractor had considered doing so, but the percentage varied from 19% for those with some college education to 9% for those with a high school education or less.

A survey of 500 randomly selected Connecticut households conducted by the Institute of Social Inquiry at the University of Connecticut (Wardwell, 1988) obtained results comparable to earlier studies plus additional findings regarding the attitudes of nonusers of chiropractic. Although 28% of the respondents stated they were not familiar with chiropractic, 21% had visited a chiropractor at least once in the past, and 40% of the respondents or a member of their family had been to a chiropractor. Of the respondents who went, 78% rated the treatment as effective, 89% were satisfied with the amount of personal attention they received (compared with 82% for MDs), 72% were satisfied with the cost of the treatment (compared with 64% for MDs), and 72% said they would go again for the same or similar problem. When those familiar with chiropractic were asked for their overall opinion of it, 78% of those who expressed a definite opinion were favorable; however, only 61% of this group thought that "most people in Connecticut" have a favorable opinion of chiropractic. When those familiar with chiropractic but who have never been to one were asked if they would go for a problem chiropractors treat, 59% said they would go, and 68% said they would encourage a friend to go. These favorable attitudes toward chiropractors by those who have never used them should be encouraging to chiropractors.

However, there was also a lot of ignorance and misinformation: 26% thought that chiropractors prescribe drugs, perhaps because some sell vitamins and food supplements. And 70% said that chiropractors *should* be able to prescribe pain relievers and muscle relaxers, something that has recently been legalized in several states, but not Connecticut, for over-the-counter medications. Only 27% of the total sample stated that they have insurance covering chiropractic treatment; 48% didn't know, including 26% of those who had gone to a chiropractor (perhaps many years ago). Of those who had gone to a chiropractor, 51% had insurance that paid for it. Forty-five percent of those familiar with chiropractic agreed with the statement: "Insurance companies discriminate against chiropractors." Only 34% thought their MD would approve of their going to a chiropractor, and 82% of those expressing an opinion agreed that "most MDs look down unfairly on chiropractors," and 73% agreed that "a lot of the problems physicians try to treat with medication or surgery could be handled better by chiropractors." Finally, 83% disagreed with the statement: "Most of the improvement patients get from chiropractic treatment is really only in their minds."

The most thorough survey of the public's attitudes and reasons for using or not using chiropractors was reported by sociologist Jose E. Sanchez (1991). Telephone interviews with 693 randomly chosen New Jersey residents confirmed the findings from other state surveys regarding satisfaction with treatment, attitudes among nonusers, and the demographic similarities between users and nonusers (Table 4). Only 13% of nonusers held an unfavorable opinion of chiropractors, whereas the other nonusers either had not had a condition they thought chiropractors could help or were ignorant of the conditions that chiropractors treat. Sanchez concluded that the most important problem faced by chiropractors is educating the public about its scope and establishing itself as a " 'primary care specialty,' neither in competition with general medical care nor an alternative to it, but as an integral and organic part of the health professions network." Inasmuch as only 10% of users had responded to any type of advertising, he recommended that chiropractors concentrate on referrals from family and friends of users and "capitalize on the public belief that they bring quick and effective relief to pain resulting from various conditions that affect the spine," and that they work to improve interprofessional relations with other health care practitioners.

Two medical school professors (Cherkin and MacCornack, 1989) examined 457 patients with low back pain in the well-known Washington health maintenance organization (HMO), the Puget Sound Group Health Cooperative. All patients were between 18 and 64 years of age and had chosen whether to go to a family physician or a chiropractor. Although "chiropractor patients reported significantly more episodes of pain and had experienced pain for a longer period of time, . . . the percentage of chiropractor patients 'very satisfied' with the care they received was triple that for patients of family physicians (66% vs. 22%)." Chiropractic patients were about three times more satisfied with the information given them by their provider, twice as satisfied with the level of concern for them, and nearly three times as likely to perceive the provider as confident and comfortable in dealing with low back pain. These results do not surprise those who (like me) have interviewed many chiropractic patients. This carefully executed study obviously was done by researchers without a promedical bias.

A "National Opinion Study" prepared for the ACA by the Gallup Organization (1991) produced results comparable to those of the state surveys.

For the record, chiropractor Clinton A. Clauson was elected governor of Maine in 1958, Anthony Tauraello was elected to Congress from New York, and Jim Glisson was a member of the Florida House of Representatives and a candidate for Lieutenant Governor. Other chiropractors have held political offices as state legislators, mayors, and councilmen. A chiropractor was appointed to the State Board of Health

TABLE 4.

Characteristics of Chiropractic Users and Nonusers in New Jersey Survey*

	Nonusers† (n = 449, 65% of total) (%)	Users† (n = 240, 35% of total) (%)	Total sample (n = 693) (%)
Gender			
Male	42	38	41
Female	58	62	59
Education			
Less than high school	10	8	9
High school graduate	27	38	31
Some college	26	21	24
College graduate	24	23	24
Some graduate or professional school	3	2	2
Graduated from graduate or professional school	10	8	10
Ethnicity/race			
White (non-Hispanic)	69	73	71
African American	16	14	15
Hispanic	8	11	9
Asian	6	1	4
Other	1	1	1
Reported state of health			
Poor	2	3	2
Fair	10	16	12
Good	49	50	49
Excellent	39	31	37
Reported annual income			
No income–unemployed	1	1	1
< $10,000	26	28	27
$10,001–$20,000	17	13	16
$20,001–$30,000	25	28	26
$30,001–$40,000	14	15	14
$40,001–$50,000	7	4	6
>$50,000	10	11	10

*From Sanchez JE: *J Manipulative Physiol Ther* 1991; 14:165–176. Used by permission.
†Four responses missing.

in Illinois in 1932, in South Dakota in 1949, and in Washington in 1959 (Smallie, 1990b, pp 12, 18, 22). In the Washington legislature in the 1970s chiropractors were chairmen of the Health and Human Resources Committee of both the Senate and the House, one of whom, ICA President William Day, previously had been Speaker of the House of Representatives. Chiropractors in that state benefited politically from staffing a room at the capitol where courtesy adjustments were offered to legislators. Ratledge (1971, p 79) wrote that he had done the same thing before leaving Oklahoma in 1912, where he treated 125 members of the first Oklahoma legislature and their families and friends in "a free chiropractic 'adjustery' near the State Capitol Building." (He, like B.J., had been appointed an honorary lieutenant colonel on the governor's staff.)

Under the now defunct National Health Planning and Resources Development Act of 1974 many chiropractors were elected or appointed to Health Systems Agencies (HSAs) and even to Statewide Health Coordinating Councils (SHCCs), for example, Stephen E. Owens in Connecticut. New York Governor Nelson Rockefeller appointed chiropractor Albert Cera to his Medical Advisory Committee (Goldschmidt AM, 1973), and in 1980 Governor Edmund Brown appointed 12 chiropractors to regional committees associated with the California Board of Medical Assurance. In 1991 the first chiropractor was appointed to the Kansas Blue Cross/Blue Shield Board of Directors, as required by law.

At the national level, R. Nelson Bakke was appointed by Congressman Dan Rostenkowski of Illinois to the Advisory Panel for National Health Insurance in 1975, and in 1982 Ronald P. Beideman, dean at the National College of Chiropractic (NCC), was appointed to the National Professional Standards Review Council of the Department of Health and Human Services.

Treatment of chiropractors in the popular press, drama, and jokes has become less critical and more factual. The best known unflattering portrayal was the 1959 Broadway play and movie "Come Back Little Sheba" by William M. Inge (1959), for which Shirley Booth received an Academy Award and in which Burt Lancaster played an alcoholic husband forced to drop out of medical school and become a chiropractor. However, the popular 1990 film "Jacob's Ladder" portrayed a chiropractor in a favorable light compared with hospital treatment. Although jokes and cartoons showing chiropractors (and osteopaths) mauling contorted bodies have become stereotypes, they usually are not so offensive as they once were. Having a chiropractic adjustment seems to have become a more normal option than formerly.

Public opinion studies demonstrate how well chiropractors are now accepted. The proportion of the population who use chiropractors continues to rise, and satisfaction with treatment is high. Even among nonusers, chiropractors' public image has improved. It is difficult to tell whether this is the result of more chiropractors being in practice, their increased professional competence, or the weakening of the AMA campaign against them. Several telephone companies have begun listing them under the heading "Physicians DC (Chiropractic)" rather than simply as "Chiropractors." Change in the public attitudes has been slow but positive.

Section 2

Remuneration

Average income and total amount of money paid for chiropractic services are the best indicators of chiropractors' progress in the economic area. Because chiropractors, even more than MDs, mainly are in independent fee-for-service practice, they are more "client dependent" than "colleague dependent," in Friedson's sense (1970b, p 107). Patients freely decide whether to consult a chiropractor and which one to see. Chiropractors' incomes therefore depend on whether they satisfy patients' needs.

Historically most chiropractors were solo practitioners. When they were not, their colleagues most frequently were spouses, siblings, children, or other family members. About 70% still practice solo (Brennan, 1991). Partnerships and salaried associates have become more common as the economies of scale become more important. For-profit corporations employing chiropractors also have appeared.

In 1969 the New York City Commissioner of Health (Bellin, 1973) appointed Julius Dintenfass, D.C. (1970, 1973) Director of Chiropractic in the New York City Medicaid program, which in 1 year disbursed in excess of $1 million for chiropractic treatments based on 48,010 invoices. The largest number were for "arthritis, myositis, neuritis, cervical sprain, and low back pain." (As a cost-cutting measure, chiropractors were eliminated from the Medicaid program in New York state in 1978.)

In 1979 Congress mandated a national survey of the utilization of chiropractic services, expenditures for them, and supply of and demand for chiropractic services (Von Kuster, 1980). Replies to mailed questionnaires were obtained from 1,638 practitioners (adjusted response rate 53%) and from 2,221 recent graduates of 13 colleges (adjusted response rate 68%). The study estimated that a total of 23,000 practitioners provided 130 million patient treatments in 1979, at a cost of approximately $1.3 billion. "New" patients paid an average of about $53 for a first visit, which included $30 for x-ray studies and $23 for the treatment. "Old" patients paid on average $15 for a spinal adjustment, and $16 for a spinal adjustment and one physiotherapy treatment. Precise income data were not obtained, but average annual gross income was estimated to be approximately $50,000 per year. When incomes under $10,000 or over $200,000 were excluded, the average gross income was estimated at $63,400.

There is some discrepancy when data are gathered from the public rather than from chiropractors. A survey conducted for the National Center for Health Statistics (Mugge, 1986), based on data from 17,123 household interviews, estimated that 9 million Americans visited a chiropractor during 1980, for a total of 75 million visits, on average 8.3 visits per patient. They paid chiropractors a total of $1,186 billion; 49.5% paid by self or family, 35% by insurance, 5.2% by Workers Compensation, 3.8% by Medicaid, and 3% by Medicare. The average charge per visit was $12, and the average total per patient for the year was $132. Only 6% of visits included an x-ray examination. Brennan's 1991 survey of a random sample of 549 ACA members found that the median fee for an initial visit, probably including x-ray films, was $128, for a routine visit $26, and $41 for a routine visit plus physiotherapy. With health care costs more than double what they were in 1980, total expenditure for chiropractic care in the United States in 1990 was estimated at between $2.7 billion and $4.5 billion, which can be contrasted with federal expenditures for medical education and research alone of nearly $7 billion (Durenberger, 1988; Taksel, 1989).

A 1983 Florida survey found that on average chiropractors treated 110 patients per week and 235 new patients each year (Mittan, 1985). Brennan's 1984 survey of a sample of 712 ACA members estimated 163 million office visits to chiropractors, of which 10,700,000 were new patients. The average number of patients treated per week was 115, while the average number of treatments that each patient received in a year was 15. Chiropractors employed on average 1.5 full-time assistants per chiropractor. Eighty-six percent of chiropractors' offices had x-ray units. Brennan's 1988 ACA survey produced comparable results, except that offices with x-ray units had dropped to 81% while those using computed tomography (CT) or magnetic resonance imaging (MRI) had risen to 62%. Eighty-five percent used at least one physiotherapy machine, the average being 3.8 machines; only 16% used thermography. His 1989 survey of 534 ACA members showed an increase in those using CT and MRI to 69%, a continuing increase in the proportion of fees paid by private insurers to 47.9%, a decrease in the proportion paid out-of-pocket by patients to 28.2%, and an increase in the proportion of neuromusculoskeletal cases to 87.7%.

In a secondary analysis of the "RAND Health Insurance Experiment," which examined 5,279 insurance claims submitted between 1974 and 1982 from six cities, Paul G. Shekelle and Robert H. Brook (1991) found that "395 different persons (7.5%) made at least one visit to a chiropractor: 7,873 visits in all, or 41 chiropractic visits per 100 person-years." The data, which excluded the elderly and patients without insurance, revealed that the median number of chiropractic visits per year was seven, and the mean eleven. The most common patient complaint was pain in the back or neck (52.4%), followed by headache (9.6%).

In 1991 the ACA reported that approximately 12% of the U.S. population receives chiropractic services each year. It is not surprising that MDs have become alarmed over chiropractors' competition, especially after a 1982 "Patient Attitude Survey" conducted for *Medical Economics* (White JS, 1983) discovered that more than one third of those responding had sought treatment from a non-MD and that more than two thirds of those chose a chiropractor. In another *Medical Economics* article Mark Holoweiko (1987) reported that in 1986 spinal manipulation was "the ninth most frequently billed procedure under Medicare."

Brennan's 1991 survey of 549 ACA members found that chiropractors' median gross income in 1989 was $177,500 (mean $216,360), and median net income was $80,091 (mean $98,088, vs. MD's mean net income of $155,800). Hence chiropractors' incomes have become adequately rewarding.

Section 3

Acceptance as Professionals

The main criterion of chiropractors' success as professionals is acceptance as competent colleagues by the scientific community, especially MDs and other health practitioners. Joseph Janse's judgment in 1952 (1976, p 10), "We stand on the verge of professional equality," was somewhat premature. I have already noted the Congressional appropriation of $2 million for research on chiropractic, which produced the Bethesda conference (Goldstein, 1975); the first federal research grant (to Professor Suh at the University of Colorado); the beginning of collaborative MD-DC research (e.g., Kirkaldi-Willis and Cassidy, 1985); and joint membership in the American Back Society and other interdisciplinary organizations. Changes in the Code of Medical Ethics, adopted soon after the antitrust suit was entered, have helped make interprofessional relationships possible. Chiropractors now have relatively easy access to medical specialists and hospitals for consultation and diagnostic assistance. College accreditation has been authorized by the U.S. Office of Education, and most chiropractic colleges now also are regionally accredited, which permits them to grant accredited B.S. and M.S. degrees and to transfer credits to other academic institutions.

Another advance occurred in 1983 when the American Public Health Association (APHA) adopted a resolution nullifying its 1969 resolution (urged on it by the AMA) condemning chiropractic ("Board Votes for Limited Chiropractic Role," 1983). Unlike other medically oriented organizations, the APHA structure permits chiropractors to participate fully; hence they have organized in it a Special Professional Interest Group called the Chiropractic Forum. By 1985, 235 chiropractors had joined APHA and had elected chiropractors as officers of the Radiological Health Section and of APHA Governing Council. At APHA annual meetings chiropractors have organized three regular sessions, at which a dozen or more professional papers are presented. In 1985 the American Cancer Society reversed its previous policy that banned distribution of its educational materials to chiropractic colleges, in response to "pressure placed on the ACS by the Association of Chiropractic College Presidents and fears generated by the Wilk anti-trust suit" ("American Cancer Society reverses Anti-Chiropractic Policy," 1985). In 1990 Ohio made chiropractors eligible to be district health commissioners ("Another Legislative Win for Ohio Doctors of Chiropractic," 1990).

Chiropractors have always freely referred patients to cooperating MDs and in return received a few patients from them. Some MDs would suggest that patients see a chiropractor but not name a particular one. It is no surprise that some referrals turned out to be problem patients (known as "crocks" or "deadbeats"). The Saunders (1954) report found that 5% of patients had been referred by an MD. However, Kleiman (1979), in a survey of chiropractors in 12 states, found that chiropractors referred approximately 2% of their patients to MDs in a specified month, but that only a negligible percentage were referred to them by MDs. Although 84% expressed willingness to participate in a team or clinic practice with nonchiropractors, only 17.6% rated the cooperation they received from MDs as good or excellent.

Several of the opinion studies cited in Section 1 of this chapter reported that about 10% of chiropractic patients had been referred by an MD. In Canada, Kelner et al. (1980, p 227) found that 97% of chiropractors referred patients to MDs, 84.5% had patients referred to them by MDs, and 78% shared patients with MDs. Brennan's

1980 survey of 837 ACA members reported that 96% of the chiropractors had referred patients to MDs, and that 49% had MDs as patients. In his 1984 survey he found that 92.3% perceived relations with "other health providers" as improved. In his 1989 survey of 534 ACA members, which inquired about referrals to and from other health providers, in every case more chiropractors referred *to* other providers than *received* patients from them (Table 5).

Medical researchers Cherkin et al. (1988; 1989, p 637) reported that 57% of family physicians in Washington State had encouraged patients to see a chiropractor, and found evidence that these physicians "were not merely 'dumping' difficult patients but actually expecting these patients to receive potentially effective care that they themselves could not provide." Mootz and Meeker (1990), using questionnaires returned by 25% of 2,000 California chiropractors, found that 84.5% had received direct referrals from other health providers; however, 36.5% had received only two or fewer referrals in the previous year. In Canada, on the other hand, Patel-Christopher (1990), a medical resident at the University of Toronto, found that 62 of the 99 MDs she questioned referred patients to chiropractors, with relatively more coming from those who were in solo practice and had been in practice more than 10 years.

There are other indications of MD willingness to cooperate with chiropractors. In 1985 a Preferred Provider Organization (PPO) in New York City advertised for chiropractors as participating providers ("New PPO Solicits Chiropractic Doctors," 1985). (Recently several chiropractic PPOs have been organized.) HMOs increasingly offer chiropractic services to members (see Cherkin et al., 1988), and some states require it, although regulations for federal HMO qualification do not. Not only do some MDs now employ chiropractors, but some chiropractors even employ MDs, according to *Medical Economics* (Holoweiko, 1985):

> Physicians practically beat down the door of chiropractor David A. Underwood in Lincoln Park, Michigan, after he ran a newspaper ad offering a $50-an-hour, part-time position. "I took between 40 and 60 applications, then started turning doctors away," he says. "A lot of them were newly out of school, and a lot were foreign-born. But many weren't. They had their own practices and just wanted extra work."

Another first is that in 1991 Terry R. Yokum, co-author of the two-volume *Essentials of Skeletal Radiology* (1987), was appointed assistant professor in the radiol-

TABLE 5.

Referrals Among Health Care Providers

	Referrals To (%)	Referrals From (%)
MD	96	79
DO	40	25
DC	80	73
DPM	52	31
PT	24	16

ogy department of the University of Colorado Medical School, on the basis of his chiropractic credentials and publications.

Hospitals more strongly resisted providing services to chiropractors after the AMA antichiropractic campaign heated up in the 1960s, because of the requirement of strict adherence to the Code of Medical Ethics as a condition of accreditation. In earlier years not only could some chiropractors admit patients to hospitals and treat them there, they even ran hospitals themselves, usually with MDs on staff. The Attorney General of Michigan in 1950 and of South Dakota in 1965 ruled that chiropractors could practice in county hospitals (Smallie, 1990b, pp 18, 26). Under Joint Commission on Accreditation of Hospitals (JCAH) regulations the privilege of treating patients in hospitals became a closely guarded medical prerogative. Dentists and podiatrists gradually won the right to those privileges, with varying degrees of freedom from medical supervision. Chiropractors currently are pressing for these privileges through both the legislative and judicial routes, and are making inroads. They want hospital privileges for two classes of patients: those admitted for medical treatment who want chiropractic care continued, and those whom the chiropractor wants to admit for supportive care while the patient is receiving chiropractic care. Chiropractors have the law on their side, concludes a law journal article titled "Denial of Hospital Admitting Privileges for Non-Physician Providers: A Per Se Antitrust Violation" (Christie, 1985).

The first hospital to open its doors to chiropractors in recent years was Lindell Hospital in St. Louis, where in 1984 "thirty-one chiropractors gained the privilege and responsibility of caring for patients in tandem with MDs and podiatrists" (King, 1984). In 1985 it established the first chiropractic hospital residency program (Carmichael, 1988). Soon three other hospitals followed suit: Doctor's Hospital in Detroit, Seattle Osteopathic Hospital, and Scottsdale (Arizona) Community Hospital. Shorewood Osteopathic Hospital in Seattle had 32 chiropractors on staff in 1984 and 92 applications pending ("An Interview at Shorewood Osteopathic Hospital," 1984; "Rules and Regulations of the Chiropractic Service of the Surgery Department, Shorewood Osteopathic Hospital," 1985). According to *Newsweek* ("A New Medical Marriage," April 12, 1985), chiropractors brought in "about 25 percent of Lindell's business." The hospitals most receptive to chiropractors initially were those struggling to survive; indeed, Lindell Hospital went bankrupt and closed in 1988. It may seem ironic that osteopathic hospitals were among the first to accept chiropractors, considering the fact that osteopaths provide osteopathic manipulative therapy (OMT). Aside from the fact that they may have been weak financially and seeking additional patients, another reason may be osteopath Frederick Leweranz's contention (see Chapter 2, Section 4) that chiropractic adjustments do not duplicate OMT but have a different purpose and achieve different goals.

At New Center Hospital in Detroit "twenty-two DCs on staff . . . can refer a case that requires emergency care to the hospital, and continue chiropractic care within the hospital setting" ("Rep Appointed Hospital Chief of Chiropractic," 1985). *Medical Economics* (Thomas, 1988) quotes New Center's chief-of-staff as saying:

> Overall, the medical staff has *accepted* the chiropractic program, but not everyone has
> *embraced* it. . . . No physician left the hospital over the issue. As a result of our coop-
> eration with chiropractors, patients are getting better care. . . . The DCs are specialists
> in their area, just like other specialists.

And in "Chiropractors Invade Doctors' Domain" (1989):

> Alfred Moore, administrator at New Center Hospital, said that to survive, his hospital
> began "diversifying the use of our beds." Sixty chiropractors are now on staff, and
> Moore estimated that they have boosted the hospital's income by 10 percent annually.

Unlike some of the other hospitals that have awarded admitting privileges to chiropractors, New Center Hospital authorizes them to "order x-ray examinations of the
spine, perform spinal adjustments with or without apparatus, provide nutritional advice, and prescribe rehabilitative exercises and physical measures" without the need
for co-signing by the co-admitting MD or DO.

Chiropractors usually have criticized MDs for doing spinal manipulation under
anesthesia (MUA; also called manipulation under sedation treatment, or MUST) but
Texas Chiropractic College Dean Robert S. Francis (1991), on the medical staffs of
four Texas hospitals, defends the practice (always done in a hospital) as especially
useful in rare cases of "severe antalgia" or "chronic intra-articular adhesions and fibrosis of supporting soft tissues."

In 1990 chiropractor Joan Davis joined the staff of the San Francisco Magnetic
Resonance Center, which co-sponsored with Palmer College of Chiropractic—West
a "complimentary seminar" on "MRI for the Chiropractor: Spine and the Peripheral
Joints."

By 1990 at least 60 hospitals and ambulatory surgical centers had chiropractors
on staff. The variety of chiropractors' relationships with hospitals is covered in the
August 1991 issue of the *ACA Journal of Chiropractic*. Books have been published,
titled *Chiropractic and Hospital Privileges Protocol* (Kranz, 1987) and *Credentialing
the Chiropractor: Specific Mechanisms and Clarifications for the Chiropractic Applicant* (Thompson and Trickel, 1989). The most thoughtful analysis of the impact of
hospital privileges on chiropractors, MDs, hospitals, and patients is an article by
Rand Baird (1990).

It is not likely that chiropractors will want to treat many patients in hospitals, but
they believe it important to be able to do so when their patients need hospital care. Their
more important need is for laboratory and diagnostic services and clinical opportunities
for students. But the status significance of hospital staff privileges is so great that chiropractors can be expected to push strenuously for wider acceptance in that area.

The most impressive evidence that chiropractic has evolved into a reputable profession is that *Jobs Related Almanac* (1988), using six criteria, rated chiropractic
tenth best of 250 jobs in the United States, and the student-oriented periodical *Moving Up* (1988) listed chiropractic as one of the top professions for the 1990s, the
fourth highest paying profession, and the eleventh highest paying career; exclusive of
sports it ranked seventh!

Chapter 12

WHY HAS CHIROPRACTIC SURVIVED?

Chiropractic will always survive; the question is,
Will Chiropractors?

B.J. Palmer (1985a)

From a sociohistorical point of view there are lessons to be learned from chiropractic's remarkable evolution. It has not only survived but has truly prospered over the past century, growing literally from nothing to a legitimate health profession—politically, economically, socially, and professionally (Wardwell, 1978; 1980a; 1980b; 1982b; 1989). Approximately 50,000 chiropractors currently serve at least one tenth of the American population on a regular basis, and perhaps one fourth to one third occasionally, and even more in some states (e.g., Oklahoma). If the public opinion surveys are correct, somewhere around three fourths of Americans would seriously consider going to a chiropractor if an appropriate occasion arose. What such an occasion would be is not easy to determine. Most first approaches would probably be for a musculoskeletal condition. Many would be conditions that medicine had failed to help. And almost certainly the path to a chiropractor will continue to be the recommendation of a friend or relative rather than an advertisement.

A comparative approach suggests questions about the evolution of chiropractic. Why did it not disappear? Why has it not followed the path of osteopathy, toward fusion with medicine? Why has it been so much more successful than naturopathy, a term and a philosophy that should have been more attractive, since things natural have become so highly respected, indeed revered in our society? And why was organized medicine's aggressive campaign unable to prevent *The Rise of Chiropractic,* as Turner titled his 1931 book?

Four sociologic concepts are particularly relevant to these questions. One is that of a "social movement," in which a new political, religious, or other group grows from small beginnings to social prominence, success, or power. Second is the importance of what Max Weber (1947) called "charismatic authority" in the leaders of such a movement, enabling them to persuade followers to move in the direction they set; their closest followers, like Christ's disciples, often accrue some of a leader's charisma. Third, absolutely required for perpetuation of the movement is what Weber called the "routinization of charisma" into stable, often bureaucratic organization. Fourth is a seedbed of social conditions receptive to the leader's new "definition of the situation for action," another sociologic concept. In the case of chiropractic the new definition of the situation was provided by its philosophy of the cause and cure of illness.

Social movements are most likely to arise during periods of social unrest, turmoil, or change, when people are open to new ideas because of perceived problems with the status quo and the need for new solutions. Such was the case with medicine at the end of the 19th century. Flexner had not yet been commissioned to prepare his famous 1910 report, but the conditions requiring it were apparent. Medical education was still in a sorry state, with little standardization, inadequate laboratories and clinical facilities, and entrepreneurial schools competing for students and tuition money. In a period of great scientific advance, medicine was stagnating. The proverbial American optimism about attaining the good life was being sabotaged by contagious diseases not yet conquered, surgical procedures not yet entirely antiseptic, and hospital care best avoided. Jealous rivalries still divided allopathic, homeopathic, and even eclectic MDs. Christian Scientists and spiritualist healers were challenging orthodox therapies. New ways of improving health that had been propounded by laymen such as William Andrus Alcott, Sylvester Graham, John Harvey Kellogg, Alexander Haig, Horace Fletcher, and Bernarr MacFadden (Roth, 1976; Whorton 1982, 1988) featured such natural remedies as fresh air, cleanliness, exercise, nutrition, abstinence, vegetarianism, and fruitarianism.

Late 19th century European medical literature contained ample evidence of the benefits of correcting subluxations using manipulation, and regarding bonesetters, but according to Gaucher-Peslherbe (1992):

> People's judgment was, it still is, distorted by the deliberate exclusion of any data relating to a body of knowledge that was rejected less because it was empirical than because of its low origins. . . . It is clear that at the beginning Palmer overturned too many accepted beliefs and posed too many new problems for his method to be easily integrated. Besides, the biomechanical approach to the human body had no place in mainstream medical research at the time. Attention was focussed almost exclusively on Pasteur's discoveries and the new microbiology.

Freidson (1970a, pp 150–151, 155) made this more general observation:

> Physicians are likely to be very poorly informed about any institutional and occupational resources that lie outside their own jurisdiction. And, as is quite natural for people who have developed commitment to their work, they are likely to be suspicious of the value that lies outside their domain, including the competence and ethicality of those working outside. Their commitment leads them to deprecate the importance of extramedical services, and their position as professionals encourages them to restrict their activities to the medical system they control. . . .

And when outsiders doing work related to his espouse a mission predicated upon a different set of paradigms than that of his profession, the professional rather naturally feels that they and their occupation should either be converted and controlled (as medicine seems to be doing to osteopathy), or, if not destroyed, excluded from any significant interaction. And so it is that the thrust of professional activity is to seek to build barriers that keep the profession and its clientele safe from those beyond the pale while at the same time seeking jurisdiction over all that cannot be excluded.

I like what Freud said (Viereck, 1957, p 5): "History, the old plagiarizer, repeats herself after every discovery. The doctors fight every new truth in the beginning. Afterward they try to monopolize it."

Into this confused situation plunged A.T. Still, and later D.D. Palmer. Both were charismatic leaders who attracted many loyal followers. Both were cantankerous, opinionated, and inconsiderate, and hence they alienated other potential followers, as is often the case with charismatic personalities. However, important differences between the two men significantly influenced subsequent developments. D.D. was always an outsider to the medical profession in a way that Still was not. Still conceived of osteopathy as a reform of medicine, not its opposite, as was shown clearly in the 1894 charter he obtained for his American School of Osteopathy (later the Kirksville College of Osteopathy) in Kirksville, Missouri. Its stated objective, as Northup (1972, p 16) highlights in the subtitle of his book *Osteopathic Medicine: An American Reformation,* was

> to establish a college of osteopathy, the design of which is to improve our present system of surgery, obstetrics and treatment of diseases generally, and place the same on a more rational and scientific basis, and to impart information to the medical profession, and to grant and confer such honors and degrees as are usually granted and conferred by reputable medical colleges.

Twenty years earlier, in 1874, Still tried to present his ideas to the faculty at Baker University but was turned away. Although he was a "frontier doctor" with minimal medical education, he had registered as a doctor in 1874 when the Missouri law allowed him to do so, which permitted him to practice the full range of medical therapies available at the time. He had previously served as an Army steward during the Civil War, when much of the surgery practiced involved amputations.

D.D., on the other hand, had practiced only as an unlicensed magnetic healer. Both he and B.J. Palmer considered themselves outsiders to medicine. Although Still severely criticized medicine, he proposed its reformation, not its extirpation. With its head start, osteopathy more quickly became licensed and began improving its colleges. After the turn of the century and incorporation of more of the standard medical curriculum, its graduates could claim to be the most comprehensive physicians, able to use drugs and surgery as well as manipulation.

B.J., by contrast, convinced by the arguments used so persuasively in the 1906 Morikubo trial, determined that chiropractic was the opposite, the antithesis of medicine, and insisted they could never coexist. Although his motivation may have been largely political, as a strategy to gain licensure, his unceasing rejection of medicine both orally and in print and his insistence on a new terminology ("subluxation," "analysis," "adjustment") polarized chiropractic and medicine. Gaucher-Peslherbe (1992) contends that B.J. made chiropractic into a cult, whereas D.D. would have kept it a science:

> Under B.J. Palmer chiropractic became a closed shop, cut off from developments in the world of science, and it is not surprising that it began to develop a special chiropractic physiology, histology, etc.; and that emphasis was placed on clinical results, at the expense of basic research. What B.J. Palmer preached was none other than an anti-medical crusade.

Lerner (1954, p 716) provides the somewhat different insight that by adding "philosophy" to the science of chiropractic "the Chiropractor took upon himself the impossible task of solving nearly every problem in the field of general science." Ian Coulter (1990) argues that B.J. made chiropractic anti-intellectual as well as antimedical: "There has been a long history within chiropractic of anti-intellectualism, and again this was heavily influenced by B.J. Palmer (his quotes often capture this, e.g., we can't give you brains but we can give you a diploma)."

A particularly good example of adulation of B.J. as a charismatic figure was written by James Greggerson (n.d., p 12):

> It remained for B.J. to take the pitifully small something, and slowly add fact after fact to the science, move after move to the art, and thought after thought to the philosophy until it reached its present status. The power that armed him with intellect, wisdom and spirit, that shielded him from ridicule and calumny, that enabled him to carry the new discovery through the curse of bell, book, and candle, past the door of college and university, across the battlefields of vested privilege, into the legislative halls and finally upon the statute books of state after state, unmixed, undefiled and unadulterated; the power that endowed his body, mind and soul with an unswerving strength of purpose, and made him the living personification of the qualities that conquer was the *inside power* some call centrifugal force and which *we* call Innate Intelligence.

Turner (1931, pp 232–233), a critic of B.J., also waxed almost poetic about the loyalty of B.J.'s followers:

> The "Fountain Head" holds an abiding interest in the absent sons and daughters, and as faces turn toward Mecca at the muezzin's call, so the Palmer graduates faithfully retrace their steps yearly to the great assembly known as the Lyceum, a gala event for the Iowan city. There the full significance of the common cause is renewed, fresh objectives are clarified, old loyalties dramatized. To have fought the fight of chiropractic, to have endured imprisonment—ignominy—this breathes vitality into organization. Here is no musty chronicle of annual meetings, but a vast modern epic, whose stage has been set and whose drama has been lived in every clime under the sun.

Chiropractors became antimedical in the eyes of organized medicine and isolated from it, even from much medical literature in the earliest days. The medical historian Henry Sigerist (1934, p 199) noticed this: "Chiropractic has held fast to its original faith and so far has resisted every temptation to make concessions. This has added to its strength, and thanks to this alone it is today the most powerful medical sect in America."

With B.J. even more charismatic than his father, chiropractors remained mostly "straight." As Lerner (1954, p 708) put it, "a *principle* of science became a *platform* to fight for." Despite early attempts, especially in California, to add pharmacology and surgery to the chiropractic curriculum, even most mixers preferred not to engage in obstetrics, setting of fractures, or surgery of any kind, even in the few states where they could do so legally. Hence chiropractic did not follow the historic path of osteopathy, even with the projected time lag of 20 years or so. B.J. constantly warned against that path, attacked mixers without mercy, and worked to obtain licensing laws that would keep chiropractic as straight and narrow as possible. Consequently the majority of chiropractors retained the traditional "one cause–one cure" philosophy of disease and its cure despite their increasing use of physiotherapeutic methods, which were justified as *adjuncts* to chiropractic. This kept straight chiropractic "separate and distinct" not only from medicine and osteopathy but also from naturopathy, which might otherwise have held greater attraction. Although Morinis (1980, p 118) and Barge (1990, 146) argue that chiropractors will lose their uniqueness if they relinquish their philosophy, there is no empirical evidence that this is so. Bachop (1991, p 36) instead states: "Chiropractors will have to choose which they want to survive: chiropractic or chiropractic philosophy, the profession or the creed."

In 1946 Bernard Baruch commissioned a $1 million study of physical medicine including osteopathy and chiropractic (Wilbur, 1946), which recommended that

> one of the centers of physical medicine devote its major attention to the preventive and manipulative aspects of the structural mechanics of the human body; . . . promote research on non-medical therapeutic procedures of Osteopathy, Chiropractic and Naturopathy; . . . investigate by means of extremely careful analysis by experts, the diagnoses and results of treatment by persons considered most skilled in these procedures.

Apparently the report made little impact on the medical profession, although it may have stimulated early efforts by the American Medical Association (AMA) to bring osteopathy within the fold.

Inasmuch as back pain is the most common complaint in office practice after upper respiratory infection, there have been plenty of clients for all types of practitioners, and much unneeded surgery has been performed. In an article in *The Atlantic* Ellen Shell (1988) wrote:

> With the advent of penetrating imaging devices like the CAT scanner it gradually became clear that as many as a fifth of people between the ages of thirty and fifty have abnormal disks, yet most of them do not experience pain as a result.

She quoted orthopedist Rowland Hazard:

> The fact is, science is absolutely stretched when it comes to the diagnosis and treatment of back pain. . . . A lot of people are operating way beyond anything they can prove.

and also neurologist-researcher Gerald Leisman:

> I saw at least three thousand patients who suffered from low back pain. . . . Generally the diagnosis was radiculopathy, or irritation of the nerve roots. But there is no scientific way to establish what such a diagnosis means, because irritation, per se, cannot be measured. Subluxation and irritation are not the same, but they are related concepts. There are demonstrable physical states associated with subluxations, and it is possible to show that after a manipulation these states are changed.

Shell concluded:

> If, as the medical community claims, the success of chiropractic is due to good politics rather than to good health care, then it is certainly of the grass-roots variety. Chiropractic will not go away. Nor does it seem in the public's best interest that it should.

Other idiosyncratic factors helped, as Inglis (1964, p 113) noted: "It has been fortunate that two of the fields where chiropractors' services are most often required are sports and show business—both admirable for publicity purposes." The recent favorable publicity regarding chiropractic's benefits to Joe Montana and the San Francisco Forty-Niners football team could not have been purchased for millions of dollars. Every Olympiad and international championship sporting event now features athletes receiving chiropractic therapy as an important ingredient for success.

In an investigation of whether patients were using chiropractors as alternatives to MDs in rural Iowa, Yesalis et al. (1980, p 416) found that between 1972 and 1977 chiropractor use increased rather than decreased as the number of MDs increased from 11 to 25 during the same period, and suggested that patients "were actually triaging themselves to different kinds of health practitioners for different complaints or problems. . . . Perceived access to physician services did not correlate with chiropractic utilization." I agree with his conclusion (see also Cleary, 1982; Schmitt, 1978).

Why did naturopathy not keep pace with chiropractic? Or at least become as strong? One reason is that chiropractic's emphasis on correcting subluxations, to the exclusion of most other therapeutic modalities, gave chiropractic a focus and an identity that naturopathy, best defined residually as employing all healing methods except drugs and major surgery, did not have. The second main reason was organizational. A leader's charisma must eventually be transmuted into an organization if a new social movement is to endure. A successful movement requires stability, access to financial resources, and replaceable leaders if it is to become a permanent social institution. B.J.'s invaluable contribution was to accomplish this for chiropractic. He first made the Palmer School of Chiropractic (PSC) a flourishing enterprise. Then he united most chiropractors into a national organization (the Universal Chiropractors

Association [UCA]) that struggled for separate licensure against the medical "monopoly." He innovated annual "homecomings" of PSC alumni, which kept them and their families involved in what anthropologists call "rites of intensification"; these reunions reaffirmed chiropractors' identity and strengthened their determination to continue in practice and to defend chiropractic against its oppressors. And he maintained contact with "the field" by marketing millions of tracts, bulletins, and books, which also helped financially. He was truly high priest of chiropractic, and PSC was its Mecca.

Mixers had their own schools and organizations (the National Chiropractic Association [NCA], that later became the American Chiropractic Association [ACA], which enhanced their social solidarity as they fought B.J., the International Chiropractors Association (ICA), and organized medicine. Their leaders also exhibited sufficient charisma to recruit and inspire followers. For B.J. the mixers were another enemy to rail against, as both straights and mixers found the other group almost as suitable an enemy as the AMA. Internal and external conflicts kept most of them actively involved in chiropractic's political and legal conflicts (Palmer BJ, 1951b). Every chiropractor could find other chiropractors with whom to identify and ally, and they knew who their enemies were. Chiropractic has had a lively history!

Luce (1978, p 17) pointed out that chiropractors "serve several social and medical functions. One obvious function is to act as whipping boys and thereby to allow physicians to overlook problems in their own profession. Another function is to remind doctors of their deficiencies in the diagnosis and treatment of musculoskeletal disorders." Other functions served by chiropractors are summarized by Firman and Goldstein (1975). Gaucher-Peslherbe (1992) added: "No doubt the American medical world's preoccupation with its own reorganization in the period after 1910 gave chiropractic a breathing space."

In my doctoral dissertation (1951, pp 411–427; 1955) I used the phrase "ideology of an oppressed minority" to characterize chiropractors' explanations for their anomalous situation and what they should do about it. An ideology comprises ideas and beliefs that define the situation and predispose to action. Chiropractors' ideology provided them with five rationalizations (justifications) that facilitated adjustment to their marginal status:

1. It blamed biased medical researchers for chiropractic's not being accepted as a valid system of healing.

2. It blamed organized medicine's dominance of the health care system for chiropractors' marginal status in society.

3. It morally justified the chiropractors' cause as based on patient rights to a doctor of their choice and on their own right and duty to provide patients with a successful method of healing that eliminates the *cause* of illness.

4. By defining their situation for action, it motivated them to fight oppression in

the political sphere (as an alternative to focusing on research) and if necessary to "go to jail for chiropractic."

5. It justified combatting medicolegal opposition by any means, including even the same kind of "dirty fighting" that medicine was believed to use against them.

Their ideology helped chiropractors "understand" their situation, better contend with it, and hence better accept it. Even chiropractic patients, as Riesman (1939, p 133) observed, may "feel a certain moral exaltation in espousing the cause of a supposed underdog."

Naturopathy, on the other hand, lacked a truly charismatic leader and was organizationally weak. The "Father of Naturopathy," Benedict Lust, may have been handicapped by not being American born. Although he founded and presided over four closely related colleges (American School of Naturopathy, American School of Chiropractic, American School of Physiotherapy, and American School of Massage), founded the American Naturopathic Association (1896) and was its president until 1921, and published several naturopathic journals (*National Cyclopedia of American Biography,* 1945), he is hardly remembered today. After his death in 1945 the American Naturopathic Association split into *six* different organizations (Cody, 1985, p I-22). The chiropractic colleges that offered N.D. degrees ceased doing so by the middle of the century. Naturopaths are now licensed in very few states, and the two small colleges in Seattle and Portland graduate fewer than 100 students a year. However, naturopathy has experienced a mild resurgence of interest in recent years. My earlier prediction (Wardwell, 1978) of its impending demise clearly was premature, but naturopaths are not serious rivals to chiropractors today, although chiropractors continue to share with them a strong attachment to drugless healing methods.

The separate but related small group of naprapaths are in more serious difficulty as a result of court-ordered changes in the Illinois licensing law and the closing of their Chicago National School of Naprapathy. The National College of Chiropractic (NCC) is legally now its owner, and has enrolled as chiropractic students those who have 2 years of preprofessional college credit.

To conclude, chiropractic has followed its own distinctive course. It has neither completely disappeared nor been absorbed into orthodox medicine. Elimination of chiropractic is what the AMA wanted but did not get. Chiropractic not only has survived, but has prospered. The alternative of becoming more medical, like osteopathy, also did not happen, although it was what B.J. and the straights feared that the mixers wanted and was what many predicted would happen. Chiropractic has maintained its own independent course, at least so far. The prediction that if chiropractic gave up its cultist philosophy it would disappear clearly has not happened, despite the fact that mixers now greatly predominate and that some of the formerly very straight colleges (e.g., the two Palmers and the two Clevelands) now teach relatively little traditional philosophy. All is not roses, however. In Chapter 13 I examine chiropractic's present status as a health profession and the serious problems and dilemmas that still confront it. In Chapter 14 I evaluate the future possibilities available to chiropractors.

Chapter 13

CONTINUING PROBLEMS AND DILEMMAS

As a rule the practitioner is very much a zealot, in
whose philosophy Innate Intelligence remains fun-
damental.

Chittenden Turner (1931, p 281)

The principal dilemma facing chiropractors is the same that has plagued it since its beginning, succinctly summarized in the question: What is a chiropractor? It reminds me of the question frequently posed in Jewish circles: "What is a Jew?" It is inevitable perhaps that a culturally distinct minority of any type will be continually faced with the dilemma of defining how different it is from the dominant majority. Is it fundamentally different? What makes it different? Is it becoming less different? Will it disappear as a distinct group?

The straight-mixer division within chiropractic is the crux of the dilemma. Although it is not difficult to demonstrate that chiropractors do not exhibit a bimodal distribution but a "normal," or gaussian, distribution, with most somewhere in the middle rather than at the poles, chiropractic ideology has implied otherwise. Words have tended to obscure the facts and to magnify the differences between them, especially in the matter of using adjunctive modalities. While most chiropractors continue to rely on spinal manipulation as their primary therapeutic remedy, most also use some adjunctive methods, such as ultrasound and microcurrent, orthotics, corrective exercises, heat and cold applications, and dietary and life-style counseling. These chiropractors can be considered relatively straight. Others also use nutritional supplements, traction, additional electrical modalities, and sometimes acupuncture and homeopathic remedies. Very few include vegetarianism, fasting, or high colonic irrigations.

The split between straights and mixers creates most of the problems and dilemmas that chiropractors face: at the national level competing associations are unable to unite; in the legal and political areas licensing laws and scopes of practice vary widely from state to state; in education, despite increased agreement on a core of basic science, diagnostic, and clinical courses, schools are still ideologically and philosophically divided; in the economic area there is excessive variability in what chiro-practors can be reimbursed for; and in the area of public relations and marketing the public is confused by inconsistent messages (mostly advertisements) as to what chi-ropractors are, what conditions they treat, and how they treat them, while some of these messages attack and criticize other chiropractors for the way they practice.

Section 1

Differences in Mode of Practice

Wilcher (1989b) summarizes well the continuing variability in chiropractic licensing laws:

> Some states allow chiropractors to do minor surgery; others don't. Some consider ob-stetrics within the chiropractic scope; others specifically forbid it in their laws. In some states it is illegal to draw blood; in others it is not. Chiropractors may use acupuncture needles in some jurisdictions, but it is illegal in others. Some allow colonics under the chiropractic scope of practice; others disallow them. Some permit the use of nutrition, and still others outlaw its use by the doctor of chiropractic. Some states have limited pharmaceutical privileges, and others do not. Some permit the use of homeopathy; oth-ers aren't even sure what homeopathy is. Some accept physiological therapeutics within the chiropractic scope; in others they are illegal. Hypnosis is okay in some states and not in others. Others allow adjustment of extremities and soft tissues; in still others you are in trouble if you adjust them. Need we go on! Total chaos reigns in the so-called chiro-practic profession. . . . With 50 different definitions of chiropractic in the United States and still different ones in the Canadian provinces, and yet different ones in each of the other foreign countries where it is practiced, chiropractic can have only minimal in-traprofessional relations. Until we figure out what chiropractic legally is, there is little hope that we can ever be united.

Furthermore, according to Holoweiko (1987), Utah doesn't even define chiropractic by statute, fewer than half the statutes ban obstetrics, Oregon prohibits chiropractors from practicing naturopathy, and Hawaii prohibits chiropractors from giving mas-sages; 21 states permit chiropractors to sign death certificates; 34 permit them to do school examinations.

Aitkin et al. (1989) point out that the definition of "drug" used by the Food and Drug Administration is so comprehensive that much of what chiropractors do even for diagnostic purposes could be ruled illegal in some states:

> According to the Food, Drug, and Cosmetic Act the term "drug" means "(a) articles recognized in the official United States Pharmacopoeia, official Homeopathic Pharmaco-poeia of the United States, or official National Formulary, or any supplement to any of them; and (b) articles intended for use in the diagnosis, cure, mitigation, treatment, or prevention of disease in man or other animals; and (c) articles (other than food) intended to affect the structure or any function of the body of man or other animals." . . . The

authors feel that the chiropractic profession must make changes in the scope of practice laws to take into account the greater diagnostic accuracy that can be obtained with the use of pharmaceutical compounds. Fluori-Methane spray is being widely used within the profession despite its questionable legal status. The same is true for iontophoresis and phonophoresis. The state boards must acknowledge these uses and make appropriate legislative changes.

Most leaders recognize the need for agreed-on standards of practice, and the profession has contracted for assistance in achieving them from the Rand Corporation, which also has been helping the medical profession achieve the same goal. Other contributions are Herbert Vear's *Guidelines to Quality Assurance and Standards of Practice* (1992) and the volume edited by Scott Haldeman, *Guidelines to Chiropractic Quality Assurance and Standards of Practice* (1992b), based on a consensus of the profession's most knowledgeable and influential leaders.

The differences between straights and mixers are not so great as ideology and legal definitions suggest. Using data from the first survey sponsored by the federal government, which was based on mailed questionnaires covering practice characteristics of a random sample of 1,638 chiropractors (Von Kuster, 1980), I developed two scales of the straight-mixer dimension: one was a Guttman-type scale (Stoufer et al., 1950); the other was based on factor analysis. I then ran Pearson correlation coefficients between the scales and other practice characteristics. There was a built-in high correlation between mixing and the number of different modalities used, number of different services provided per visit, and percentage of patients treated with modalities of all types, but these correlations were expected and served only to confirm the validity of the scales.

My most significant finding was a *lack* of correlations between the straight-mixer dimension and most basic practice characteristics: sex of practitioner, years in practice, hours per week spent in patient care, weekend or evening hours worked, number of weeks worked in 1978, number of different patients treated per week, number of new patients treated per week, number of visits per patient per week, percentage of patients aged 65 and older, percentage of patients who are male, female, black, or Hispanic, percentage of patients referred by MDs or DOs, and feeling that the public is well informed about chiropractic services. There were a few weak positive correlations: being toward the mixer end of the scale was correlated with doing more urinalyses and blood counts in the office, doing more physical examinations on new patients, taking more (but not full spine) x-rays, earning a little higher income, and being reimbursed slightly more by third-party payors.

There were several other interesting correlations. Although income was positively correlated with using a larger number of modalities, it also was correlated with giving spinal adjustments to a larger proportion of patients, which was inversely correlated with age of practitioner, suggesting that younger chiropractors are more likely to do adjustments and hence that chiropractors are not following the path of osteopaths by doing less adjusting as time passes. It came as no surprise that income was positively correlated with working longer hours and more weeks per year, treating more patients and more patients per hour, seeing more new patients per week, and seeing the same patient more times per week, but all of these correlations were weak. Higher income also was correlated with practicing in a larger group, seeing more patients aged 17 or younger, seeing fewer patients aged 65 or older, receiving a higher proportion of income from third-party payers, saying that more chiropractors are not needed in their area, and not wanting more patients or more hours of work. There was no correlation with percentage of patients treated for acute, chronic, or maintenance conditions.

To repeat, the most important finding was the absence of significant correlations with most practice variables. Therefore it seems safe to conclude that differences between straights and mixers in mode of practice do not constitute a serious barrier to uniting the profession in one national association, despite conflicts over philosophy.

Section 2

Dilemmas in Education

The philosophic split within the profession has always "swirled around the schools." Although they now teach a standard core curriculum, they continue to differ in philosophic emphasis. This is true especially of the superstraight colleges accredited by the Straight Chiropractic Academic Standards Association (SCASA), which minimize diagnostic techniques, unlike such mixer colleges as National College of Chiropractic (NCC), Los Angeles College of Chiropractic (LACC), and Western States Chiropractic College (WSCC), which emphasize diagnostic sophistication and what Gibbons (1980a) called "broad scope" chiropractic. Students at Sherman College of Straight Chiropractic, for example, hear frequent lectures on chiropractic philosophy beginning in their freshman year. Although all colleges teach the original chiropractic philosophy in conjunction with history and theory, some minimize or even belittle it.

A more serious dilemma was created when the schools began hiring M.S. and Ph.D. recipients to teach the basic sciences, because these scholars naturally present their subjects as they have been trained to do, rather than from a chiropractic perspective; a significant number previously have taught in medical schools (Coulter, I, 1981). Ratledge (1971, p 93) had warned about this:

> Chiropractic Colleges should not permit any person who believes any part of medical theory to attempt to teach undergraduates. Such instructor just gets the student confused so that he never really gets the science of chiropractic and its universal applicability to every condition of the human body.

After the preprofessional requirement became universal and many students had 3 or even 4 years of "premedical" education prior to 2 years of basic sciences in chiropractic colleges, students became less willing to accept chiropractic dogma unsupported by scientific evidence. This schism in chiropractic education has been exacerbated because the clinical instructors often lack an advanced degree in one of the basic sciences and are unable to hold their own when challenged by their best students. One college administrator stated in 1989: "The clinical faculty is being 'eaten alive' by the students." Another said, "Not only the faculty but also the students are becoming demoralized." The schism within the faculty and the lack of conceptual integration between the basic and clinical components of the curriculum has produced a kind of schizoid split in the self-image of many students. It is difficult to judge whether this is a more serious problem in the straight schools or in those that deemphasize traditional chiropractic philosophy. Although the contradictions should be more apparent in the straight schools, the stronger indoctrination received there seems to resolve or suppress them. In earlier days basic science teachers were encouraged to pursue a D.C. degree concurrently with teaching. Alternatively, admitted students who were already qualified to teach a basic science course often were invited and given academic and/or financial credit to teach them. Both courses of action tended to reduce discrepancies between the basic science and chiropractic courses. These alternatives occur less frequently today because, first, the level at which the basic sciences is taught is higher, and second, teachers already holding a Ph.D. are less likely to seek another doctorate and are under increased pressure to devote more time to research.

An interesting example is Robert Anderson, an anthropologist at Mills College, who was appointed part-time Director of Research at Life Chiropractic College— West. He earned a D.C. degree while there, then an M.D. degree at the Universidad Autonoma de Ciudad Juarez, Mexico, which provides an accelerated program for those already possessing a Ph.D. He continues as Professor of Anthropology at Mills College while collaborating in research on back pain with MDs at St. Mary's Hospital in San Francisco. He has been especially active in publishing research papers and in the American Back Society.

The principal question about chiropractic education today is: How good is it? Does it produce competent chiropractors? Keating and Mootz (1989, p 395) argue that in response to pressures for accreditation and in order to prepare students to pass National Board and state licensing examinations, "Chiropractic education developed its basic science training at the expense of developing the clinical (applied) science," and that the way for the profession to escape the burden of its unproved dogma is to provide better training in and appreciation of clinical research. They believe that such training would help resolve the dilemma faced by faculty and students resulting from the schism between the basic sciences and chiropractic practice. The schools have begun teaching courses in research, and some of the excellent foreign colleges (e.g., Canadian Memorial Chiropractic College [CMCC] and Anglo-European College of Chiropractic [AECC]) require a research thesis from all students. The Australian School of Chiropractic and Osteopathy of LaTrobe University also places more emphasis on research in its academic programs than do most U.S. colleges.

Efforts of the Foundation for Chiropractic Education and Research (FCER) to upgrade education and research have progressed all too slowly. However, under

Steve Wolk it sponsored in 1989 its first annual interdisciplinary International Conference on Spinal Manipulation, in Washington, D.C. And in 1988 it received its first million dollar grant for research, which it allocated to NCC. Almost simultaneously it granted $20,000 a year for 3 years to Palmer College of Chiropractic (PCC) to establish the profession's first research professorship. So some progress has been made. Whether it will reduce the ideological split between straights and mixers remains to be seen.

There are still too many weak colleges and too little chiropractic research being done. Quite apart from the superstraight objections to better education in medical diagnostic techniques, student clinical training needs vast improvement. The principal deficiency is that college clinics do not attract patients with as wide a range of diseases as students will confront in practice. Hospital-based clinical training is beginning in a few schools. Without such training students cannot become as competent in differential diagnosis as they should be. Consequently they must continue to learn as they practice (as their predecessors and MDs did in earlier times), which is the trial-and-error learning that the schools are intended to replace. A national "Survey on Straight Chiropractic Completed" (1989) of 500 straight chiropractors (return rate 41%) found that only 47% felt adequately prepared for practice when they left school. Incidentally, 23% used ancillary modalities in their "straight" practices, and a nearly unbelievable 18% carried no malpractice insurance.

Nevertheless all schools continue to improve, especially as hospital rotations become available. As chiropractic becomes a more desirable profession, it attracts students who are better prepared and better able to pay the higher tuition associated with improved education. With greater income the colleges can further improve their faculties, facilities, and research capabilities and thus continue to upgrade the profession. The cycle is on an upward swing.

Section 3

Organizational Problems

"Organized chiropractic is a shaky structure," concluded Geiger (April 1942, p 104). As important as ideology is, much of chiropractic's internal conflict is ascribed to fights over territoriality or to the egos of leaders. With defeat of the merger effort the straight-mixer division widened organizationally in the late 1980s. In addition to the International Chiropractors Association (ICA) and the American Chiropractic Association (ACA), new national organizations appeared at each pole of the straight-mixer continuum. The superstraight Federation of Straight Chiropractic Organizations (FSCO) is at the extreme conservative pole, and the even smaller National Association of Chiropractic Medicine (NACM) is in one sense at the opposite pole; it does not advocate the use of more adjunctive modalities, but accepts the idea that chiropractic is part of the practice of medicine, not opposed to it, and should find its proper niche and collaborate with MDs, perhaps even in an ancillary role. Doing so might severely narrow chiropractors' scope of practice by limiting the types of conditions they treat and the methods they use. For example, Samuel Homola wrote to me in 1987:

> I simply agree with NACM's view that chiropractic treatment should be limited to musculoskeletal conditions. . . . My experience tells me that chiropractic would be better off as a profession if it would limit its field and describe its practitioners as musculoskeletal specialists who use spinal manipulation in conjunction with physical therapy. My opinions have not changed much since I wrote my *Bonesetting* book in 1963.

An even larger group, sometimes called "medipractors" or "ultraliberals," comprises those who favor changing state laws to permit at a minimum prescription of over-the-counter drugs, especially analgesics and muscle relaxers; Florida, Idaho, Indiana, Maine, Nevada, and Vermont have done so. According to Lamm and Wegner (1989), of the 42 licensing boards reporting (i.e., 70% of the 60 states and Canadian provinces written to), "over 70% of the states and provinces provide by statute for the inclusion of botanical remedies, homeopathic preparations, patient counseling and rehabilitation programming." A new brand of ibuprofen, called Chirofen, has been marketed to chiropractors in at least six states. A survey by Gemmell and Jacobson (1989) of 273 chiropractors in Oklahoma (a strong mixer state) found that three fourths of them prescribe over-the-counter drugs: 34.6% do so sometimes, 28.9% seldom, and 10.6% often. Apparently 45.6% inject vitamins. Homeopathic remedies are considered by some chiropractors "an extremely valuable adjunctive therapy consistent with the chiropractic view of encouraging the body's intrinsic healing resources" (Miller, JD, 1989). Texas Chiropractic College has sponsored a 200-hour certification course in homeopathy ("Homeopathy Series Continues," 1989). Straights recoil in horror at these developments, which they see as the nose of the medical camel entering the chiropractic tent. Such developments have widened the straight-mixer split, and were used in the ICA as their strongest argument to defeat the proposed merger in 1989.

There is overlap between the national associations in that some chiropractors belong to more than one. However, no longer does each association provide malpractice insurance. The NCA-established National Chiropractic Mutual Insurance Company (begun in 1946), which now insures about 21,000 chiropractors, offers liability insurance to all licensed chiropractors, fearing antitrust litigation if it refuses. And the ACA and ICA now cooperate in most political activity and lobbying at state and national levels. But because the efforts to merge into a single national organization failed in 1930, 1963, 1974, and 1989, the profession remains organizationally fragmented, despite the desire for merger of the majority of chiropractors, even within the ICA. In several states there are as many as four rival associations. A serious problem is that approximately half of practicing chiropractors belong to no chiropractic association. A fundamental cause of chiropractic's organizational weakness is that, unlike medicine, in which membership in the local medical society has been essential for maintaining hospital privileges, chiropractors can function perfectly well without belonging to any association. However, in 1991 efforts to merge into a single national association began again.

I earlier predicted that even if efforts to merge into one national association should bring some of the straights into the dominant broad-scope association (now the ACA), as occurred in 1963 and 1989, there would probably always remain a hard core of straights dedicated to traditional chiropractic. That is what has happened. The current situation is unstable because the three national associations do not really represent the left, middle, and right of the chiropractic spectrum. The superstraight FSCO and the ICA together claim far fewer members than the ACA does; and despite the differences between them over education for diagnosis, they are at this writing in many ways closer to each other philosophically than to the more permissive ACA, which tolerates as broad a scope of practice as state laws permit. I can conceive of several possible solutions to this dilemma, but shall refrain from trying to predict what will happen.

At the international level there has been somewhat greater organizational success. An enterprising chiropractor, Gary Auerbach, succeeded in organizing a World Federation of Chiropractic at the 1988 International Chiropractic Congress in Sydney, Australia, "an umbrella organization to coordinate international programs of the chiropractic profession alongside other international health agencies such as the World Health Organization" (Tamulaitis, 1988, 1989). Its Secretary-General is David Chapman-Smith, the New Zealand attorney who represented chiropractors in the hearings for *Chiropractic in New Zealand: Report of the Commission of Inquiry* (1979). Its office is located in Toronto, Ontario, Canada, where in 1991 it held its first World Chiropractic Congress of representatives from 40 countries.

Section 4

Remuneration

Because of differences in licensing laws and modes of practice, third-party payers are uncertain about what chiropractors should be reimbursed for. If it is less costly to reimburse chiropractors than MDs, insurance companies should not be reluctant to reimburse them for almost anything they do. Even if they believe that chiropractic benefits are due only to a placebo effect, they should find it advantageous to reimburse. (While it may not be a flattering comparison, some insurance companies have even reimbursed Christian Science practitioners for their services, presumably because it saved them money. One wonders what diagnoses they put on their claim forms, since their religious beliefs discourage even the naming of a disease!)

Numerous studies have shown that the total cost per patient is less for chiropractic treatment even when more office visits are needed, in part because patients lose less time from work. Most such studies have examined comparable nonsurgical Workers' Compensation cases involving trauma or other work-related disability. Although insurance companies should be able to make similar studies comparing MD and DC treatment, I have not been able to locate any. The most comprehensive study was conducted by Steve Wolk (1988) using statistics supplied by Florida's Division of Workers' Compensation in 10,233 closed cases of patients not requiring surgery who had a "temporary total disability" but recovered and returned to work. Chiropractic patients had a 48.7% shorter period of disability and an average cost for professional services of more than 50% less. Those treated by an MD had an average *total* cost, including compensation for lost work days, 83.8% higher than those treated by a chiropractor. A Utah study produced similar findings (Jarvis et al., 1991).

Regulations governing reimbursement of chiropractors under Medicare have created special problems because Congress limits the total amount of money available. Many of the private insurance companies that administer Medicare in the various states use a 12-visit screen for chiropractic treatment, which means that documentation and paperwork are required to get additional treatments authorized. Because insurance company auditors usually are medically oriented, and often are nurses, chiropractors consider them unqualified to evaluate their therapy and deny them reimbursement for treatment they believe their patients need. Although less than 7 % of all chiropractors' fees are derived from Medicare (Brennan, 1991), denial of reimbursement has become one of chiropractors' most irritating problems. The U.S. Health Care Financing Administration asked ACA to submit information for its new "resource-based relative value scale fee schedule" as the basis for reimbursing chiropractors' Medicare claims, and on November 15, 1991, Secretary Sullivan announced increases of 26% to 28% in chiropractors' reimbursements by 1996.

Even when "peer review" decisions regarding claims are made by other chiropractors, the pressure to deny claims is sometimes great if they wish to continue in that remunerative work or to perform independent medical examinations (IMEs) on other chiropractors' patients. Although peer review is an important function and is vitally needed for patient protection, those who do it are often despised by their colleagues and are sometimes considered traitors to the profession. Following is an extreme example of a chiropractor's grievance ("Chiro Consultant Irks DC," 1989):

> One of our Workers' Compensation patients went to a chiropractic insurance consultant in Queens for an examination. This patient was totally unable to work, almost unable to walk, in constant pain, with massive muscle spasms and rigidity, positive on most all of the usual and customary orthopedic and neurological tests, and definitely not a malingerer.

> The patient reported the examination was not a pleasant experience, with the veteran chiropractor forcing him down and having him get on and off the examination table several times.

This consultant's report said that the patient is capable of returning to work immediately and that all chiropractic care should stop. This implies that not only is the patient a malingerer, but that we are performing unnecessary treatments on a patient who doesn't need them.

This patient was subsequently examined by six different MDs over a period of months who pronounced him totally disabled and recommended continued chiropractic care. Nevertheless, the insurance company used the DCs report to deny the patient disability benefits, so that his car was sold, his telephone disconnected, and he borrowed thousands of dollars to pay his rent.

It is unfortunate when money drives any profession, as it increasingly does our health care system. The best critical analysis of the devastating consequences of economic competition for both the quality of medicine and access to it by the underprivileged is Lindorff's *Marketplace Medicine: The Rise of the For-Profit Hospital Chains* (1992). It is ironic, now that chiropractors have won licensure in all states and the universal right to reimbursement by third-party payers, that they have become subject to many new limitations and restrictions. The most stringent regulations are those of Medicare, because current law permits reimbursing chiropractors only for adjustment of a vertebral subluxation demonstrated by x-ray diagnosis. Yet Medicare does not pay for the x-ray examination. (In New York the 1963 licensing law, now changed, prohibited chiropractors from even taking x-rays of the lower spine!) Consequently Medicare still does not reimburse chiropractors for much of their work (e.g., manipulating other parts of the musculoskeletal system and physiotherapy treatments), yet the ruling subjects some patients to unnecessary ionizing radiation. This archaic regulation should be changed, but the American Medical Association (AMA) and related interests oppose that. The insurance companies often apply these Medicare restrictions in their other health insurance programs.

In 1990 Congress mandated a study of the availability of chiropractic services under Medicare. However, even if chiropractors were to persuade Congress to change the Medicare law, they have little influence on how insurance companies manage their business. The committees on insurance of all of the state and national associations work incessantly to persuade companies to pay more claims. Chiropractors believe they are being unfairly treated compared with MDs, and are frustrated that they can do so little about it. Lawsuits have been filed in Georgia against insurance companies for arbitrarily reducing chiropractors' reimbursement claims (Day, 1989). In 1991 the California Chiropractic Association won a $2.1 million settlement with an insurance company that had failed to pay chiropractors' liability claims.

A new problem concerns the Employee Retirement Income Security Act (ERISA), which exempts from state regulation companies that establish their own employee health plans, including laws requiring equal access to chiropractors. Possible solutions to this problem would be to change the law so as to remove that provision and leave state regulations in effect, or to obtain federal legislation guaranteeing equal access for all licensed practitioners in all health plans. Again chiropractors find themselves allied with other health professions (e.g., psychologists) also affected.

Chiropractors constantly seek to be included in the legal definition of "physician," and often have been successful at state levels. In Sweden, ironically, the term "chiropractic physician" is authorized and protected, but the designation "chiropractor" can be used by anyone with little or no training.

Keating and Mootz (1989, p 396) refer to chiropractors' "realistic paranoia born of nine decades of confrontation with medical orthodoxy." Such paranoia is pervasive as chiropractors continue to feel discriminated against by insurance companies unwilling to reimburse them fairly for their services, and they see the hand of organized medicine influencing third-party payers, which was one of the AMA's stated goals from at least 1962 (Null, 1986, 20). Ronald Caplan (1991) points out that with 80% of chiropractors' reimbursement now coming through insurance companies, the financial squeeze on chiropractors has intensified.

Congress asked the Von Kuster survey (1980) to study the supply and demand for chiropractors. It correctly projected future *supply* from college enrollments as a 35% to 48% increase over the following 5 years. But as is well known, it is nearly impossible to predict *demand* for any health profession, since "members of the health professions have significant abilities to generate demand for their services" (Von Kuster, 1980, pp xvii–xix). The report concluded:

> The subjective evidence developed by this study suggests, however, that substantially more D.C.s could be absorbed in the existing D.C. labor market. . . . We suggest a national survey of actual and potential customers to determine (1) the proportion of the population using chiropractic care services and (2) the characteristics of those who do and do not use these services and some of the determinants why people use this service, and (3) measurement on as many dimensions of the effectiveness of chiropractic care as one can from the patients themselves.

Although 26% of 506 ACA members responding to Brennan's 1991 survey thought there were too many chiropractors in their communities, my conclusion is that the potential demand for chiropractors has not yet been met. Public opinion surveys (e.g., Gallup Organization, 1982; Wardwell, 1989) document the readiness of those who have never used a chiropractor to go to one if they perceive the need. And the wide variation in ratios of chiropractors to population in different states and in different regions of the country (see Table 2 and Chapter 11, Section 1) shows that it would require many more chiropractors to bring the states with the lowest ratios up to the levels of states with high ratios.

Section 5

Political Action

Some of the economic problems that chiropractors face can be improved by political action. North Dakota was the first state to pass a nondiscriminatory insurance bill.

Equal access laws have been passed in 46 states (Bureau of Health Professions, 1990). A few states require that all health insurers reimburse for "chiropractic services" without specifying that a chiropractor must provide them, so presumably either an MD or a physical therapist can fulfill the requirement. On the other hand, Washington's attorney general ruled in 1965 that a physical therapist could not do spinal adjusting even under medical prescription (Smallie, 1990b, p 26).

Some states include Health Maintenance Organizations (HMOs) under the equal access requirement; others do not. If an HMO of the Independent Practitioner Association (IPA) type requires referral by an MD (the "primary care provider") before a patient can go to a medical specialist, hospital, or chiropractor, then the chiropractic patient faces a barrier. Very few HMOs permit access to a chiropractor without some restriction, such as MD referral or a maximum payment limitation. However, a few HMOs (e.g., the Group Health Cooperative of Puget Sound) have learned to appreciate chiropractors and to utilize them. It is relevant that the Puget Sound HMO, which also owns its own hospital, is considered one of the best in the United States. A most helpful political change would be greater uniformity in state laws governing licensure and scope of practice.

Other political issues continue to trouble chiropractors. The state associations (like all professional associations) must be constantly alert to ensure that no adverse legislation is passed. If a state has two or more rival associations, each must be alert and watch the other(s) and protect its interests. The straight-mixer split is the main source of these problems, inasmuch as most state contests involve the superstraights. FSCO wants its graduates able to be licensed in more than the dozen or so states where they now are. Recognition of its accrediting agency Straight Chiropractic Academic Standards Association (SCASA) by the U.S. Office of Education in 1989 permits their graduates to sit for examination in states that require only graduation from an accredited college, not from one accredited by the Council for Chiropractic Education (CCE). Legislative proposals and lawsuits over this issue continue to cause confusion and frustration for students, licensing boards, legislatures, and the public at large.

Two other branches of the federal government in which chiropractors seek recognition are the Armed Forces, where they want commissions awarded on the same basis as other health professions, and the Veterans Administration (VA), where they want chiropractic authorized for those who desire it whether outpatient or inpatient. In 1944 Representative J.H. Tolan of California introduced in Congress a bill to establish a Chiropractic Corps in the Medical Department of the Army; it was reintroduced by Senator Frank Case of South Dakota in 1957 (Smallie, 1990, pp 16, 21). And Senator Claude Pepper introduced a bill in 1949 to authorize the VA to utilize chiropractors' services. All of these bills failed. Congress mandated a Department of Defense study in 1985, and again in 1990 a bill to commission chiropractors in the Armed Forces was introduced by Senator Strom Thurman. Senator Sam Nunn promised to hold hearings on such a bill in 1992.

In 1985 President Reagan signed a law directing the VA to carry out a "Chiropractic Services Pilot Program" (1990) with veterans receiving VA treatment "for a neuromusculoskeletal condition of the spine within the 12-month period immediately preceding the commencement of the furnishing of such services." That restriction greatly limited the number of veterans eligible to be included, many of whom had chronic conditions that had not been helped by previous VA care. It is not surprising that of the 204 patients who completed the study, 154 chose chiropractic care and only 50 chose VA care. With such small numbers the results could not be conclusive (Stano, 1990). Although chiropractic patients were incapacitated or confined to bed fewer days, their treatment costs were greater than the estimated costs of VA treatment because the normal pattern of chiropractic care is to provide more frequent treatments. The Chief Medical Director of the VA then announced, "No additional actions are envisaged by the Department to make chiropractic care more widely available to veterans," beyond the existing fee basis, that is, only when an MD decides that chiropractic care is "medically necessary," which happens rarely.

In 1984 Congress mandated that the Department of Defense conduct a demonstration project to evaluate the cost effectiveness and clinical benefits of chiropractic care (MacDonald MJ, 1988). After several years delay involving a preparatory study and the resolution of difficult questions regarding location of treatment and responsibility for liability, a research design for the CHAMPUS Chiropractic Care Project was adopted and a third-party payer selected. The study began April 1, 1990, in Colorado and Washington, with $2.5 million allocated for the remainder of fiscal year 1990. At this writing the results have not been announced.

A broader question concerns chiropractic representation at the highest political levels. Chiropractors have been excluded from most policy-making and advisory boards at the federal level. They want to be included not merely for the symbolism but to influence decisions affecting them and their profession. They constantly exert pressure on the Secretary of the Department of Health and Human Services (DHHS) to appoint chiropractors to such federal policy boards and commissions. On July 11, 1991, the Senate Appropriations Committee, in "report language" accompanying H.R. 2707, the FY 1992 appropriations bill, directed DHHS to correct the longstanding inequity.

When and if the United States establishes a national health service, chiropractors want to be sure they are included in it. They probably don't want national health care, but they know that they must prepare for that possible future development. Encouraged by the Health America Act introduced in 1991 by Senate Majority Leader George Mitchell and others ("Senate Leadership Unveils National Health Care Plan: Chiropractic Included," 1991), chiropractors are somewhat reassured, but at the same time they are fearful because they remember the problems that the 1965 Medicare law created for them. The ACA was pleased to be invited to join and serve on the board or executive committee of the Health Care for America coalition lobbying for passage of the bill.

Section 6

Public Relations and Marketing

Whether it is called "public relations" or "public education," chiropractors always have been concerned about their public image, both individually and collectively. B.J. Palmer took the lead, or rather copied his father, in publicizing chiropractic. In lectures, pamphlets, and radio he pioneered chiropractic advertising. Later, when other health professions began abiding by their ethical codes restricting advertising, chiropractors continued to advertise profusely and blatantly, arguing that an unknown and disparaged profession has no alternative.

After the Supreme Court decided in Goldfarb vs. Virginia Bar Association in 1975 that most controls on advertising by professional associations violate antitrust laws, MDs and other health practitioners began and chiropractors continued to advertise. The profession finds it difficult to restrain the worst offenders: those who use bait-and-switch tactics or who promise free examinations or x-ray studies to attract patients and then pressure them to undergo an expensive course of treatments (Barrett, 1990). In 1988 the Connecticut Chiropractic Association took the rare action of expelling a member for just such unethical advertising. Another disciplined Connecticut member appealed to the Federal Trade Commission, which exonerated him! Leaders of the profession increasingly are concerned over ethical violations involving solicitation of patients, and are working hard to discourage it. Several state licensing boards have limited advertising in yellow pages of telephone directories, but other segments of the profession still encourage it (London, 1991, p 26).

Excessive treatment always has been a leading ethical offense of chiropractors. In their defense, some argue that even a patient who feels no pain or disability needs regular adjustments ("checkups") to maintain health and prevent future illness, euphemistically called "reconstructive and wellness care," but it is impossible to convince insurance companies that such maintenance care is "medically necessary" and deserves to be reimbursed.

Most chiropractic leaders agree that the bane of the profession is the "practice-building" entrepreneurs who prey on chiropractors wanting more patients. Almost every state or national convention features one of their "seminars," often billed as "office management" sessions. Indeed, the complexity and quantity of paperwork required today to run any health care office efficiently so as to garner third-party reimbursements is staggering. The seminars provide excellent and needed training in office procedures and reimbursement regulations to chiropractors and their office assistants and update attendees concerning new techniques of diagnosis and treatment. But the implicit and hardly veiled message is that these seminars will help chiropractors attract more patients and keep them coming back. For many years the colleges resisted permitting practice builders to offer seminars to their students, but they have caved in because of student demand for them. Like the graduating seniors of every profession, students are burdened with debt, anxious about the uncertainties and hazards of practice, and want reassurance. The practice-building seminars also can be called "morale-building" sessions, because that is one of the major functions they serve, not just for novices but also for older chiropractors who need reassurance that what they are doing is an important and legitimate calling that deserves to be generously remunerated (see Wardwell, 1955). The Saunders (1954) report concluded that their gross effect was "not educational but inspirational. They are glorified 'pep talks.' " Sometimes the exhortations of the practice builders are so emotional and persuasive in their Palmer-like appeals to save the world through chiropractic that they are referred to condescendingly as "that old-time religion."

Devotion to traditional chiropractic philosophy can lead chiropractors to treat some cases they probably should not, as well as to excessive treatment. "The early chiropractor's motto was, 'If they are breathing adjust them' " (Mawhiney, 1984). At the 1978 annual meeting of the ICA in Charlestown, South Carolina, President Sid Williams, President of Life College, stated, "A chiropractic case is one with a subluxation. . . . We take a case even though our instrumentation doesn't show a subluxation because *we know it's there*." At the 1989 ICA convention in St. Louis, President Fred Barge (1987), who heads a large clinic in La Crosse, Wisconsin, stated in a lecture:

> Don't refer. . . . Every case is your case if there is a subluxation. In twenty years I never saw my father refuse a case. He'd say: "We'll do everything possible to help you." . . . The difference between doctors with high-maintenance and low-maintenance practices is the doctor's belief system. *Charisma runs on the fuel of commitment* [italics supplied].

Such committment can transform chiropractic "philosophy" into an *ideology,* defined as a set of beliefs, whether valid or false, that govern action. Perhaps it is not surprising that the ideologically committed straights are those most likely to argue that spinal manipulative therapy will help O-type (organic) conditions (DeGiacomo, 1979, 1989). In any case, the most popular slogan for many years was, "It's not true to say 'We did everything possible' unless chiropractic was included."

Some chiropractors still subscribe to the idea that germs play an insignificant role in causing disease, and oppose fluoridation of public water supplies. Scientific judgment and public opinion condemn such chiropractors. A vote in 1989 to instate fluoridation in La Crosse, Wisconsin, was successful only because the chiropractors were, unlike previously, at least divided on the issue (Jones R et al., 1989).

Practice builders often boast about the large increases in numbers of patients and income that their graduates obtain. No doubt their seminars produce results. One motivating technique reportedly used at a school and in seminars is to have all the participants simultaneously hum: "M-M-M-M" (for "money")! The most successful practice-builder over many years was unquestionably Jim Parker, a role model since 1951 who still attracts thousands (in 1991, more than 2,200) of eager, paying clients to one of his seminars offered several times a year in different parts of the country. (Many years ago a certificate from one of his seminars was falsely used by a medical critic as evidence that a chiropractic degree could be obtained for only a few days of instruction.) In 1981 he founded the Parker College of Chiropractic in Dallas, which quickly became a popular school. The best defense of the practice builders who marketed their own technique of adjusting was provided by Joseph Donahue (1991, p 99):

> I believe clinical entrepreneurs have historically filled a void. Considering the poor state of our colleges over most of the profession's history, chiropractic would not have survived without technique systems. . . . Without a technique system to guide him/her, the chiropractor was very likely to fail in practice. In many ways, chiropractic technique systems are necessary heuristic devices.

A study by Cowie and Roebuck (1975), titled *An Ethnography of a Chiropractic Clinic: Definitions of a Deviant Situation* portrayed in embarrassing detail how the techniques taught by a practice-builder were implemented in a chiropractic office in Louisiana. The authors wrote that they "unashamedly made use of the conceptual framework of Erving Goffman," whose book *The Presentation of Self in Everyday Life* (1959) is the classic analysis of how people manipulate settings, props, and most of all their own personalities to produce the effects they desire. Cowie became "a participant observer" clerk-receptionist in the chiropractor's office for 3½ months. The chiropractor, apparently perceiving him as a potential future practitioner, took him into his confidence more than he did other members of what Cowie called the chiropractor's "dramaturgical team." Cowie thus became privy to the team's "backstage conversations," "staging of the front," and "impression management" designed to (1) portray the chiropractor as a competent professional despite hostile medical propaganda, (2) reassure the patient that the treatment will not be painful or harmful, and (3) persuade the patient that chiropractic adjustments will benefit him. The principal deficiency of the book is that the chiropractor studied was not representative of most chiropractors but was a superstraight guided wholly by Stephenson's "Thirty-three Principles of Chiropractic Philosophy" (1927), which the authors published as an appendix in the book, implying that most chiropractors subscribe to them. Such portrayals perpetuate the stereotype that most chiropractors still believe in a "one cause–one cure" theory of disease, that they are dedicated to convincing patients to become lifetime clients, and (by omitting mention in the book of any benefits received by patients) that chiropractic provides patients only with psychologic support and placebo effects. I was embarrassed that a fellow social scientist would offer such a biased portrayal, even though antichiropractic medical propaganda was pervasive at the time. The authors missed an excellent opportunity to gather systematic data on the personal and demographic characteristics of chiropractic patients, their symptoms, diagnoses, results of treatment, and interrelationships between these variables. Negative stereotypes remain one of the most critical problems facing the profession. Leaders who try to counter them face hostility and resistance from the minority of extreme straights for whom adherence to traditional dogma is the acid test of a true chiropractor. (Compare Still's phrase, "a tried and true osteopath.")

Major efforts continue to educate the public about chiropractic. It is obvious to everyone that the profession would benefit more from an institutional program of public education than from advertising by individuals touting their own brand of chiropractic and claiming superiority over that of other chiropractors. The most impressive national public education effort was the placing of two ACA-sponsored pull-out advertisements in *Readers' Digest* in 1989, at a reported cost of $0.5 million each, respectively titled "Which of These Doctors are Chiropractors?" and "Is a Chiropractor Really a Family Doctor?"

Section 7

Conclusion: Continuing Problems and Dilemmas

Even if there were no straight-mixer split, the chiropractic profession still would face serious problems, because its theoretical and research bases still are tenuous, especially at the basic science level. There is little doubt that spinal manipulative therapy and chiropractic "work," as clinical research, much of it medical and osteopathic, shows. The New Zealand study (1979) decided to focus on what Willis (1983, p 193; 1991) in his study of chiropractic acceptance in Australia calls its "political-legal legitimation" based on "clinical legitimacy"—that is, that it works—rather than on the question of its "scientific legitimacy," which organized medicine denies to it. Why chiropractic works remains a matter of dispute, with numerous theoretical possibilities needing further investigation. Until far more research has been done chiropractic will continue to be attacked by its medical critics.

Although chiropractic seems secure today in regard to its legal status and public support, the vagaries of politics keep it vulnerable to opportunities for its enemies—and they are still many—to harm it. Constant vigilance is needed to preserve its hard-won privileges. Changes in the political sphere can influence much of what happens in the economic sphere. Some of the newer problems regarding reimbursement may presage even more stringent future restrictions as appropriated funds for health care dwindle in the face of increasingly expensive high-tech medical care and an ever higher societal ratio of dependent aged to able-bodied wage earners.

Competition for the health dollar is intensifying. Although chiropractors are experienced in techniques for attracting and retaining patients, other health professionals are using more practice builders and health administrators to help them compete more effectively. If it isn't already "a jungle out there," as some say, it soon may become one. Chiropractors could be hard put to hold on to the political, economic, and professional gains they have won over the last two decades. Full acceptance by organized medicine remains unachieved. Victories in the courts and in hospitals facing bankruptcy generate resentment by MDs forced to share power and patients with competitors. Much depends on future developments, especially on those internal to the profession, which is the topic of Chapter 14.

Chapter 14

THE FUTURE OF CHIROPRACTIC

Chiropractic does not and should not belong to chiropractors, to MDs or to anyone else except to the sick. . . . It is finally a question of who is and who will render the most efficient service with it.

R.W. Sandoz (1978, p 32)

Section 1

Possible Outcomes

The classification of health professions presented in Chapter 3 outlines the possible directions in which chiropractic could evolve in the future (Figure 30). We shall now explore them more fully and suggest reasons why each is more or less likely to occur. Doing so also illustrates the usefulness of the classification.

Since chiropractic is clearly not a *quasi-profession* dependent only on suggestion or religious faith, the other possible options, other than for it to disappear completely, are for chiropractic to regress to an *ancillary* status; to follow the path of osteopathy toward *fusion* with medicine; to evolve to a *limited medical* status comparable to dentistry, podiatry, optometry, or psychology; or simply to remain in the somewhat marginal status it occupies today, challenging fundamental medical theories of illness and therapy and continuing to claim the ability to treat a wide range of human disorders, both musculoskeletal and organic (i.e., M-type and O-type illnesses). I disagree with Caplan (1991) that the only future possibilities for chiropractic are cooptation by (i.e., disappearance into) the medical profession or subordination to it, with or without the nationalization of health care.

Figure 30 shows the possible changes in category for chiropractic and physical therapy and the change that osteopathy already has made to a status parallel with medicine. Other than disappearing, chiropractic could follow one of the four following scenarios: (1) remain unchanged in its relations with medicine and the rest of the health care system, (2) become ancillary to medicine, (3) follow osteopathy by expanding its scope of practice to include the use of as many drugs and as much sur-

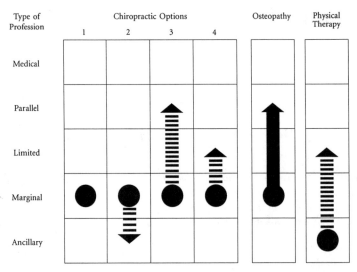

FIGURE 30.
Possible ways in which chiropractic can evolve in the future.

gery as states and hospitals will permit, or (4) evolve to the status of a limited medical profession. Since there are no other logical possibilities, I will consider each of these in turn. My starting point is the conclusion of two medical researchers (Tobis and Hoehler, 1986, pp 67, 81):

> Spinal manipulation works. . . . One can with confidence predict that manipulation will continue to be employed in the vast array of musculoskeletal complaints for which it has been used for centuries. . . . In addition, the risk of complications or harmful effects is small indeed. . . . In the light of the fact that medical care is costly, that physicians are generally very busy with relatively less time available per patient than other groups of health care providers and that the use of pharmaceutical agents is potentially more toxic with greater risk of complications than manual therapy, it is likely that manipulation will grow in popularity in America in the remainder of this century.

Section 2

Will Chiropractic Remain Marginal?

Although some writers (e.g., Coulter I, 1983; Rosenthal, 1981) insist that chiropractic no longer is a marginal profession, they are clearly wrong. Chiropractors like to hear that, but they know in their hearts that it is not true. Wild (1978, p 43) suggests an interesting qualification:

> Perhaps the marginality of the chiropractor ought not be viewed as a social or social psychological marginality, with social and social psychological causes and effects but rather as political marginality, with political causes and effects.

I do not agree, because political marginality always produces social and social psychologic effects, as was decided by the U.S. Supreme Court in the case of legal racial segregation in 1954. Straights seem to object more strongly than mixers to the term "marginal," probably because their ideology tells them that chiropractic is diametrically opposed to medicine, equal or better than it, even if not equal in social standing. However, they *know* that their professional stance is not accepted by society at large and that their one cause–one cure theory of disease is their most marginal attribute. G.D. Evans (1973) and others have argued that chiropractic's full professional acceptance depends on achieving "an effective and scientifically proven technology," which should lead to public and legislative support. However, George McAndrews (1989), attorney for the chiropractors in the Wilk antitrust suit and later General Counsel of the American Chiropractic Association (ACA), makes the following astute observation:

> The dogma or "Captain of the Ship" mentality is not necessarily based on knowledge or science . . . but rather is necessary as an embellishment to status and makes up one of the benefits of having crossed the "entry barrier." No typical medical physician will ever surrender that status voluntarily. . . .
>
> Quality and patient benefit are not the real issues. The medical profession reacts like Pavlov's Dog to competition from without. The medical profession has been conditioned to spout altruistic slogans and reasons for its arrogance in claiming the natural right to be "Captain of the Ship.". . .
>
> Don't even concentrate on gaining acceptance; there are factors beyond the limits of health care that dictate against acceptance. Try to gain respect. Beat the hell out of them in the marketplace. Let them worry about being hanged at dawn.

Hence the many statements that better research will vastly improve chiropractors' standing may be somewhat overoptimistic.

However, several factors are mitigating chiropractors' marginality: the increased amount of research demonstrating the limited (though certain) pathologic effects of the vertebral subluxation complex (VSC) and the benefits derived from "adjusting" it; the new developing relationships with MDs and hospitals; and the shifting scientific conceptions of disease cause and therapy, including what third-party payers will pay for. Chiropractic probably will not remain in its status quo ante. So much for Scenario 1.

Section 3

Chiropractic Won't Become an Ancillary Profession

It should be obvious that chiropractic is not, never was, and likely never will become an ancillary profession. Although that was and still is a logical possibility, and indeed a few chiropractors have become employees of medical clinics, especially in some foreign countries (e.g., Italy; see Mazzarelli, 1982), American chiropractors have never accepted such subordination. They have insisted on and enjoyed "independent access" without the need for a referral by an MD.

Even physical therapists, who historically have been ancillary (i.e., dependent on MD prescription), no longer are willing to accept that relationship and are succeeding in getting state laws changed to permit independent access (Kranz, 1986; Manceaux, 1987; Paris, 1983). There is little question that the medical profession, given a choice, prefers physical therapists to chiropractors as their assistants in rehabilitative and spinal manipulative therapy (SMT)—so much so that they often join chiropractors in opposing changes in state laws giving physical therapists independent access. An unconscious bias influencing this preference may have derived from the fact that the majority of physical therapists are women, whereas the majority of chiropractors are men. However, events may be passing everyone by, because it will be patients who will eventually decide whether they will choose to go to physical therapists or chiropractors.

If and when physical therapists gain the right to independent access in all states, MDs still will be able to choose which profession they will refer to. Probably they will choose physical therapists for the routine cases that chiropractors do not usually treat (e.g., post-stroke and post-surgical cases). If physical therapists move generally into chiropractic-type SMT, as urged by James Cyriax, Stanley Paris, and G.D. Maitland (1964), it remains to be seen how skilled they will become and whether MDs will send most patients with back pain to them or to chiropractors. The problem is that the average MD is not really qualified to judge when SMT is indicated or contraindicated; and the same will continue to be true of physical therapists as long as they remain less well trained than chiropractors. James Cyriax (1975a, pp 43–45) has written:

> It is slightly ridiculous that, at a time when deep massage and manipulative methods are beginning to be recognized as complementary, two professions should exist side by side, the one laying the greater emphasis on exercise therapy and massage, the other on forced movements. Clearly all physiotherapists should—and some of them do—know how to perform the various manipulations that are asked of them. Similarly every bone-setter and osteopath should be an expert masseur. . . . We should have one set of medical auxiliaries of acceptable ethics and educational standards, expert in every type of manual treatment. . . . Any patient curable by manual treatment given by an osteopath or a bone-setter should already have been cured by the same measures, carried out by a physiotherapist.

His slighting reference to "bone-setters" is not lost on chiropractors! So much for Scenario 2.

Section 4

Will Chiropractic Follow Osteopathy?

When chiropractic began it was not much different from or much inferior to osteopathy; indeed, it was alleged to have been "stolen" from osteopathy. A.T. Still established his college in Kirksville only in 1892, and Palmer began teaching students in 1898. Although Still's curriculum was much strengthened when he was joined by MDs William Smith, James Littlejohn, and Andrew P. Davis, the Palmer School also had MDs on its faculty and as directors of its student clinic. That which most differentiated chiropractic and osteopathy was the incorporation of surgery into the osteopathic curriculum in 1897 and the gradual inclusion of "comparative therapeutics," "supplementary therapeutics," and finally (without equivocation) pharmacology in 1929 (Gevitz, 1988b, pp 35–40). From then on, the differences between osteopathic and medical education and practice became minimal, resulting in gradual rapprochement of the two professions and finally the complete reversal of American Medical Association (AMA) policy in 1961, which could best be described as "cooptation."

However, Louis Reed (1932, pp 58–59) missed the mark in his conclusion regarding chiropractic for the Committee on the Costs of Medical Care:

> Chiropractic is rapidly changing. The rigid, "pure" dogma of the sect is becoming loose and broad, and softening into conformity with the ideas of medical science. The "straight" chiropractic treatment is losing prestige, and all sorts of auxiliary methods of treatment, some of them endorsed by medicine, are being adopted. The chiropractors are beginning to work for laws granting them a wider scope of practice. In short, the chiropractors now are like the osteopaths of fifteen or twenty years ago. Quite probably they will undergo a similar evolution. Their schools will become fewer in number but larger and better, and they will give a general medical course. In a word, we shall have half a dozen more inferior medical or near-medical colleges, and in the twilight of this sect a host of poorly qualified men will become fused into the general body of medical practitioners. The prospect is not a happy one. It will have to be endured unless the life process of this sect can be aborted by bringing into play forces which will strike at the root of the sect and cause it to wither for lack of patrons.

We know that the AMA already had begun its campaign to accomplish precisely that.

Chiropractic often was viewed from both within and outside the profession as following the course of osteopathy with a delay of 15 to 20 years. If one considers only progress in obtaining licensing legislation and raising licensing and educational standards, that may be correct. However, regarding scope of practice, despite a few futile attempts by some California colleges to add pharmacology and surgery to the curriculum in the 1930s, chiropractors in general have resisted the temptation to expand into those areas. And times, they were a-changing! After the impact of Flexner's (1910) exposé of medical education, the levels of expertise required to practice modern medicine rose rapidly. A thorough grounding in biochemistry and cellular biology became more and more necessary. Osteopaths, at least in the United States, copied medicine, whereas the chiropractic colleges concentrated on neurophysiology and spinal biomechanics. Although osteopathy in other countries remained much like chiropractic, focused on musculoskeletal problems and manipulation (Baer, 1984, 1987), U.S. osteopaths became hardly distinguishable from allopaths. The "National Ambulatory Medical Care Survey" (1987) found that only 13% of patient visits to osteopaths involved osteopathic manipulative therapy (OMT). Inasmuch as OMT is now given little more recognition in osteopathic colleges than homeopathy was given in the later stages of its schools, there is hardly any justification for retaining the word "osteopathic." The principal remaining difference between osteopathy and medicine is that, because medical specialty boards and hospitals sometimes still discriminate against osteopaths (McAndrews, 1989, p 41), they are more likely than MDs to specialize in family medicine, and they have disproportionately entered the military.

An MD-DC (Gilley, 1989) wrote: "The most valuable degree is one I don't have: D.O. . . . They have it all: pharmacology, surgery, and manipulation." But chiropractors seem now less likely than ever to follow the osteopathic route. If they were to try to do so, they would meet as much or more resistance than ever from MDs and DOs. The niche they have carved out for themselves is far more satisfying than the status they formerly held. They have a vested interest in what they have gained, and more to lose than earlier: licensure in all states and provinces in the United States and Canada (as well as in Australia, New Zealand, England, Ireland, Switzerland, Sweden, Norway, South Africa, and Panama; Tamulaitis, 1989); third-party reimbursement; academic accreditation; and increasing professional acceptance for their limited scope of practice. Despite problems with Medicare, which, after all, finances mainly treatment for the elderly, insurance companies pay chiropractors for a reasonably well-accepted range of treatments. What would motivate them today to try to become MDs? Indeed, there is little indication that they will do so in the foreseeable future. We have now discussed Scenario 3.

Section 5

A Limited Medical Profession?

Scenario 4 would be for chiropractic to evolve into a limited medical profession. It then would not oppose most of the fundamental tenets of medical science and practice regarding disease cause and treatment. Chiropractors already recognize the need for some surgery (but not so much for the spine) and for some medications and inoculations when appropriate, sometimes in conjunction with chiropractic adjustments. Chiropractors agree that the VSC is only one of several factors in the cause of disease. They agree that chiropractic adjustments are limited in the range of conditions they are appropriate for, and that even in those conditions medical supplementation is sometimes required. None of these compromises prevent chiropractors from continuing to treat diseases using alternative paradigms (e.g., homeostasis, holism, prevention, health maintenance). There already is more variability in the medical models of disease and therapy than chiropractors' stereotyped view of medical practice admits, and there is adequate room under the umbrella of medicine for chiropractic models of health care when grounded in scientific research rather than in outdated ideology.

Limited medical professions are like that. They do not advance theories of disease cause and therapy contradictory to those of medicine, as chiropractors earlier did. However, they are limited in two ways: in the range of illnesses they treat and in the range of diagnostic and therapeutic methods they use (e.g., scalpel, injections, controlled drugs, anesthetics). Usually they limit their involvement to one part of the body (e.g., teeth, feet, eyes). However, psychologists have different limitations, because behavior and personality are not spatially circumscribed. And much the same is true of chiropractic. Limited professions are permitted independent access without medical referral, a responsibility that requires sufficient training in differential diagnosis to enable them to distinguish the cases they are qualified to treat from those they should not, and know when to refer the latter to another practitioner, more often to a medical specialist than to a general practitioner. When limited practitioners are demonstrably qualified to diagnose, then organized medicine should have no fear (other than that of economic competition) that patients will be at risk if they go to them without referral.

The medical profession already is so preoccupied and fractionated into specialties that it ought not oppose full utilization of the limited professions in areas where they are needed. Dental caries, vision deficiencies, hearing problems, pedal diseases, and mental illnesses exceed in vast numbers what MDs can or will treat, certainly at comparable fees. That is the principal reason why the limited medical professions appeared in the first place. The same is true of back pain.

Chiropractic would fit reasonably well into the status of a limited medical profession. It always has offered independent access. And despite what some ideologues claim, it is, more now than previously, limited in the range of illnesses it is considered appropriate for and in the range of therapies it is licensed to use. A recent defense by superstraights (*Position Paper on the Acceptance of SCASA-School Graduates,* 1990, p 9) argues that chiropractors should "limit their diagnoses to the spine as podiatrists limit themselves to the feet." To the disappointment of many senior chiropractors who attest to chiropractic's benefits with somatovisceral conditions, the curricula of chiropractic colleges are far more focused today on musculoskeletal conditions. If chiropractors gain the right in all states to prescribe over-the-counter analgesics, muscle relaxers, and a few other mild medications, such expansion of their mode of practice would be no more, and probably less, than the way optometrists are beginning to practice in about half of the states, including the use of prescription medicines to dilate pupils for better diagnosis, analgesics to permit painless glaucoma tests, and the therapeutic administration of anti-glaucoma medications. However, medical researchers Cherkin and Berg (1989, p 637) found that the proportion of chiropractic patients seen with nonmusculoskeletal problems decreased from 21% in 1979 to 13% in 1985, and concluded:

> If this trend continues, and if the more accommodating attitudes of rank-and-file family physicians in the State of Washington prevail over those who speak for medicine, physicians and chiropractors may reach a point of peaceful coexistence.

David Chapman-Smith (1991), the attorney who represented chiropractors in the *Chiropractic in New Zealand* study (1979), appears to agree when he lists chiropractors' requirements for professional success in the next 10 or 20 years:

1. Skilled manipulative care for neuromusculoskeletal disorders.
2. As part of the basic accepted health care team, cooperating with medicine rather than as an alternative and adversary.
3. On a model similar to dentistry and optometry, a major profession, primary care, diagnostic rights and duties, but acknowledged limitations in scope.

The pressures pushing chiropractors toward becoming limited medical practitioners can be summarized as follows: (1) interdisciplinary research, which reduces the knowledge gap separating medicine and chiropractic and achieves one of the goals of the Wilk antitrust suit—"a common lexicon," intended to promote interprofessional exchanges of scientific knowledge; (2) the strong trend in the colleges (despite the ideology of the superstraights) toward a standardized curriculum incorporating improved skills in differential diagnosis and clinical hospital experience; (3) concerted efforts within the profession to establish "standards of care," which should help reduce conflicts over scope of practice; (4) pressures from third-party payers for agreement on the proper scope of chiropractic; (5) political pressures for chiropractic to fit into the national health care scene and into plans for reorganizing the health care system; and (6) a more sophisticated chiropractic leadership aware of all these pressures and trends and able to make more enlightened decisions regarding chiropractic's goals and strategy.

Section 6

What Can Organized Medicine Do?

Although Nortin Hadler, M.D., earlier wrote (1979), "The battle organized medicine needs to rejoin relates first to the ethic of licensure of chiropractors," he acknowledged that it was already a fait accompli that "chiropractors are licensed and seeing patients."

Despite the fact that chiropractors are the principal decision makers regarding their own professional fate, they cannot decide it alone; federal policy makers and organized medicine also are involved. The AMA is reeling still from the Wilk antitrust suit. Not only did it have to revise its Code of Medical Ethics to permit full professional association with chiropractors, but it had to raise millions of dollars to pay its lawyers' fees, court costs, and settlements with the chiropractic plaintiffs for their legal expenses. As early as 1981 one of its best known anti-chiropractic activists (Stephen Barrett) was quoted as saying, "The anti-chiropractic movement is rudderless and leaderless." After the AMA recovers from losing one of its major political battles of the century, it should consider its long-range goals and how best to achieve them.

The historical precedents set by homeopathy and osteopathy provide only limited guidance. The AMA goal of absorbing these groups into medicine has been substantially achieved. Inasmuch as neither chiropractors nor organized medicine want chiropractic to become fused into or parallel (as is osteopathy) to medicine, the AMA must consider other alternatives. Recognizing that chiropractors clearly are not destined to become ancillary practitioners, there remain only two realistic possibilities from the scenarios presented: (1) the status quo of marginality, or (2) limited medical status. Organized medicine should consider the implications of each for itself and for the health of the American people, and choose between them.

The status quo is destabilizing for chiropractors, organized medicine, and the entire health care system. The more marginal chiropractic remains the more it will attack organized medicine, politically and professionally. The more isolated chiropractors are made to feel the more they will concentrate on their differences from medicine, the failures of medicine and its iatrogenesis, and their own propaganda regarding chiropractic's miraculous cures of medical failures and their persecution by organized medicine, which they will continue to accuse of seeking only to protect its narrow economic interests.

On the other hand, if organized medicine should decide that a limited medical status is appropriate for chiropractic, it could help to bring it about in three important ways:

1. It could collaborate with chiropractors in research on illnesses and disabilities in which it shares a vital interest, not only on the neuromusculoskeletal and biomechanical conditions that chiropractors most frequently treat (about 85% of all chiropractors' practices), but also the O-type illnesses (both somatovisceral and viscerosomatic), which chiropractors have historically treated with considerable success. If carefully controlled research is never done on these cases, it will never be known how effective spinal manipulative therapy (SMT) is in treating them.

2. Organized medicine could help improve chiropractic education in several ways. Because it is weakest in providing students with opportunities to view the most serious diseases (because they seldom arrive at a school clinic), nearby hospitals should provide such clinical training. Scott Haldeman (1982, p 139) has said, "What we physicians need to do is work to see that all chiropractors have enough training to diagnose illnesses and diseases for which manipulation isn't indicated." Cheek-by-jowl participation with medical students on hospital rounds reduces suspicion and paranoia on both sides and promotes future professional collaboration, as has hap-

pened with new programs in clinical pharmacology. Chiropractic postgraduate specialization in diagnostic imaging, orthopedics, neurology, sports medicine, and diagnosis and internal disorders would be upgraded by exposure to management of appropriate hospitalized patients. Admission to postgraduate medical seminars and workshops also would help.

3. The ultimate goal should be full professional collaboration in patient treatment: consultations, referrals, and joint management both in and out of hospitals. The last will be the most difficult to achieve, partly because of economic competition for the patient's (and the insurance company's) dollar. Researchers and educators are not primarily money oriented, but practitioners are. For the AMA to admit a rival group of practitioners into the sacred medical fold would require a supreme act of good judgment, not an unselfish but a wise one. It made that judgment earlier in the case of homeopathy, and later in the case of osteopathy, with results quite satisfactory to the medical profession, if not to the others. A decision for full professional cooperation with chiropractors could be beneficial to all parties in the long run.

What would such a decision do for organized medicine that could be interpreted to be in its enlightened self-interest? It would reduce much of the negative criticism that MDs are motivated by fear of losing patients and more concerned with money than with providing the best possible care to their patients. It would improve their relations with patients who have conditions that medicine, drugs, and surgery often do not handle well. It would remove the frustration most MDs feel in attempting to treat back problems. MDs would receive more referrals and consultation requests from chiropractors more willing to collaborate and share responsibility for patient care. Everyone agrees that optimum health care today requires the cooperation of several types of specialists. Chronic pain clinics would seem to be an especially promising area for future collaboration. Patient care would improve, and would be less costly, because the best of chiropractic and medicine would be readily available to every patient. Hence the goal of both professions could be achieved: better health care for the American people.

Section 7

Conclusion

Historically there have been only two outcomes for sectarian medicine: die out completely or be absorbed into the medical mainstream. Homeopathy and osteopathy illustrate the second alternative. Despite osteopaths' protests, there is little that they offer that allopaths do not also do, including SMT. The word "osteopathy" may persist, but reality is what counts. With no formal professional barriers between them, the remaining stigma associated with the word "osteopathy" offers little incentive to potential recruits to enter the profession and compete with allopaths in the health marketplace. The osteopath nearest my home told me that he uses SMT only if a patient specifically requests it. I would expect that in the future his patients might be more likely to go to a chiropractic specialist in SMT, who would probably be a more proficient manipulator than an allopathic osteopath.

Examples of medical sects that have disappeared are not hard to find. Thomsonism is one. Most of whatever there was of value in botanical medicine has been incorporated into orthodox medicine as pharmaceutical chemists identified the active ingredients in "simples" and synthesized them. Since there was little philosophic difference between thomsonism and orthodox medicine, except the desire to escape the horrors of heroic medicine with its bleeding and toxic medications, medicine has been able, as those offensive practices were dropped, to clean its skirts, to incorporate what was of value, and thus to deal thomsonism a lethal blow.

There remains the final question of why chiropractic has not suffered one of these fatal outcomes. Why has it followed a different historical course? One main reason certainly was the isolation that orthodox medicine imposed on chiropractors throughout their nearly a century of existence. Their isolation was probably due as much, perhaps even more, to the stance adopted by B.J. Palmer. Whether B.J.'s motives were legal and political, he developed a chiropractic philosophy that was, as he said, the exact opposite, "antipodal," to medicine. He also invented his distinctive terminology, encouraged his colleagues to author a parallel set of textbooks, and attacked medicine in a never-ending stream of lectures, pamphlets, and books. When he employed MDs for his clinic and faculty, he required them to adhere to his "party line" so as not to contaminate student minds. Although many graduates of the Palmer School of Chiropractic later wandered afield from straight chiropractic and its narrow scope of practice, that did little to change the ideologic climate of the profession.

On the other hand, organized medicine made few overtures to chiropractic. Those individual MDs who studied it were scorned and/or ostracized. The Massachusetts MD who was sympathetic to chiropractic was deathly afraid of losing his hospital appointments if his "failing" became known to his colleagues. The AMA stigmatized chiropractors, especially B.J., as cultists, quacks, buffoons, "mad dogs," or unscrupulous charlatans. It focused on the low social origins of the Palmers and their followers and on their limited educational backgrounds. It made no effort to examine chiropractic's claims seriously. The few studies that were favorable were ignored or buried (Wilk, Plaintiffs Exhibit No. 241). As Mootz and Keating (1989) so aptly put it: "In rejecting spinal adjusting without hard data, political medicine provided the chiropractor with a perfect example of the very activity it condemned: the making of unsubstantiated claims." Simultaneously chiropractors were denied the research facilities and subsidies that would have tested their claims. As a result, chiropractic and medicine traveled on parallel tracks, with minimal input from medicine into chiropractic education and almost no reciprocal influence from chiropractic on medicine.

The legal and political areas remained arenas of constant hostility. Battles over legislation and arrests for practicing medicine without a license were in vogue by 1906 and lasted into the 1960s. Culmination of the hostility came in the 1970s and 1980s when the Wilk antitrust suit halted the AMA campaign to "contain and then eliminate chiropractic," forced the AMA to change its Code of Medical Ethics, and won court settlements permitting unlimited professional interaction with MDs and admission of chiropractors to hospital staffs.

The overall result of the long history of chiropractic's enforced isolation and of the barriers between chiropractic and medicine was to entrench chiropractic in our legal, political, and social institutions as a separate system of healing. Legislatures and courts often accepted the argument that chiropractic was a "separate and distinct" theory and therapy and therefore entitled to separate licensure procedures (i.e., separate boards of registration) and that citizens' freedom of choice would be infringed on if they could not go to a chiropractor. Only in a federated system like ours, with 51 different legal and political jurisdictions, could such great variability in licensing laws and scope of practice have developed. Although the variability created problems, it permitted chiropractors to ratchet up legal advantages, as gains in the most favorable states were used as leverage in other states. Chiropractors used to advantage this well-known feature of our federated system. (Of course, the AMA tried to work it in the reverse direction.) Thus the long period of chiropractors' isolation permitted them to gain footholds and beachheads separate from the stricter and more hostile locales of medical regulation.

Now that barriers to professional intercommunication and cooperation are reduced, it remains to be seen what will be the impact of future changes in the health care system on chiropractics' fairly well-established status. With the vested interests that chiropractors now have in their system of higher education and their separate laws and licensing boards, and considering their practice limitations in relation to the sacrosanct areas of controlled drugs and major surgery, it seems to me very unlikely that chiropractic will ever evolve toward fusion with the medical mainstream, as has osteopathy. It also seems certain that chiropractic will not simply fade away, considering its currently entrenched legal status, its solid acceptance by the public, and its developing collegial relations with MDs.

Although many chiropractors have expressed the fear that medicine will take over chiropractic once it discovers how effective it is, it also seems to me unlikely that any significant number of orthopedists, neurologists, or physiatrists will adopt SMT extensively, considering how much easier it is to earn good money using surgery or drugs.

As for physical therapists, a problem of competition with chiropractors could develop, as is already the case in places where they and osteopaths use SMT extensively: Australia, New Zealand, England, Scandinavia, and to a lesser extent Canada. In the United States physical therapists are more concerned with upgrading their entry-level education to a masters degree and obtaining the right to independent access than becoming specialists in SMT. It is difficult to predict how physical therapy will evolve in the future. If it fully incorporates SMT, that could have a serious impact on chiropractic, but that seems now to be in the quite distant future. Physical therapists continue to receive relatively little training in diagnosis for the entire range of disorders that patients present with, and in interpreting laboratory tests, x-rays, and other types of diagnostic imaging, all of which are needed today for competent differential diagnosis. Hence physical therapists have a long way to go before they will be able to compete effectively with chiropractors. As long as they continue to work in medical settings and on referral from MDs and DOs (in actuality even if it ceases to be a legal requirement), those in the United States will probably not use much SMT. Some of those who have studied it under Cyriax, Paris, or Maitland seem more impressed with its limitations than are most chiropractors. Hence physical therapists seem not likely to move so wholeheartedly into SMT as many chiropractors fear.

My overall conclusions are that the role of chiropractors in the U.S. health care system will continue to change, that chiropractors will probably not remain in as marginal a social and professional role as they have known for nearly a century, that they will not track osteopaths into the medical mainstream, and that they will most likely evolve slowly into a "limited medical" status comparable to that of dentists, podiatrists, optometrists, and psychologists. Even if the United States should adopt some form of national health system or service, I would expect the other current realities I have discussed to continue to govern chiropractors' status in U.S. society.

BIBLIOGRAPHY

"A New Medical Marriage." 1985. *Newsweek* April 12.

Abbott, Andrew. 1988. *The System of Professions: An Essay on the Division of Expert Labor*. Chicago: University of Chicago Press.

Abrams Albert. 1910. *Spondylotherapy: Spinal Concussion and the Application of Other Methods to the Spine in the Treatment of Disease*. San Francisco: Philopolis Press.

———1912. *Spondylotherapy; Physio-Therapy of the Spine Based on a Study of Clinical Physiology*. San Francisco: Philopolis Press.

———1914 (1915). *Progressive Spondylotherapy*. San Francisco: Philopolis Press.

ACA Council on Technic. 1986. "The Evaluation of Chiropractic Technic: An Analysis with Recommendations." *ACAJ* 23(3):64–73.

Aitken, Steven T., et al. 1989. "The Use of Pharmaceutical Compounds for Diagnostic and Limited Therapeutic Procedures in Chiropractic Practice." *DC* 7(23):38–39.

"Amendment to the Medical Registration Law." 1915. *Boston Medical and Surgical Journal* 173:23. July 1.

"American Cancer Society Reverses Anti-Chiropractic Policy." 1985. *ICA Today* 22:1.

"An Interview at Shorewood Hospital." 1984. *ACA Journal of Chiropractic* 21(12):38–47.

Anderson, Robert. 1981. "Bonesetting: A Medical Bone of Contention." *ACAJ* 18(10):S91–S100.

———— 1982. "Hawaiian Therapeutic Massage." *World-Wide Report* 24(5):4A.

———— 1983a. "On Doctors and Bonesetters in the 16th and 17th Centuries." *Ch Hist* 3:11–15.

———— 1983b. "An American Contribution to Third World Medicine: Spinal Manipulative Therapy." In John H. Morgan (Ed.). *Third World Medicine and Social Change: A Reader in Social Science and Medicine.* Lanham, Md: University Press of America.

———— 1987. "The Treatment of Musculoskeletal Disorders by a Mexican Bonesetter (Sobador)." *Social Science and Medicine* 24:43–46.

———— 1989. "One of My Favorite People: Aubrey A. Swartz." *DC* 7(15):31.

Anderson, Steven E. 1991. "Chiropractic's First Steps in Hungary." *DC* 9(16):1,33.

"Annual Report of the Council on Chiropractic Education." 1984. Des Moines, Ia.: CCE.

"Another Legislative Win for Ohio Doctors of Chiropractic." 1990. *DC* 32(5):122.

Aquilina, Anthony D. 1990. "General Practice Residency Training and the Osteopathic Profession: Issues for the 1990s." *JAOA* 90:161–178.

Assendelft, Willem J.J., Lex M. Bauter, and Alphons G.H. Kessels. 1991. "Effectiveness of Chiropractic and Physiotherapy in the Treatment of Low Back Pain: A Critical Discussion of the British Randomized Clinical Trial." *JMPT* 14:281–286.

Attitudes Toward Health Care in Oklahoma. 1984. Oklahoma City: Chiropractic Association of Oklahoma.

Bachop, William. 1991. "The Warfare of Science with Philosophy in Contemporary Chiropractic." *Philosophical Constructs for the Chiropractic Profession* 1:33–36.

Baer, Hans A. 1984. "A Historical Overview of British and European Chiropractic." *Ch Hist* 4:11–15.

———— 1987. "The Divergent Evolution of Osteopathy in America and Britain." In Julius A. Roth (Ed.). *Research in the Sociology of Health Care.* Vol. 5. Greenwich, Conn.: JAI Press.

———— 1989a. "Divergence and Convergence in Two Systems of Manual Medicine: Osteopathy and Chiropractic in the United States." *Medical Anthropology Quarterly* (New Series) 1:176–193.

———— 1989b. "The American Dominative Medical System as a Reflection of Social Relations in the Larger Society." *Social Science and Medicine* 28:1103–1112.

———— 1991. "The Sociopolitical Development of British Chiropractic." *JMPT* 14:38–45.

Baird, Rand. 1990. "Benefits of Chiropractic Integration of Hospitals." *California Chiropractic Journal* 15(8):29–37.

Baker, W. Joseph. 1985. "A Clinical Reformation in Chiropractic." *Ch Hist* 5:59–62.

Barge, Fred H. 1987. *Life without Fear*. Eldridge, Ia: Bowden Bros.

———— 1989. " 'Thots': A Call to Close Ranks." *ICA Review* 45(2):7.

———— 1990. *One Cause One Cure: The Health and Life Philosophy of Chiropractic*. LaCrosse, Wisc: LaCrosse Graphics.

Barker, Sir Herbert Atkinson. 1927. *Leaves from My Life*. London: Hutchinson and Co., Ltd.

Barrett, Stephen. 1980. *The Health Robbers*. Philadelphia: George Stickley Co.

———— 1990. "Views of a Chiropractic Critic: Your Real Enemy Is Yourself." *ACAJ* 27(11):61–64.

Bayer, Charles M. 1945. *Medicine Men and Men of Medicine*. New York: Medical Society of the State of New York.

Bealle, Morris. 1939. *Medical Moussolini*. Washington, D.C.: Columbia Publishing Co.

Beatty, Homer G. 1939. *Anatomical Adjustive Technique*. Denver.

Bechgaard, Paul, and Ole Bentzen. 1966. "Auditory Disturbances Originating in Columna Cervicalis" (translated from Danish). *Journal of the Canadian Chiropractic Association* 10(4):5ff.

Beck, Brian L. 1991. "Magnetic Healing, Spiritualism, and Chiropractic: The Union of Methodologies." *Ch Hist* 11(2):11–16.

Becker, Howard S. 1961. *Boys in White*. Chicago: University of Chicago Press.

Beideman, Ronald P. 1983. "Seeking the Rational Alternative: The National College of Chiropractic from 1906 to 1982." *Ch Hist* 3:16–22.

———1990. "A Short History of the Chiropractic Profession." In Dana J. Lawrence (Ed.). *Fundamentals of Chiropractic Diagnosis and Management*. Baltimore: Williams & Wilkins.

Bellin, Lowell E. 1973. "Should a Paper on the Administration of Chiropractic have been published in *Medical Care?* With Comments on Derivative Questions." *Medical Care* 11:441–448.

Bennett, George Matthews. (1884) 1981. *The Art of the Bonesetter: A Testimony and a Vindication*. London: Tamor Pierston.

Berk, Marc L. 1985. *Nonphysician Health Care Providers: Use of Ambulatory Services, Expenditures, and Sources of Payment*. Item 491-B-16. National Center for Health Services Research and Health Care USPHS. Washington, D.C.

Berlant, Jeffrey L. 1975. *Profession and Monopoly: A Study of Medicine in the United States and Great Britain*. Berkeley, Calif.: University of California Press.

Bernard, Claude. 1861. "Lectures on the Spinal Cord." *Medical Times and Gazette* 1:547ff.

———1865 (1927). *An Introduction to the Study of Experimental Medicine*. Translated by H.C. Greene. New York: Macmillan.

Biedermann, Freimut. 1959. *Fundamentals of Chiropractic from the Standpoint of a Medical Doctor*. Translated by L.C.J. Iekeler. Davenport, Ia.: International Chiropractic Research Committee.

Bierring, Walter L. 1948. "An Analysis of Basic Science Laws." *JAMA* 137:111–112.

Biggs, Errol L. 1975. "Allopathic, Osteopathic Hospitals Unite." *Hospitals* 49(9):45–47.

Blackstone, Erwin A. 1977. "The A.M.A. and the Osteopaths: A Study of the Power of Organized Medicine." *Anti-Trust Bulletin* 22:405–440.

"Board Votes for Limited Chiropractor Role." 1983. *The Nation's Health* Aug.

Bolton, S.P. 1987. "Similarities and Differences between Chiropractic and Osteopathy." *Journal of the Australian Chiropractors' Association* 17:90–93.

Booth, Eamons R. 1905. *History of Osteopathy and Twentieth Century Medical Practice.* Cincinnati: Jennings and Graham.

Bourdillon, John F. 1973. *Spinal Manipulation.* New York: Appleton-Century-Crofts.

Bowers, Walter B. 1935. "Educational Symposium: The Massachusetts Board of Registration in Medicine." *NEJM* 213(1):3.

Boyle, Wade. 1989. "Our Naturopathic Heritage." *AANP Quarterly Newsletter* 4(4):8.

Bradbury, Parnell. 1957. *Healing by Hand.* London: Harwell Press.

Brantingham, James W. 1986. "Still and Palmer: The Impact of the First Osteopath and the First Chiropractor." *Ch Hist* 6:19–22.

———— 1988. "A Critical Look at the Subluxation Hypothesis." *JMPT* 11:130–132.

Brennan, Matthew J. 1980. *Opinion Survey II: Advertising, Education, Referrals, Insurance Equality, and Other.* Des Moines, Ia.: ACA.

———— 1983a. "Perspectives on Chiropractic Education in Medical Literature." *Ch Hist* 3:25–30.

———— 1983b. "A Comparison of D.C.s and M.D.s. *ACAJ* 20(3):32–35.

———— 1983c. "CMCC Leads the Way in Chiropractic Research." *ACAJ* 20(8):100–103.

———— 1984. 1988. 1989. 1991. *Demographic and Professional Characteristics of ACA Membership: Annual Survey and Statistical Study.* Arlington, Va.: ACA.

Brigman, Linda. 1983. "Survey Results: North Carolina Opinion Poll." W.H. Long Marketing, Inc.

Brockington, Yvonne L. 1987. *A Comparison of the Personality Traits of Three Student Groups as Measured by the Edwards Personal Preference Schedule.* Doctoral Dissertation in Education. International Graduate School (St. Louis).

Brunarski, David J. 1984. "Clinical Trials of Spinal Manipulation: A Critical Appraisal and Review of the Literature." *JMPT* 7:243–249.

Budden, William A. 1928. *Physiotherapy, Technique and Treatment*. Chicago: Published by the author.

Buerger, A.A. and J.S. Tobis (Eds). 1977. *Approaches to the Validation of Manipulative Therapy*. Springfield, Ill.: Charles C Thomas.

Buerger, A.A. and Philip E. Greenman. 1985. *Empirical Approaches to the Validation of Spinal Manipulation*. Springfield, Ill.: Charles C Thomas.

Bureau of Health Professions. 1990. *Seventh Report to the President and Congress on the Status of Health Personnel in the United States*. Washington, D.C.: DHHS.

Burich, Stephen J. 1919. *A Textbook on Chiropractic Chemistry*. Davenport, Ia.

Cabot, Hugh. 1940. *The Patient's Dilemma*. New York: Reynall and Hitchcock.

"California Chiropractic Association: The First 50 Years." 1978. *California Chiropractic Association Journal* Sept., pp. 8–29.

Campbell, Louis K., C. Jacob Ladenheim, Robert P. Sherman, and Louis Sportelli. 1990. *Risk Management in Chiropractic: Developing Malpractice Prevention Strategies*. Fincastle, Va.: Health Services Publications, Ltd.

Cannon, Walter B. 1934. "President Eliot's Relations with Medicine." *NEJM* 210:730–738.

———— 1939. *The Wisdom of the Body*. New York: W.W. Norton.

Canterbury, Robin, and Gary Krakos. 1986. "Thirteen Years after Roentgen: The Origins of Chiropractic Radiology." *Ch Hist* 6:25–29.

Caplan, Ronald L. 1987. "The Clash over Quackery." *Health/PAC* Winter:22–26.

———— 1991. "Chiropractic in the United States and the Changing Health Care Environment: A View from Outside the Profession. *JMPT* 14:46–50.

Carmichael, Joel P. 1988. "Chiropractic Residency at Lindell Hospital: A Program Description." *JMPT* 11:177–180.

Carrick, Frederick Robert. 1990. Letter in *ACA/FYI*, Sept. , p. 6.

Carr-Saunders, A.M., and P.A. Wilson. 1933. *The Professions*. London: Oxford University Press.

Cartman, Thabiti H.N. 1988. "American Black Chiropractors Association." *DC* 6(14):27.

Carver, Willard. 1909. *Carver's Chiropractic Analysis as Applied to Anatomy, Physiology, Chiropractic Principles, Symptomatology and Diagnosis*. Oklahoma City: Warden-Elbright Printing Co.

———1936. *History of Chiropractic*. Mimeographed, 196 pp.

Cassidy, J. David, and W.H. Kirkaldi-Willis. 1988. "Manipulation." In W.H. Kirkaldi-Willis (Ed.). *Managing Low Back Pain*. New York: Churchill Livingstone.

———1990. Letter. *JMPT* 13:40–41.

Chapman-Smith, David. 1989. "Commentary: The Wilk Case." *JMPT* 12:142–146.

———1990. "Medical Referrals: Signs and Symptoms of a New Era." *The Chiropractic Report* Nov. 1990.

———1991. "Perspective on the Future of Chiropractic." *California Chiropractic Association Journal* 16(2):31,49–50.

Cherkin, Daniel C., and Frederick A MacCornack. 1989. "Patient Evaluations of Low Back Pain from Family Physicians and Chiropractors." *Western Journal of Medicine* 150:351–355.

———F. MacCornack, and A.O. Berg. 1988. "The Management of Low Back Pain: A Comparison of the Beliefs and Behaviors of Family Physicians and Chiropractors." *Western Journal of Medicine* 149:475–480.

———1989. "Family Physicians' Views of Chiropractors: Hostile or Hospitable?" *AJPH* 79:636–637.

Chinnicci, Leonard J., vs. Central DuPage Hospital et al. 1990. Civil Action No. 89 C 7752 filed February 9 in the United States District Court for the Northern District of Illinois, Eastern Division.

"Chiro Consultant Irks DC." 1989. *New York State Chiropractic Association Newsletter* 17(2):5.

"Chiropractic." 1914. *JAMA* 62:1177–1178.

Chiropractic in New Zealand: Report of the Commission of Inquiry. 1979.
Wellington, New Zealand: P.D. Hasselberg.

Chiropractic Services Pilot Program Evaluation Study: Final Report. 1990. U.S.
Department of Veterans Affairs. Mimeographed, Washington, D.C.

Chiropractic: State of the Art. 1985. 1987. 1989-1990. Arlington, Va.: ACA.

Chiropractic's White Paper on Health, Education, and Welfare Secretary's Report.
1969. Cheyenne, Wyo.: ACA, ICA, and Council of State Chiropractic
Examining Boards.

"Chiropractors." 1988. *Occupational Outlook Handbook (1988-1989).* U.S.
Department of Labor Bulletin 2300. April 1988. Scottsdale, Ariz.: Associated
Book Publishers.

"Chiropractors: Healers or Quacks?" 1975. *Consumer Reports* 40:542–547,
606–610.

"Chiropractors Invade Doctors' Domain." 1989. *New York State Chiropractic
Association Newsletter* 17(2):24–25.

"Chiropractors and Low Back Pain" (Editorial). 1990. *Lancet* 336:220. July 28.

Chrisman, O.D., and R.F. Gervais. 1962. "Otologic Manifestations of the Cervical
Syndrome." *Clinical Orthopedics* 24:34–39.

————et al. 1964. "A Study of the Results Following Rotary Manipulation in the
Lumbar Intervertebral Disc Syndrome." *Journal of Bone and Joint Surgery*
46A:517–524.

Christensen, Finn. 1981. "An Updated Study of Chiropractic in Danish Medicine."
Archives of the California Chiropractic Association 5(1):67–76.

Christie, Sharon A. 1985. "Denial of Hospital Admitting Privileges for
Non-physician Providers: A Per Se Antitrust Violation?" *Notre Dame Law
Review.* 60:724–744.

Cleary, Paul D. 1982. "Chiropractic Use: A Test of Several Hypotheses. *AJPH*
72:727–730.

Coburn, David. 1991. "Legitimacy at the Expense of Narrowing of Scope of Practice: Chiropractic in Canada. *JMPT* 14:14–21.

Cody, George. 1985. "History of Naturopathic Medicine." In Joseph E. Pizzorno, Jr., and Michael T. Murray (Eds.). *A Textbook of Natural Medicine*. Seattle: John Bastyr College Publications.

Coe, Rodney M. 1970. *Sociology of Medicine*. New York: McGraw-Hill.

Cohen, Solomon Solis. 1902-1905. (Ed.). *A System of Physiological Therapeutics: A Practical Exposition of the Methods, Other than Drug-Giving, Useful for the Prevention of Disease and in the Treatment of the Sick*. Philadelphia: Blackiston's.

Cohen, Wilbur J. 1968. *Independent Practitioners under Medicare: A Report to Congress*. Washington, D.C.: U.S. Department of Health, Education, and Welfare.

Commonwealth vs. Zimmerman. 1915. 221 Mass. 184.

Commonwealth vs. New England College of Chiropractic. 1915. 221 Mass. 190.

Communications Consulting Group. 1983. "Public Attitudes and Predispositions toward the Chiropractic Profession." Mimeographed, California Chiropractic Association.

Coser, Lewis. 1956. *The Functions of Social Conflict*. Glencoe, Ill.: Free Press.

Costs of Education in the Health Professions. 1974. Washington, D.C.: Institute of Medicine, National Academy of Sciences.

Coulehan, John L. 1985. "Chiropractic and the Clinical Art." *Social Science and Medicine* 21:383–390.

————1991. "The Treatment Act: An Analysis of the Clinical Art in Chiropractic." *JMPT* 14:5–13.

Coulter, Harris L. 1970. "Homeopathy Revisited." *Scope* (Boston University Medical Center Magazine) Sept./Oct. pp. 16–21.

————1975. *Divided Legacy: A History of the Schism in Medical Thought*. Vol. 3. Washington, D.C.: Wehawken Book Co.

Coulter, Ian D. 1981. "The Chiropractic Curriculum: A Problem of Integration."
JMPT 4:147–154.

———— 1983. "Chiropractic Observed: Thirty Years of Changing Sociological
Perspectives." *Ch Hist* 3:43–48.

———— 1989. "Chiropractic Utilization: A Statistical Analysis." *AJCM* 2:13–21.

———— 1990 (Letter). "The Influence of Political Medicine on Chiropractic Dogma:
Applications for Scientific Development." *JMPT* 13:234.

———— 1991. "Sociological Studies of the Role of the Chiropractor: An Exercise in
Ideological Hegemony." *JMPT* 14:51–58.

Cowie, James B. and Julian Roebuck. 1975. *An Ethnography of a Chiropractic
Clinic*. New York: Free Press.

Cranston, Ruth. 1955. *The Miracle of Lourdes*. New York: McGraw-Hill.

Creel, George. 1915. "Making Doctors While You Wait." *Harper's Weekly*
60:319–321.

Crisp, Kathleen A. 1984. "Chiropractic Lyceums: The Colorful Origins of
Chiropractic Continuing Education." *Ch Hist* 4:17–22.

Cummings, Mark. 1990, "The Pull Toward the Vacuum: Osteopathic Medical
Education in the 1980s." *JAOA* 90:353–362.

Curtis, Peter. 1988. "Spinal Manipulation: Does It Work?" *Occupational Medicine:
State of the Art Reviews*. 3(1):31–44.

Cyriax, James Henry. 1975a (1951). *Textbook of Orthopaedic Medicine: Treatment
by Manipulation and Deep Massage*. (4th edition). London: Cassell.

———— 1975b. "Treatment of Pain by Manipulation." *NINCDS*, pp. 271–276.

Dan, N., and P. Saccasan. 1983. "Serious Complications of Lumbar Spinal
Manipulation." *Medical Journal of Australia* 2:672–673.

Daneshmend, T., et al. 1984. "Acute Brain Stem Stroke During Neck
Manipulation." *British Medical Journal* 288:189.

Davis, Andrew P. 1899. *Osteopathy Illustrated: A Drugless System of Healing*.
Cincinnati: F.L. Rowe.

———1905. *Neurology*. Cincinnati: F.L. Rowe.

———1909. *Neuropathy: The New Science of Drugless Healing Amply Illustrated and Explained, Embracing Ophthalmology, Osteopathy, Chiropractic Science, Suggestive Therapeutics, Magnetism, Instructions on Diet, Deep Breathing, Bathing, etc.* Cincinnati: F.L. Rowe.

Day, S. 1989. "Glad Ya Met Aetna?" *Georgia Chiropractor* 8(12):6, 8, 14.

"DC to Direct Medical Services for Soviet Olympic Team." 1991. *DC* 9(24):1.

DeGiacomo, Frank P. 1979. *Man's Greatest Gift to Man: Chiropractic*. Old Bethpage, New York: LSR Learning Associates.

———1989. "Where Have We Been . . . Where Are We Going?" *Transitions: A Publication of the New York College of Chiropractic Alumni Association* 15(1):4–5.

DeJarnette, Major. 1940 (1967). *Sacro Occipital Technique of Spinal Therapy*. Published by the author.

Denslow, J.S. 1944. "An Analysis of the Variability of Spinal Reflex Threshholds." *Journal of Neurophysiology* 7:207–215.

———1975. "Pathophysiologic Evidence for the Osteopathic Lesion. Data on What Is Known, What Is Not Known, and What is Controversial." *NINCDS*, pp. 227–234.

Deyo, Richard A. 1983. "Conservative Therapy for Low Back Pain: Distinguishing Useful from Useless Therapy." *JAMA* 250:1057–1062.

———and Yuh-Jane Tsui-Wu. 1987. "Descriptive Epidemiology of Low-back Pain and Its Related Medical Care in the United States." *Spine* 12:264–268.

Dintenfass, Julius. 1970. *Chiropractic: A Modern Way to Health*. New York: Pyramid House.

———1973. "The Administration of Chiropractic in the New York City Medicaid Program." *Medical Care* 11:40–51.

Dishman, Robert W. 1988. "Static and Dynamic Components of the Chiropractic Subluxation Complex: A Literature Review." *JMPT* 11:98–107.

Dock, George. 1922. "A Visit to a Chiropractic School." *JAMA* 78(1):60–63.

Dods, A. 1824. *Pathological Observations on the Rotated or Contorted Spine, Commonly Called Lateral Curvature, Deduced from Practice*. London: T. Cadell.

Donahue, Joseph. 1986. "D.D. Palmer and Innate Intelligence: Development, Division, and Derision." *Ch Hist* 6:31–36.

——— 1987. "D.D. Palmer and the Metaphysical Movement in the Nineteenth Century." *Ch Hist* 7(1):23–27.

——— 1990. "Philosophy of Chiropractic: Lessons from the past—Guidance for the Future." *Journal of the Canadian Chiropractic Association* 35:194–205.

——— 1991. Letter. *Journal of the Canadian Chiropractic Association* 35:98.

Drain, James R. 1927. *Chiropractic Thoughts*. San Antonio, Texas: TCC.

——— 1949. *Man Tomorrow*. San Antonio: Standard Printing Co.

"Drug Company Tests Chiropractic Market." 1989. *CJ* 3(7):1, 7.

Duffy, Daniel, J. 1978. "Public Attitude toward Chiropractic and Patient Satisfaction with Chiropractic in the State of Wisconsin." Mimeographed. Madison, Wis.

Duke, R., and T. Spreadbury. 1981. "Closed Manipulation Leading to Immediate Recovery from Cervical Spine Dislocation with Paraplegia." *Lancet* 8246:577–578.

Durenberger, David. 1988. "Perspectives: A Senator." *Health Affairs* 7(2 suppl.):39–44.

Dvorak, Jiri. 1989. "Editorial." *Journal of Manipulative Medicine* 4(1):1.

——— and F. V. Orelli. 1985. "How Dangerous is Manipulation to the Cervical Spine?" *Manual Medicine* 2:1–4.

Dye, Abiathar Augustus. 1939. *The Evolution of Chiropractic: Its Discovery and Development*. Philadelphia: Published by the author.

Dzaman, Fern, et al. (Eds.). 1980. *Who's Who in Chiropractic International*. Littleton, Colo.: Who's Who in Chiropractic International Publishing Company.

Eddy, Mary Baker. 1875. *Science and Health With Key to the Scriptures*. Boston: Christian Science Publishing Company.

Edelstein, Marcia S. 1974. *Commonwealth vs. Zimmerman and the History of Chiropractic Registration in Massachusetts*. Senior Honors Thesis in History and Science, Harvard University.

Eisenberg, Abne M. 1990. "Medicine vs. Chiropractic: A Rhetorical Analysis." *DCE* 33(2):106–117.

Elkind, David. 1971. "Wilhelm Reich—the Psychoanalyst as Revolutionary." New York *Times* Magazine: April 18, pp. 25ff.

Emerson, L. Eugene (Ed.). 1929. *Physician and Patient*. Cambridge, Mass.: Harvard University Press.

Etzel, Sylvia I., et al. 1990. "Graduate Medical Education in the United States." *JAMA* 262:1029–1037.

Evans, David P., and Victor M. Hawthorne. 1985. "The Design and Results of Clinical Trials of Lumbar Manipulation: A Review." In A.A. Buerger and P.E. Greenman (Eds.). *Empirical Approaches to the Validation of Spinal Manipulation*. Springfield, Ill.: Charles C. Thomas.

Evans, G.D. 1973. "A Sociology of Chiropractic." *Journal of the Canadian Chiropractic Association* 17(3):6–18.

Evans, Harold W. 1978. *Historical Chiropractic Data*. Stockton, Calif.: World Wide Books.

Fager, C. 1984. "The Age Old Back Problem: New Fad, Same Fallacies." *Spine* 9:326–330.

Farfan, H.F. 1973. *Mechanical Disorders of the Low Back*. Philadelphia: Lea & Febiger.

Farrell, J., and L. Twomey. 1982. "Acute Low Back Pain." *Medical Journal of Australia* 1:160–164.

Fay, Leonard E., 1986. "The 1986 Lee-Homewood Award: John B. Wolfe." *Ch Hist* 6:85–86.

"Federal Grant for Disadvantaged Students." 1990. *DCE* 33(2):104–105.

Ferguson, Alana. 1984. " 'The Sweetheart of the PSC'—Mabel Heath Palmer: The Early Years." *Ch Hist* 4:25–28.

Fine, Judylaine. 1987. *Conquering Back Pain.* New York: Prentice Hall.

Firman, G.J., and M.S. Goldstein. 1975. "The Future of Chiropractic: A Psychosocial View." *NEJM* 293:639–642.

Firth, James N. 1914. *A Textbook on Chiropractic Symptomatology; or the Manifestations of Incoordination Considered from a Chiropractic Standpoint.* Rock Island, Ill.: Driffill Printing Co.

Fishbein, Morris. 1925. *The Medical Follies.* New York: Boni and Liveright.

———1932. *Fads and Quackery in Healing.* New York: Blue Ribbon Books.

Flexner, Abraham. 1910. *Medical Education in the United States and Canada.* New York: Carnegie Foundation for the Advancement of Teaching.

———1914. "A Layman's View of Osteopathy." *JAMA* 42:1831–1833.

Ford, Clyde W. 1989a. "The Psychodynamics of Human Touch." *DCE* 32(3):43–46.

———1989b. *Where Healing Waters Meet: Touching Mind and Emotion Through the Body.* Barrytown, N.Y.: Station Hill Press.

Foreman, Stephen M., and Arthur C. Croft. 1988. *Whiplash Injuries, the Cervical Acceleration/Deceleration Syndrome.* Baltimore: Williams & Wilkins.

Forster, Arthur Leopold. 1915. *Principles and Practice of Spinal Adjustment.* Chicago: NCC.

Francis, Robert S. 1991. "A Different Perspective of Manipulation under Anesthesia." *DC* 9(13):34–35.

Frank, Jerome. 1961. *Persuasion and Healing: A Comparative Study of Psychotherapy.* New York: Schocken.

Freeman, Michael D., et al. 1990. "The Superior Intracapsular Ligament of the Sacroiliac Joint: Presumptive Evidence for Confirmation of Illi's Ligament." *JMPT* 13:384–390.

Freidson, Eliot. 1970a. *Professional Dominance: The Social Structure of Medical Care*. New York: Atherton Press.

———1970b. *Profession of Medicine: A Study of the Sociology of Applied Knowledge*. New York: Dodd, Mead.

Frigard, Ted. 1970. *The Whiplash Injury*. Richmond Hill, New York: Richmond Hall Inc.

Gallagher, Harry. 1930. *History of Chiropractic: A History of the Philosophy, Art, and Science of Chiropractic and Chiropractors in Oklahoma*. Guthrie, Okla.: Cooperative Publishing Co.

Gallinaro, P., and M. Cartesegna. 1983. (Letter.) "Three Cases of Lumbar Disc Rupture and One of Cauda Equina Associated with Spinal Manipulation (Chiropraxis)." *Lancet* 8321:411.

Gallup Organization. 1982. *A Survey of New York State Adults Measuring Public Awareness, Utilization, and Acceptance of Chiropractic Care in New York State*. Report of a Survey Prepared for the New York State Chiropractic Association. Princeton, N.J.

———1991. *National Opinion Study*. Prepared for the ACA. Princeton, N.J.

Garceau, Oliver. 1941. *The Political Life of the American Medical Association*. Cambridge, Mass.: Harvard University Press.

Gates, Douglass. 1987. "Focus on Philosophy." *Triune* ("The Official Publication of the FSCO"). 9(2):15.

Gatterman, Meridel I. 1982. "W.A. Budden: The Transition Through Proprietary Education." *Ch Hist* 2:21–25.

Gaucher-Peslherbe, Pierre-Louis. 1983. " 'The Doctress of Epsom Has Outdone. . .' a Chiropractor." *European Journal of Chiropractic* 31:13–16.

———1991. "La Médicine a l'Epreuve du Reboutage." *Cahiers de Sociologie Economique et Culturelle (Ethnopsychologie)*. June, pp. 105–119.

———1992. *Chiropractic Early Concepts in their Historical Setting*. Lombard, Ill, NCC. (Translated by Elizabeth Weeks from *La Chiropractique: Contribution à l'Histoire d'Une Discipline Marginalisée*. 1985, LeMans, France: Jupille.)

Geiger, Arthur J. 1942. "Chiropractic: Its Cause and Cure." *Medical Economics* Feb., April, June, Aug.

Gemmell, Hugh. 1990. "An Academic Quality Ranking of the Oklahoma Regional Chiropractic Schools." *Oklahoma Chiropractic Journal* 2(1):12–13.

————and Bert H. Jacobson. 1989. "Practice Methods and Procedures of Chiropractic Doctors in Oklahoma." *Oklahoma Chiropractic Journal* 1(2):6–7.

George, Phillip E., et al. 1981. "Identification of the High Risk Pre-Stroke Patient." *ACAJ* 18(3):S26–S28.

Gevitz, Norman. 1982. *The D.O.'s: Osteopathic Medicine in America*. Baltimore: Johns Hopkins University Press.

————1988a. "A Coarse Sieve: Basic Science Boards and Medical Licensure in the United States." *Journal of the History of Medicine and Allied Sciences* 43:36–63.

————1988b. (Ed.). *Other Healers: Unorthodox Medicine in America*. Baltimore: Johns Hopkins University Press.

————1989. "The Chiropractors and the AMA: Reflections on the History of the Consultation Clause." *Perspectives in Biology and Medicine* 32:281–299.

Gibbons, Russell W. 1976. "Chiropractic History: Lost, Strayed, or Stolen." *ACAJ* 13(1):18–24.

————1980a. "The Rise of the Chiropractic Educational Establishment, 1897-1980." In Fern Dzaman (Ed.). *Who's Who in Chiropractic International*. Littleton, Colo.: Who's Who in Chiropractic International Publishing Company, pp. 339–352.

————1980b. "The Evolution of Chiropractic: Medical and Social Protest in America." In Scott Haldeman (Ed.). *Modern Developments in the Principles and Practice of Chiropractic*. New York: Appleton-Century-Crofts.

————1981a. "Physician-Chiropractors: Medical Presence in the Evolution of Chiropractic." *Bulletin of the History of Medicine* 55: 233–245.

————1981b. "Solon Massey Langworthy: Keeper of the Flame During the 'Lost Years' of Chiropractic." *Ch Hist* 1:14–21.

——— 1982. "Forgotten Parameters of General Practice: The Chiropractic Obstetrician." *Ch Hist* 2:26–34.

——— 1983. "Chiropractors as Interns, Residents and Staff: The Hospital Experience, 1910-1960." *Ch Hist* 3:50–57.

——— 1985. "Chiropractic's Abraham Flexner: The Lonely Journey of John J. Nugent, 1935-1963." *Ch Hist* 5:44–51.

——— 1987. "Assessing the Oracle at the Fountainhead: B.J. Palmer and His Times, 1902-1961." *Ch Hist* 7(1):9.

——— 1989. "Fred Collins and His New Jersey 'Mecca.' " *Ch Hist* 9(1):41.

Gibson, Mike. 1989. "American Legion Endorses Chiropractic Care for Vets." *ACAJ* 26(11):39–41.

Gielow, Vern. 1981. *Old Dad Chiro: Biography of D.D. Palmer Founder of Chiropractic*. Davenport, Ia.: Bawden Bros.

Gilb, Corinne L. 1966. *Hidden Hierarchies: The Professions and Government*. New York: Harper & Row.

Gilchrist, Iain C. 1976. "Psychiatric and Social Factors Related to Low-Back Pain in General Practice." *Rheumatology and Rehabilitation* 15:101–107.

Gillet, Henry. 1973. "A Definition of the Subluxation." *Digest of Chiropractic Economics* 15(6):14–17.

——— 1983. "The History of Motion Palpation." *European Journal of Chiropractic* 31:196–201.

——— n.d. "A Hundred Holes in One." Mimeographed.

——— and M. Liekens. 1951 (1973). *Belgian Chiropractic Research Notes*. Davenport, Ia.: PCC.

Gilley, L.D. 1989. "An M.D.-D.C. Tells What You Can Learn from Chiropractic." *Medical Economics* 66: May 15, pp. 136–143.

Gilman, Greg, and John Bergstrand. 1990. "Visual Recovery Following Chiropractic Intervention." *Journal of Behavioral Optometry* 1(3):73–74.

Goddard, H.H. 1899. "The Effects of Mind on Body As Evidenced by Faith Cures." *American Journal of Psychology*. 10:431–502.

Goffman, Irving. 1959. *The Presentation of Self in Everyday Life*. New York: Doubleday.

Goldberg, Milton M. 1941. "A Qualification of the Marginal Man Theory." *American Sociological Review* 6:52–58.

Goldschmidt, Arnold M. 1973. "New York." *DCE* 15(6):37.

Goldschmidt, Sol. 1970. *A Brief History of Chiropractic in New York State, 1902-1963*. New York State Chiropractic Association.

Goldstein, Murray (Ed.). 1975. *The Research Status of Spinal Manipulative Therapy*. Workshop Held at the National Institutes of Health, February 2–4, 1975. National Institute of Neurological and Communicative Disorders and Stroke (NINCDS). Bethesda, Md.: DHEW Pub. No. (NIH76–998).

——— 1978. "Foreword." In Irwin M. Korr, *The Neurobiologic Mechanisms in Manipulative Therapy*. New York: Plenum.

——— 1990. "War, Politics, and Osteopathic Medicine." *JAOA* 90:157–160.

Goldthwaite, Joel E. 1941. *Body Mechanics in Health and Disease*. Philadelphia: Lippincott.

Goodheart, George J. 1970. *Applied Kinesiology*. Detroit: Published by the author.

Gort, E.H., and D. Coburn. 1988. "Naturopathy in Canada: Changing Relationships to Medicine, Chiropractic, and the State." *Social Science and Medicine* 26:1061–1072.

Green, F.H. 1919. *State Regulation of the Practice of Medicine*. Chicago: American Medical Association.

Greenman, Philip E. (Ed.). 1984. *Concepts and Mechanisms of Neuromuscular Functions: An International Conference on Concepts and Mechanisms of Neuromuscular Functions*. New York: Springer-Verlag.

——— 1989. *Principles of Manual Medicine*. Baltimore: Williams & Wilkins.

Gregg, Alan. 1956. *Challenges to Contemporary Medicine*. New York: Columbia University Press.

Greggerson, James G. (n.d.; before 1950) *Seven Essays*. Pamphlet.

Gregory, Alvah A. 1912. *Spinal Adjustment*. Oklahoma City: Palmer-Gregory College.

———1913. *Rational Therapy: A Manual of Rational Therapy Methods Embracing a Brief Description of the Etiology, Pathology, and Symptomatology of Disease Written with Special Reference to the Application of Rational Therapy Methods in the Treatment of Disease*. Oklahoma City: Palmer-Gregory College.

Griffin, Leonard K. 1988. "Merger Almost: ICA Unity Efforts and the Formation of the American Chiropractic Association." *Ch Hist* 8(2):19–22.

Groddeck, Georg. 1933. *Exploring the Unconscious; Further Exercises in Applied Analytical Psychology*. London: C.W. Daniel Co.

Gromala, Theresa. 1983. "Women in Chiropractic: Exploring a Tradition of Equity in Healing." *Ch Hist* 3:59–63.

———1984. "Broadsides, Epigrams, and Testimonials: The Evolution of Chiropractic Advertising." *Ch Hist* 4:41–45.

———1986. " 'Bees in His Bonnet': D.D. Palmer's Students and Their Early Impact on Chiropractic History." *Ch Hist* 6:57–62.

Grossman, Carl M. 1965. *The Wild Analyst: The Life and Work of Georg Groddeck*. New York: Braziller.

Gunby, Phil. 1983. "Study to Evaluate Manipulative Therapy." *JAMA* 249:3148–3150.

Hadler, Nortin M. 1979. "The Sociopolitical Climate Surrounding Low Back Pain (LBP)." *Journal of Occupational Medicine* 21:681–682.

———1988. "Industrial Rheumatology: A Challenge for Primary Care and Clinical Investigation." *Occupational Problems in Medical Practice* 3(1):1–8.

———et al. 1987. "A Benefit of Spinal Manipulation as Adjunctive Therapy for Acute Low-Back Pain." *Spine* 12:703–706.

Hahnemann, Samuel Christian. 1833. *The Homeopathic Medical Doctrine, or, "Organon of the Healing Art."* Dublin: W.F. Wakeman.

———1846. *Materia Medica Pura*. New York: W. Radde.

Haldeman, Scott. 1975. "The Pathophysiology of the Spinal Subluxation." *NINCDS* pp. 217–226.

———— 1978. "The Clinical Basis for Discussion of Mechanisms of Manipulative Therapy." In Irvin M. Korr (Ed.). *The Neurobiologic Mechanisms in Manipulative Therapy*. New York: Plenum.

———— 1980. (Ed.). *Modern Developments in the Principles and Practice of Chiropractic*. New York: Appleton-Century-Crofts.

———— 1982. "How Being a Chiropractor Makes Me a Better MD." *Medical Economics* 49(October 25):132–139.

———— 1983. "Spinal Manipulative Therapy: A Status Report." *Clinical Orthopedics* 179:62–70.

———— 1988. "How To Make DC/MD Relations Work After Anti-Trust." *ICA Review* Sept./Oct. pp. 19–21.

———— 1992a. (Ed.). *Principles and Practice of Chiropractic*. Norwalk, Connecticut: Appleton and Lange.

———— 1992b. (Ed.). *Guidelines to Chiropractic Quality Assurance and Standards of Practice*.

Hale, Annie R. 1926. *These Cults*. New York: National Health Foundation.

Harding, Randolph, et al. 1977. "CHP Task Force Surveys Chiropractic Utilization in a Florida County." *ACAJ* 14(7):26–27.

Hariman, George E. 1970. *A History of the Evolution of Chiropractic Education*. Grand Forks, N.D.: Knutson Printing Company.

Harris, James D. 1985. "History and Development of Manipulation and Mobilization." In John V. Basmajian (Ed.). *Manipulation, Traction and Massage*. Baltimore: Williams & Wilkins.

Harrison, Edward. 1827. *Pathological and Practical Observations on Spinal Diseases: Illustrated with Cases and Engravings. Also an Inquiry into the Origin and Care of Distorted Limbs*. London: T. and G. Underwood.

Harrison, James D. 1989. "Legal Corner: Standards of Practice." *ICA Review* 45(6):11–13.

————1990. *Chiropractic Practice Liability: A Practical Guide to Successful Risk Management*. Arlington, Va.: ICA.

Hartmann, J.J., Jr. 1984. *Chiropractic in Alabama: A History—1918 to 1984*. Montgomery: Alabama State Chiropractic Association.

Hassenger, Edward W., et al. 1975. "Changes in Number and Location of Health Practitioners in a 20-County Rural Area of Missouri." *Public Health Reports* 90:313–318.

Hearne, Lisa R., and Janet L. Smalley. 1985. *The Role and Image of Chiropractic Services in Pennsylvania: 1985 and 1981*. Presented to the Pennsylvania Chiropractic Society, under the supervision of Arno J. Rethans, Associate Professor of Marketing, The Pennsylvania State University. Mimeographed.

Henderson, L.J. 1932. "An Approximate Definition of Fact." In Bernard Barber (Ed.). 1970. *L.J. Henderson on the Social System: Selected Writings*. Chicago: University of Chicago Press.

————1935. "Physician and Patient as a Social System." *NEJM* 212:819–823.

————1936. "The Practice of Medicine as Applied Sociology." *Transactions of the Association of American Physicians* 51:8–15. Also in Bernard Barber (Ed.). 1970. *L.J. Henderson on the Social System: Selected Writings*. Chicago: University of Chicago Press.

Hendricks, Arthur G., and Earl A. Rich. 1947. *X-Ray Technique and Spinal Misalignment Interpretation*. Indianapolis: Lincoln Chiropractic College.

"High Cost of Back Pain." 1991. *ACAJ* 28(7):13.

Hilary, C.P. 1948. "Lecture Given by Father Hilary, C.P., in the B.J. Palmer Chiropractic Clinic Assembly Hall," Davenport, Ia. Pamphlet.

Hildreth, Arthur Grant. 1938. *The Lengthening Shadow of Dr. Andrew Taylor Still*. Kirksville, Mo.: Published by the author.

Hill, Napoleon. 1937. *Think and Grow Rich*. Meriden, Conn.: The Ralston Society.

Hinz, David G. 1987. "Diversified Chiropractic: Northwestern College and John B. Wolfe, 1941-1984." *Ch Hist* 7(1):35–41.

Hoehler, Fred K., Jerome S. Tobis, and A.A. Buerger. 1981. "Spinal Manipulation of Low Back Pain." *JAMA* 245:1835–1836.

Holbrook, Stewart H. 1959. *The Golden Age of Quackery*. New York: Macmillan.

Holmes, Oliver Wendell. (1842) 1849. "Homeopathy and Its Kindred Delusions." *Medical Essays 1842-1882*. Boston: Houghton, Mifflin.

———1857 (1904). *The Autocrat of the Breakfast Table*. Cambridge, Mass, Houghton Mifflin.

Holoweiko, Mark. 1985. "The New Health Care Partnership: M.D.s and D.C.s." *Medical Economics* 62(May 27):80–86.

———1987. "Is Anyone Serious About Chiropractic Policing?" *Medical Economics* 64(Sept. 7):68–84.

"Homeopathy Series Continues." 1989. *CJ* 4(3):24.

Homewood, Albert Earl. 1962. *Neurodynamics of the Vertebral Subluxation*. Thornhill, Ontario: Published by the author.

———1965. *The Chiropractor and the Law*. Toronto: Chiropractic Publishers.

———1982. *75 Years of Tenacity, Challenge and Progress: A History of Western States Chiropractic College, 1907-1982*. Mimeographed. Portland, Oregon: WSCC.

———1988. "What Price Research?" *DC* 6(6):32–33.

Homola, Samuel. 1963. *Bonesetting, Chiropractic, and Cultism*. Panama City, Fla.: Critique Books.

Hood, W. 1871. *On Bone-Setting, So-Called, and Its Relation to the Treatment of Joints Crippled by Injury*. London: Macmillan.

"Houston DC Addresses Naprapathic Convention." 1989. *DCE* 32(2):140.

Howard, John Fitzalan. 1912. *Encylcopedia of Chiropractic (The Howard System)*. 3 Vols. Chicago: NCC.

Howells, William. 1948. *The Heathens: Primitive Man and His Religions*. New York: Doubleday.

Hubbard, Elbert. 1913. *The New Science, or the Fine Art of Getting Well and Keeping So*. East Aurora, N.Y.: The Roycrofters.

Hughes, Everett C. 1945. "Dilemmas and Contradictions of Status." *American Journal of Sociology* 50:353–359.

Hviid, H. 1955. "A Consideration of Contemporary Chiropractic Theory." *JNCA* 25(January): 17–18.

Hyde, David R., and Payson Wolff (Eds.). 1954. "The American Medical Association: Power, Purpose, and Politics in Organized Medicine." *Yale Law Journal* 63:938–1022.

ICA Review. 1990. 46(3):28.

Illi, Frederick W.H. 1940. *The Sacro-Iliac Mechanism Keystone of Body Balance and Body Locomotion*. Chicago: NCC.

———1951. *The Vertebral Column, Life Line of the Body*. Chicago: NCC.

———1965. "Morbid Predisposition of a Mechanical Origin Inherent to the Phylogenesis of Man." (Part 1 of 3 parts). *ACAJ* Sept.

———1971. *High Lights of 45 Years of Experience and 35 Years of Research*. Geneva, Switzerland: Institute for the Study of the Statics and Dynamics of the Human Body.

Imrie, David, and Lu Barbuto. 1988. *The Back Power Program*. Toronto: Stoddart.

"Inevitable Decline of Chiropractic." 1973. *New York State Journal of Medicine* 73:324–328.

Inge, William M. 1959. *Come Back, Little Sheba*. New York: Random House.

Inglis, Brian. 1964. *Fringe Medicine*. London: Faber and Faber. Republished in 1965 as *The Case for Unorthodox Medicine*. New York: Putnam.

Ingram, Gladys Little. 1970. *Traveling an Uncharted Road*. Philadelphia: Dorrance and Co.

Jacobs, Hayes B. 1962. "Oral Roberts: High Priest of Faith Healing." *Harpers Magazine* 224(Feb.):37–43.

Janse, Joseph. 1975. "History of the Development of Chiropractic Concepts." *NINCDS* pp. 25–42.

————1976. *Principles and Practice of Chiropractic*. Lombard, Ill.: NCC.

————H. Hauser, and B.F. Wells. 1947. *Chiropractic Principles and Technic*. (2nd Edition). Chicago: NCC.

Jarvis, Kelly B., Reed B. Phillips, and Elliot K. Morris. 1991. "Cost Per Case Comparison of Back Injury Claims of Chiropractic versus Medical Management for Conditions with Identical Diagnostic Codes." *Journal of Occupational Medicine* 33:847–852.

Jaskoviak, P.A. 1980. "Complications Arising from Manipulation of the Cervical Spine: A Literature Review." *JMPT* 3:213–219.

Jobs Related Almanac. 1988. Chicago: American References.

Johnson, Kirk B. 1988. "Editorial Statement from AMA's General Counsel." *JAMA* 259:83.

Jones, J. Henry. 1926. *Healing by Manipulation (Bone-Setting)* London: Watts and Co.

Jones, Rhys B., et al. 1989. "Fluoridation Referendum in La Crosse, Wisconsin: Contributing Factors to Success." *JMPT* 79:1405–1408.

Joseph, Alice. 1942. "Physician and Patient: Some Aspects of Interpersonal Relations between Physicians and Patients, with Special Regard to the Relationship between White Physicians and Indian Patients." *Applied Anthropology* 1:4.

Joy, Robert T. 1954. "The Natural Bonesetters with Special Reference to the Sweet Family of Rhode Island." *Bulletin of the History of Medicine* 28:416–441.

Kane, R., et al. 1974. "Manipulating the Patient: A Comparison of the Effectiveness of Physician and Chiropractic Care." *Lancet* 7870:1333–1336.

Kaufman, Martin. 1971. *Homeopathy in America: The Rise and Fall of a Medical Heresy*. Baltimore: Johns Hopkins University Press.

————1988. "Homeopathy in America: The Rise and Fall and Persistence of a Medical Heresy." In Norman Gevitz (Ed.). *Other Healers: Unorthodox Medicine in America*. Baltimore: Johns Hopkins University Press.

Keating, Joseph. 1987. "Claude O. Watkins: Pioneer Advocate for Clinical Scientific Chiropractic." *Ch Hist* 7:11–15.

————1989a. "Beyond the Theosophy of Chiropractic." *JMPT* 12:147–150.

————1989b. "Inter-Examiner Reliability of Motion Palpation of the Lumbar Spine: A Review of Quantitative Literature." *AJCM* 2:107–110.

————and Robert D. Mootz. 1989. "The Influence of Political Medicine on Chiropractic Dogma: Implications for Scientific Development." *JMPT* 12:393–398.

Kelner, Merrijoy, Oswald Hall, and Ian Coulter. 1980. *Chiropractors: Do They Help? A Study of Their Education and Practice*. Toronto: Fitzhenry & Whiteside.

Kemper, Steve. 1989. "Eileen Denver." Hartford *Courant's* Northeast Magazine, Sept. 11, p. 5.

"Kentuckiana Children's Center Plans Large New Facility." 1989. *ACAJ* 26(11):34–36.

Kett, Joseph F. 1968. *The Formation of the American Medical Profession: The Role of Institutions 1780-1860*. New Haven: Yale University Press.

Kfoury, Peter W. 1977. (Ed.). *Catalogue of Chiropractic Techniques*. St. Louis: Logan College of Chiropractic.

King, Janet. 1984. "Hospital Privileges: Yesterday's Dream Today's Reality." *ICA Review of Chiropractic* 40(2):41–44.

Kirkaldi-Willis, William H. 1988. *Managing Low Back Pain*. New York: Churchill Livingstone Inc.

————and J.D. Cassidy. 1985. "Spinal Manipulation in the Treatment of Low-Back Pain." *Canadian Family Physician* 31:535–540.

————et al. 1989. "Health Through Activity." *AJCM* 2:101–106.

Klaes, Christopher J. 1980. "Dr. Klaes' Commencement Address." *PCC Alumni News,* Aug., pp. 14–15.

Kleiman, Michael B. 1979. *The Chiropractic Component Health Planning: A Twelve-State Survey of Practice Characteristics and Utilization Patterns*. Tampa, Fla.: Human Resources Institute, University of South Florida.

Kleynhans, Andries M. 1980. "Complications of and Contraindications to Spinal Manipulative Therapy." In Scott Haldeman (Ed.). *Modern Developments in the Principles and Practice of Chiropractic.* New York: Appleton-Century-Crofts.

Klougart, N., N. Nilsson, and J. Jacobsen. 1989. "Infantile Colic Treated by Chiropractors: A Prospective Study of 316 Cases." *JMPT* 12:281–288.

Koff, Stephen. 1988. "Chiropractors Seeking Advice Find Scientology-Influenced Seminars." *DC* 6(5):3.

Korr, Irvin M. 1974. "Proprioceptors and the Behavior of Lesioned Segments." *Osteopathic Annals* 2:12–32.

——— 1976. "The Spinal Cord as Organizer of Disease Process: Some Preliminary Perspectives." *JAOA* 76:89–99.

——— 1978a. (Ed.). *The Neurobiologic Mechanisms in Manipulative Therapy.* New York: Plenum Press.

——— 1978b. "Sustained Sympathicotonia as a Factor in Disease." In Korr (Ed.). *The Neurobiologic Mechanisms in Manipulative Therapy.* New York: Plenum.

——— 1981. "The Spinal Cord as Organizer of Disease Processes: IV. Axonal Transport and Neurotrophic Function in Relation to Somatic Dysfunction." *JAOA* 80:451–459.

Kranz, Karl C. 1986. "The Public Bootstrapping of Physical Therapy to a Provider Profession." *Ch Hist* 6:39–48.

———1987. *Chiropractic and Hospital Privileges Protocol.* Washington, D.C.: ICA.

Krueger, Bruce R., and Haruo Okazaki. 1980. "Vertebral-Basilar Distribution Infarction Following Chiropractic Cervical Manipulation." *Mayo Clinic Proceedings* 55:322–333.

Kunert, N. 1965. "Functional Disorders of Internal Organs Due to Vertebral Lesions. *Ciba Symposium* 13:85–96.

Lamm, Lester C. and Elizabeth Wegner. 1989. "Chiropractic Scope of Practice: What the Law Allows." *AJCM* 2:155–159.

Langworthy, Solon M., Oakley G. Smith, and Minora C. Paxson. 1906. *A Textbook of Modernized Chiropractic.* Cedar Rapids, Ia.: American School of Chiropractic.

Lantz, Charles A. 1990. "A Critical Look at the Subluxation Hypothesis." *JMPT* 13:42–45.

Larson, Magali Sarfatti. 1977. *The Rise of Professionalism*. Berkeley, Calif.: University of California Press.

Lauretti, Bill, et al. 1988. "WSCC History: A Proud Past, An Exciting Future." *The Axis* (Student Newspaper at WSCC). 16(6):1.

Leach, Robert A. 1981. "The Chiropractic Theories: Discussion of Some Important Considerations." *ACAJ* 18(3):S19–S25.

———— 1986. *The Chiropractic Theories: A Synopsis of Scientific Research*. Baltimore: Williams & Wilkins.

LeBoeuff, Charlotte, et al. 1989. "Chiropractic Chronic Low Back Pain Sufferers and Self-Report Assessment Methods. Part II. A Reliability Study of the Middlesex Hospital Questionnaire and the VAS Disability Scales Questionnaire." *JMPT* 12:109–112.

Lee, Herbert K. 1981. "Honoring the Founder in His Country: Conception and Struggle for Canada's Memorial College." *Ch Hist* 1:43–45.

———— 1982. "Second Honorary Membership: Albert Earl Homewood, D.C." *Ch Hist* 2:67–68.

Lensgraf, Arthur G. 1990. "The Lensgraf Chiropractors: Three Generations of Practitioners." *Ch Hist* 10(2):13–15.

Lerner, Cyrus. 1954. *Report on the History of Chiropractic*. 8 vols. Mimeographed.

Levine, Mortimer. 1964. *The Structural Approach to Chiropractic*. New York: Comet Press.

Lewis, Charles Albert. 1902. *The Only Osteopractic Way of Treating Diseases at Home: Combining Osteopathy, Magnetic Healing and Massage*. Afton, Ia.: Star-Enterprise Print.

Lewis, Donald W. 1985. *South Dakota Chiropractors Association Health Care Survey*. Vermillion, S.D.: Business Research Bureau, University of South Dakota.

Lewit, Karel. 1985. *Manipulative Therapy in Rehabilitation of the Locomotor System*. London: Butterworth.

Li, Jinxue. 1990. "A Brief Introduction to the Concept and History of Chinese Manipulative Therapy." *DCE* 33(2):24–26.

Liebl, Nancy A., and Lynn M. Butler. 1990. "A Chiropractic Approach to the Treatment of Dysmenorrhea." *JMPT* 13:101–106.

"Life Chiropractic College." 1990. *DCE* 32(4):94.

Ligeros, Kleanthes. 1937. *How Ancient Healing Governs Modern Therapeutics*. New York: Putnam.

Lin, Phylis Lan. 1972. *The Chiropractor, Chiropractic, and Process: A Study of the Sociology of an Occupation*. Ph.D. Dissertation, University of Missouri.

Lindorff, Dave. 1992. *Marketplace Medicine: The Rise of the For-Profit Hospital Chains*. New York: Bantam Books.

Lines, Dean H. 1989. "Chiropractic in the 21st Century. Part 2. The Future: Strategies for Survival, Growth and Development." *Journal of the Australian Chiropractors' Association* 19:49–54.

Ling, Per Henryk. 1853. *The Gymnastic Free Exercises of P.H. Ling. Arranged by H. Rothstein*. Trans. by M. Roth. Boston: Ticknor, Reed and Fields.

Linhart, Gordon. 1988. "Selling the 'Big Idea': B.J. Palmer Ushers in the Golden Age." *Ch Hist* 8(2):25–30.

Little, W.J. 1868. *On Spinal Weakness and Spinal Curvatures*. London: Longman, Green.

Livingston, M.C. 1971. "Spinal Manipulation Causing Injury: A Three-Year Study." *Clinical Orthopedics* 81:82–86.

Loban, Joy Maxwell. 1912. *Technique and Practice of Chiropractic*. Davenport, Ia.: Universal Chiropractic College.

———1929. *A Textbook of Neurology*. Denver: Bunn-Loban Publishing Company.

Logan, Hugh B. 1936. *Logan Basic Technique*. St. Louis: Blackwell-Wielandy.

Lomax, Elizabeth. 1975. "Manipulative Therapy: A Historical Perspective from Ancient Times to the Modern Era." *NINCDS* pp. 11–17.

——— 1977. "Manipulative Therapy: An Historical Perspective." In A.A. Buerger and Jerome S. Tobis (Eds.). *Approaches to the Validation of Manipulative Therapy.* Springfield, Ill.: Charles C Thomas, Publisher.

Lombardo, Dean M. 1990. "William H. Warner and The American Bureau of Chiropractic: Organizing a Lay Constituency." *Ch Hist* 10(1):25–29.

London, Joe. 1991. "Make Yellow Pages Advertising More Effective." *CJ* 5(8):26, 38.

"The Long Island Poll: Can Chiropractors Help When Doctors Can't?" 1976. *Long Island* Nov. 28.

Lovett, Robert W. 1922. "Quackery, Miracle Healing and Medical Cults." *Boston Medical and Surgical Journal* 187(2):53–65.

Lowen, Alexander. 1958. *Physical Dynamics of Character Structure.* New York: Grune & Stratton. Republished 1971 as *The Language of the Body.* New York: Collier Books.

Luce, John M. 1978. "Chiropractic: Its History and Challenge to Medicine. *Pharos* 41(2):12–17.

Luttges, Marvin W., and Richard A. Gerren. 1980. "Compression Physiology: Nerves and Roots." In Scott Haldeman (Ed.). *Modern Developments in the Principles and Practice of Chiropractic.* New York: Appleton-Century-Crofts.

Macdonald, Malcolm E. 1974. "1974 Congress of State Associations Establishes a Milestone in Chiropractic History." *The New England Journal of Chiropractic* 8(4):3–11.

MacDonald, Michael J. 1988. "Chiropractic Evaluation Study." (Task III Report of Relevant Literature—MRI Project No. 8533 D, Jan. 24, 1986, for Department of Defense, OCHAMPUS.) *JCR* 5(1):2–15.

MacDonald, Roderic S., and C.M. Janine Bell. 1990. "An Open Controlled Assessment of Osteopathic Manipulation in Nonspecific Low Back Pain." *Spine* 15:364–370.

Maigne, Robert. 1972. *Orthopedic Medicine*. Trans. by W.T. Liberson. Springfield, Ill.: Charles C Thomas, Publisher.

Maisel, Albert Q. 1971. "Should Chiropractors Be Paid With Your Tax Dollars?" *Reader's Digest* July, pp. 76–81.

Maitland, Geoffrey D. 1964. *Vertebral Manipulation*. London: Butterworth.

Malinowski, Bronislaw. 1948. *Magic, Science, and Religion, and Other Essays*. Glencoe, Ill.: Free Press.

Manceaux, Glenn D. 1987. "Can Physical Therapists and Chiropractors Co-Exist Despite Differences?" *JMPT* 10: 260–263.

Mannington, Jane V. et al. 1989. "Women Chiropractors: Issues of Career and Family." *JMPT* 12:434–439.

Martienssen, Jens, and Niels Nilsson. 1989. "Cerebrovascular Accidents Following Upper Cervical Manipulation: The Importance of Age, Gender and Technique. *AJCM* 2:160–163.

Martin, Steven C. 1978. *Chiropractic Licensing in the Midwest, 1910-1920*. Senior Honors Thesis in History and Science. Cambridge, Mass.: Harvard University.

——— 1989. "The Limits of Medicine: A Social History of Chiropractic, 1895-1930." Presented to the American Association for the History of Medicine, Birmingham, Ala.

Martin RJ. 1949. "Professional Mortality." *Kansas State Chiropractic Assoc Bull* 9(2):5.

Mawhiney, R.B. 1984. *Chiropractic in Wisconsin 1900-1950*. Waukesha, Wis.: Roberts Publishing Company.

Mayer, Milton. 1949. "The Rise and Fall of Dr. Fishbein." *Harpers* 199(5):76–85.

Maynard, Joseph E. 1959. *Healing Hands: The Story of the Palmer Family, Discoverers and Developers of Chiropractic*. Mobile, Ala.: Jonorm Publishers.

Mazzarelli, Joseph (Ed.). 1982. *Chiropractic: Interprofessional Research*. Torino, Italy: Minerva Medica.

McAndrews, George P. 1982. "Fighting for Chiropractic—Fighting for Justice." *ACAJ* 19(10):20–31.

———1989. "Nothing Focuses the Mind Like Knowing You Are Going to Be Hanged in the Morning." *ACAJ* 26(10):37–41.

McCorkle, Thomas. 1961. "Chiropractic: A Deviant Theory of Disease and Treatment in Contemporary Western Culture." *Human Organization (Applied Anthropology)* 20:20–23.

McGowan, Gordonne E. 1948. "Chiropractic in World Events." *The Chiropractor* 44(10):12–19.

McGregor, Marion, and J. David Cassidy. 1983. "Post-Surgical Sacroiliac Joint Syndrome." *JMPT* 6:1–11.

McNamara, Robert Emmett. 1913. *Chiropractic, Other Drugless Healing Methods, with Criticism of the Practice of Medicine.* Davenport Ia., Wagner's Printery.

McNamee, Kevin P., et al. 1990. "Chiropractic Education: A Student Survey." *JMPT* 13:521–531.

Meade, T.W., et al. 1990. "Low Back Pain of Mechanical Origin: Randomised Comparison of Chiropractic and Hospital Outpatient Treatment." *British Medical Journal* 300:1431–1437.

"The Menace of Chiropractic: Practically No Educational Requirements Necessary for Matriculation in Chiropractic Colleges." 1923. *JAMA* 80(10):715–716.

Mencken, H.L. 1924. "Chiropractic." Baltimore *Evening Sun,* Dec. Republished in *Prejudice, Sixth Series.* 1927. New York: Knopf.

Mennell, James. 1952. *The Science and Art of Joint Manipulation.* New York: Blakiston Co.

Mennell, John McM. 1960. *Back Pain; Diagnosis and Treatment Using Manipulative Techniques.* Boston: Little-Brown.

———1975. "History of the Development of Medical Manipulative Concepts; Medical Terminology." *NINCDS* pp. 19–24.

———1989. "Understanding Manipulative Medicine in General Practice." *JMPT* 12:231–235.

———— 1990. "Overview of Manual Medicine." Mimeographed.

Metz, Martha. 1965. *Fifty Years of Chiropractic Recognized in Kansas*. Abilene, Kansas: Shadinger-Wilson, Inc.

Meyer, A.W. 1925. "Chiropractic Fountain Head: An Inside View." *California and Western Medicine* 23:610–613.

Mickelson, A. 1989. "Stucky Family, 13 Strong, Named Chiropractic Family of the Year." *DC* 7(18):20.

Miller, Jonathan D. 1989. "Homeopathy." *DC* 7(23):34.

Miller, Ralph G. 1981. "History of Chiropractic Accreditation." *ACAJ* 18(2):38–44.

Miller, William D. 1975. "Treatment of Visceral Disorders by Manipulative Therapy." *NINCDS* pp. 295–301.

Minty, Leonard LeMarchant. 1932. *The Legal and Ethical Aspects of Medical Quackery*. London: William Heinemann.

Mittan, J. Barry. 1985. "Characteristics of Florida's Active Licensed Chiropractors: Results of the 1981 and 1983 Manpower Licensure Surveys." Mimeographed. State of Florida Department of Health and Rehabilitative Services.

Modde, Peter J. 1979. "Malpractice Is an Inevitable Result of Chiropractic Philosophy and Training." *Legal Aspects of Medical Practice*: Feb., pp. 20–23.

Monell, Samuel Howard. 1902. *A System of Instruction in X-ray Methods and Medical Uses of Light, Hot Air, Vibration and High Frequency Currents*. New York: E.R. Pelton.

Montagu, Ashley. 1971. *Touching: The Human Significance of the Skin*. New York: Columbia University Press.

Montenegro, Bertha. 1988. "*Dynamic Chiropractic* Pays Tribute to George H. Kopp, D.C." *DC* 6(13):3, 9.

Moore, Christine. 1989. "Chiropractors Gain Wider Acceptance." *New England Employment Review* May 1–13.

Moore, Susan. 1989. *Chiropractic: The Art and Science of Body Alignment*. New York: Harmony Books.

Mootz, Robert D. and Joseph C. Keating. 1989. "The Chiropractic Tradition: What Was Medicine's Role?" *ICA Review* 45(4):53–57.

———— and William C. Meeker. 1990. "Referral Patterns of California Chiropractic Association Members." *ABS (American Back Society) Newsletter* 6(3):17.

Morinis, E. Allen. 1980. "Theory and Practice in Chiropractic: An Anthropological Perspective." *Journal of the Canadian Chiropractic Association* 24:114–119.

Moving Up. 1988. Burbank, Calif.: Communications, Inc. Sept./Oct.

Mugge, Robert H. 1986. *Visits to Selected Health Care Practitioners: United States, 1980.* Item 512-A-29. National Center for Health Statistics. USPHS. Washington, D.C.

Myrdal, Gunnar. 1944. *An American Dilemma.* New York: Harper & Row.

Nansel, D. Dale, et al. 1989. "Interexaminer Concordance in Detecting Joint Play Asymmetries in the Cervical Spines of Otherwise Asymptomatic Subjects." *JMPT* 12:428–433.

"National Ambulatory Medical Care Survey 1985." 1987. *Advance Data from Vital and Health Statistics.* No. 138, DHHS Publ. No. (PHS)87-1250. Hyattsville, Md.:Public Health Services.

"National College of Chiropractic." 1989. *ACAJ* 26(11):80.

National Cyclopedia of American Biography. 1945, New York: James T. White.

"Naturopaths Licensed in Washington." 1970. Seattle: Washington State Department of Social and Health Services.

"NCC Announces Profile of Practice of Chiropractic." 1989. *DCE* 32(2):88–89.

New, Peter Kong-Ming. 1960. *The Application of Reference Group Theory to Shifts in Values: The Case of the Osteopathic Student.* Ph.D. dissertation, University of Missouri.

"New PPO Solicits Chiropractic Doctors." 1985. *NYSCA Newsletter* (Official publication of the New York State Chiropractic Association) March/April, p. 2.

"New Questions: Why Did D.D. Not Use 'Chiropractic' in His 1896 Charter?" 1986. *Ch Hist* 6:63.

Nimmo, R.L. 1957. "Receptors, Effectors, and Tonus—A New Approach." *JNCA* 27:21–23.

Norbeck, Timothy B. 1989. "Don't Blame the Medical Profession for Rising Costs." Hartford *Courant* Dec. 10, p. C1.

"North American Spine Society Gives Chiropractic Adjustments Top Rating." 1991. *DC* 9(24):1, 4.

Northup, George W. 1972. *Osteopathic Medicine: An American Reformation.* Chicago: American Osteopathic Association.

———— 1975. "History of the Development of Osteopathic Concepts; Osteopathic Terminology." *NINCDS* pp. 43–47.

———— 1987. (Ed.). *Osteopathic Research: Growth and Development.* Chicago: American Osteopathic Association.

Nugent, John. 1946. *Chiropractic Education: Outline of a Standard Course.* Webster City, Ia.: NCA.

Null, Gary. 1986. "War on Chiropractic." *ICA Review* 42(2):15–32, 65–69.

Numbers, Ronald L. 1977. "Do-It-Yourself the Sectarian Way." In Guenter B. Risse, Ronald L.N. Numbers, and Judith Walzer Leavitt. *Medicine Without Doctors: Home Health Care in American History.* New York: Science History Publications/USA.

The Nuprin Pain Report. 1985. New York: Louis Harris and Associates.

Nwuga, V.C.B. 1982. "Relative Therapeutic Efficacy of Vertebral Manipulation and Conventional Treatment in Back Pain Management." *American Journal of Physical Medicine* 61:273–278.

Nyiendo, Joanne A., and Scott Haldeman. 1986. "A Critical Study of the Student Interns' Practice Activities in a Chiropractic College Teaching Clinic." *JMPT* 9:197–207.

"Organization News." 1989. *CJ* 3(10):27, 33.

Orton, Ervin. 1985. *A Touching Story.* Canistota, S.D.: The Canistota Clipper.

Osler, William. 1907. *Modern Medicine.* New York: Lea Bros. and Co.

—————1910. "The Faith That Heals." *British Medical Journal* June 18:1470–1472.

"Osteopathy." 1897. *JAMA* 28:709–710.

"Osteopathy: Special Report of the Judicial Council to the AMA House of Delegates." 1961. *JAMA* 177:774–776.

Osterbauer, P.J., and A.W. Fuhr. 1990. "The Current Status of Activator Methods Chiropractic Technic, Theory, and Training." *Chiropractic Technique* 2(4):168–175.

Paget, James. 1871. "Cases That Bone-Setters Cure." *British Medical Journal* 1:1–4.

Palmer, Bartlett Joshua. 1910 (1920). *The Science of Chiropractic: Its Principles and Philosophies*. Davenport, Ia.: PSC.

—————1916. *The Tyranny of Therapeutic Transgressions; or, an Expose of an Invisible Government*. Davenport, Ia.: Universal Chiropractors Association.

—————1919. "Introduction" to E.A. Thompson, *Text on Chiropractic Spinography*. Davenport, Ia.:PSC.

—————1934. *The Subluxation Specific; The Adjustment Specific; An Exposition of the Cause of All Disease*. Davenport, Ia.: PSC.

—————1942. *Radio Salesmanship*. Davenport, Ia.: PSC.

—————1949. *The Bigness of the Fellow Within*. Davenport, Ia.: PSC.

—————1950a. *Up from Below the Bottom*. Davenport, Ia.: PSC.

—————1950b. *Fight to Climb*. Davenport, Ia.: PSC.

—————1951a. *Chiropractic Clinical Controlled Research*. Davenport, Ia.: PSC.

—————1951b. *Conflicts Clarify*. Davenport, Ia.:PSC.

—————1953. *Upside Down and Right Side Up with B.J.; Including the Greatest Mystery of History*. Davenport, Ia.: Published by the author.

—————1955. *Fame and Fortune and the Know-How and Show-How to Attain It*. Davenport, Ia.:PSC.

——1958a. *Shall Chiropractic Survive?* Davenport, Ia.:PSC.

——1958b. *Palmer's Law of Life.* Davenport, Ia.:PSC.

——1959a. *Giant Versus Pygmy.* Davenport, Ia.:PSC.

——1959b. *Inhibitions Starve History or . . . The Uninhibited Make History, or . . . Everyone Can Make History.* Davenport, Ia.:PSC.

——1961. *The Glory of Going On.* Davenport, Ia.:PSC.

Palmer, Daniel David. 1910. *The Chiropractor's Adjuster: A Textbook of the Science, Art, and Philosophy of Chiropractic for Students and Practitioners.* Portland, Ore.: Portland Printing House.

——1914. *The Chiropractor.* (Published posthumously by his wife). Los Angeles, California: Beacon Light Printing Co.

——and Bartlett Joshua Palmer. 1906. *Science of Chiropractic: Its Principles and Adjustments.* Davenport, Ia.:PSC.

Palmer, David Daniel. 1967. *Three Generations: A History of Chiropractic.* Davenport, Ia.:PCC.

——1977. *The Palmers: Memories of David D. Palmer.* Davenport, Ia.: Bawden Bros.

Palmer, Mabel Heath. 1918. *Chiropractic Anatomy.* Chicago: Rogers and Hall.

Pareto, Vilfredo. 1935. *The Mind and Society.* 4 vols. New York: Harcourt-Brace.

Park, Robert. 1928. "Human Migration and the Marginal Man." *American Journal of Sociology* 33:881–893.

Parker, Gordon B., and Hilary Tupling. 1976. "The Chiropractic Patient: Psychosocial Aspects." *Medical Journal of Australia* 2:373–378.

——1978. "A Controlled Trial of Cervical Manipulation for Migraine." *Medical Journal of Australia* 8:589–593.

Paris, Stanley. 1983. "Spinal Manipulative Therapy." *Clinical Orthopedics* 179:55–61.

Parsons, Talcott. 1951. *The Social System.* Glencoe, Ill.: Free Press.

Pascoe, Jean. 1961. "Chiropractic Is Cracking Up." *Medical Economics* August 14:181–193.

Patel-Christopher, Abdu. 1990. *"Family Physicians and Chiropractors: A Need for Better Communication and Cooperation."* Unpublished thesis, University of Toronto.

Patterson, J.K. 1988. "Spinal Manipulation: Science or Black Art." *The Practitioner* 232:289, 291.

Peabody, Francis Weld. 1927. *The Care of the Patient.* Cambridge, Mass.: Harvard University Press.

Perl, Edward R. 1975. "Pain: Spinal and Peripheral Nerve Factors." *NINCDS* pp. 173–181.

Peterson, Dennis R., and Glenda C. Wiese. 1984. "Survey of Chiropractic College Libraries in the United States and Canada 1981-1982." *PCC Research Forum* 1:24–31.

Peterson, Donald M., Jr. 1990. "What Hospitals Are Saying About Chiropractic." *DC* 8(3):3.

Phillips, Reed B. 1981. "A Survey of Utah Chiropractic Patients." *ACAJ* 15(12):S113–S134.

Pizzorno, Joseph E., and Michael T. Murray. 1985. *A Textbook of Natural Medicine.* Seattle: John Bastyr College.

Position Paper on Chiropractic. 1985. Loma Linda, Calif.: National Council against Health Fraud.

Position Paper on the Acceptance of SCASA and SCASA-School Graduates. 1990. Chandler, Ariz.: The World Chiropractic Alliance.

Quigley, William Heath. 1973. "Physiological Psychology of Chiropractic in Mental Disorders." In Herman S. Schwartz (Ed.). *Mental Health and Chiropractic.* New Hyde Park, NY: Sessions Publishers.

——— 1983. "Pioneering Mental Health: Institutional Psychiatric Care in Chiropractic." *Ch Hist* 3:68–73.

——— 1988. "The Saga of the Classroom Building Continues." *DC* 6(10): 24–25.

——— 1989a. "Early Days at Palmer: Lyceums Part III." *DC* 7(2):16–17.

——— 1989b. "The B.J. Palmer Chiropractic Research Clinic Part I." *DC* 7(6):26–27.

——— 1989c. "Last Days of B.J. Palmer: Revolutionary Confronts Reality." *Ch Hist* 9(2): 11–19.

Radis, Chuck. 1981. "Osteopathic Education: A Student Perspective." *Osteopathic Annals* 9:445–450.

Ransom, James F. 1984. "The Origins of Chiropractic Physiological Therapeutics: Howard, Forester and Schulze." *Ch Hist* 4:47–52.

Ratledge, Tullius F. 1971. *The Ratledge Manuscript* (Paul Smallie, ed.). Stockton, Calif.: World-Wide Report.

Rayack, Elton. 1967. *Professional Power and American Medicine: The Economics of the American Medical Association.* Cleveland: World.

Reagan, Ronald. 1965. *Where Is the Rest of Me?* New York: Karz Publishers.

Reed, Louis. 1932. *The Healing Cults.* Chapter 3, "Chiropractic." Publ. No. 16 of the Committee on the Costs of Medical Care. Chicago: University of Chicago Press.

Regardie, Francis I. 1948. *Some Relations between Neuropsychiatry and Spinal Asymmetry.* Doctoral dissertation, Area of the Social Sciences, Fremont University (California).

Rehm, William S. 1986. "Legally Defensible: Chiropractic in the Courtroom and After, 1907." *Ch Hist* 6:51–55.

Reich, Wilhelm. 1948. *The Function of the Orgasm.* Trans. by T.P. Wolfe. New York: Orgone Institute Press.

Report of the Special Committee on Osteopathy, Chiropractic, Foods, Drugs, and Poisons. 1939. Massachusetts House of Representatives, House No. 2151. Legislative Printers. March.

Report Submitted by the Legislative Research Council Relative to Boards of Registration for Chiropractors, Electrologists, and Sanitarians. 1956. Massachusetts House of Representatives, House No. 2725. Legislative Printers. Feb. 21.

"Rep(resentative) Appointed Hospital's Chief of Chiropractic." 1985. *ICA Today* 22(2):4.

"Requirements for Admission to Schools of Chiropractic." 1964. *JAMA* 190:763–764.

Revell, Nellie. 1923. *Right Off the Chest.* New York: George H. Doran.

Rex, Erna. 1962. *The Lengthening Shadow: The Story of Doctor Leo L. Spears.* Denver: Golden Bell Press.

Rhodes, Walter R. 1978. *The Official History of Chiropractic in Texas.* Austin: Texas Chiropractic Association.

Riadore, J.E. 1842. *Treatise on Irritation of the Spinal Nerves.* London: Churchill.

Rice, Gordon W. 1912. "Pseudomedicine." *JAMA* 58:360–362.

Riesman, David. 1939. *Medicine in Modern Society.* Princeton, N.J.: Princeton University Press.

Riley, Joe Shelby. 1918. *Zone Therapy Simplified.* Washington, D.C. Published by the author.

———1919. *Science and Practice of Chiropractic with Allied Sciences.* Washington, D.C. Published by the author.

Roberts, Richard L. 1989. "Chiropractic: A Discussion of Its Organization and Disorganization, Cause and Effect." *DCE* 31(5):14–18.

Rose, Louis. 1968. *Faith Healing.* Middlesex, England: Penguin Books.

Rosenfield, Harry N. 1986. "Planning for Chiropractic's Future." *ACAJ* 23(10):5–10.

Rosenfield, Lawrence B. 1987. "Chiropractic Versus Non-Chiropractic Patients in North Carolina: A Comparison of Demographic Characteristics and Perceptions of Health Care Providers." *DCE* 29(4):22–25.

Rosenthal, Melvin J. 1981. "The Structural Approach to Chiropractic: From Willard Carver to Present Practice." *Ch Hist* 1:25–29.

Rosenthal, Saul. 1981. "The Future of Chiropractic Is Here." *ACAJ* 18(2):19.

Roth, Julius A. 1976. *Health Purifiers and Their Enemies: A Study of the Natural Health Movement in the United States with a Comparison to Its Counterpart in Germany*. New York: Prodist.

Rothstein, William. 1972. *American Physicians in the Nineteenth Century: From Sects to Science*. Baltimore: Johns Hopkins University Press.

Ruesch, Jurgen. 1946. *Chronic Diseases and Psychological Invalidism*. New York: American Society for Research in Psychological Problems.

"Rules and Regulations of the Chiropractic Service of the Surgery Department, Shorewood Osteopathic Hospital, Seattle, Washington." 1985. *ACA Journal of Chiropractic* 22(5):34–38.

Rushmore, Stephen. 1932. "The Bill to Register Chiropractors." *NEJM* 206:614–615.

Sanchez, Jose E. 1991. "A Look in the Mirror: A Critical and Exploratory Study of Public Perceptions of the Chiropractic Profession in New Jersey." *JMPT* 14:165–176.

Sandoz, R.W. 1978. "A Perspective for the Chiropractic Profession." *ACAJ* 15(5):25–49.

———1989. "Some Critical Reflections on Subluxations and Adjustments." *Swiss Annals* 9. Abstract in *DC* 7(24):21.

Sargent, Morgan. 1946. "Psychosomatic Backache." *NEJM* 234:13.

Sarno, John E. 1984. *Mind Over Back Pain: A Radically New Approach to the Diagnosis and Treatment of Back Pain*. William Morrow.

Saunders Associates. 1954. *The Chiropractic Profession*. New York: The Public Relations Management Corporation.

Schafer, Richard C. (Ed.). 1973. *Basic Chiropractic Procedural Manual*. Des Moines: ACA.

———1982. (Ed.). *Chiropractic Management of Sports and Recreational Injuries*. Baltimore: Williams & Wilkins.

———1991a. "The Art of the Chiropractic Adjustment: Part I." *DC* 9(3):16–17.

———1991b. "The Art of the Chiropractic Adjustment: Part VII." *DC* 9(15):8–9.

———— 1991c. "The Imbroglio of the Professional Greyhound." *DC* 9(17):10.

———— and L.J. Faye. 1989. *Motion Palpation and Chiropractic Technique.* Huntington Beach, Calif.: Motion Palpation Institute.

Schaller, John M. 1911-1912. "Chiro-Practic—What Is It?" *Denver Medical Times* 2:457–466.

Schellhas, K.P., et al. 1980. "Vertebrobasilar Injuries Following Cervical Manipulation." *JAMA* 224:1450–1453.

Schiller, Francis. 1971. "Spinal Irritation and Osteopathy." *Bulletin of the History of Medicine* 45:250–256.

Schiotz, Eiler H., and James Cyriax. 1975. *Manipulation: Past and Present.* London: William Heinemann Medical Books.

Schlessing, A. 1950. "Federal, Not 'Socialized' Medicine." *Journal of the National Medical Society* 6(1&2):29.

Schmidt, Margaret J. 1948. "A Student's Approach to Chiropractic." *JNCA* 8(11):144.

Schmitt, Madeline H. 1978. "The Utilization of Chiropractors." *Sociological Symposium* 22(Spring):55–71.

Schmorl, G., and H. Junghanns. 1971. *The Human Spine in Health and Disease.* New York: Grune & Stratton.

"Schools of Chiropractic and of Naturopathy in the United States: Report of Inspections." 1928. *JAMA* 90:1733–1738.

Schwartz, Herman S. 1950. *Nervous and Mental Cases under Chiropractic Care.* Webster City, Ia.: The Chiropractic Research Foundation.

———— 1954. *The Art of Relaxation.* Elmhurst, N.J.: Sessions Publishers.

———— 1957. *Home Care for the Emotionally Ill.* London: Staples Press.

———— 1973. (Ed.). *Mental Health and Chiropractic: A Multidisciplinary Approach.* New Hyde Park, N.Y.: Sessions Publishers.

Scotton, R. 1974. *Medical Care in Australia: An Economic Diagnosis.* Melbourne: Sun Books.

Semmes, Clovis E. 1978. *Users of an Alternative Health System: Becoming a Naprapathic Patient*. Ph.D. Dissertation, Department of Sociology, Northwestern University.

———— 1990. "Non-Medical Illness Behavior: A Model of Patients Who Seek Alternatives to Allopathic Medicine." *JMPT* 13:427–436.

"Senate Leadership Unveils National Health Care Plan: Chiropractic Included." 1991. *ACA/FYI* July:1, 20.

Seyse, Arthur L. 1924. "Chiropractic from the Inside." *New York State Journal of Medicine* 24(12):550–552.

Sharpless, Seth K. 1975. "Susceptibility of Spinal Roots to Compression Block." *NINCDS* pp. 155–161.

Shears, George P. 1939. *The GPC Service Principle*. Pamphlet, 79 pp.

Shekelle, Paul G., and Robert H. Brook. 1991. "A Community-Based Study of the Use of Chiropractic Services." *AJPH* 81:439–442.

Shell, Ellen Ruppel. 1988. "The Getting of Respect: American Chiropractors Are Still Fighting for Recognition from Medical Doctors." *The Atlantic* 261:78–80.

Shryock, Richard H. 1966. *Medicine in American History*. Baltimore: Johns Hopkins University Press.

———— 1967. *Medical Licensing in America, 1650-1965*. Baltimore: Johns Hopkins University Press.

Sigerist, Henry E. 1934. *American Medicine*. New York: Norton.

Silver, B.C. 1979. "Market Research Study #9301, Conducted in Holland, Michigan." Mimeographed. Grand Rapids, Mich.: Western Michigan Research.

Silver, George A. 1980. (Editorial) "Chiropractic: Professional Controversy and Public Policy." *AJPH* 70:348–351.

Simmons, K., et al. 1982. "Trauma to the Vertebral Artery Related to Neck Manipulation." *Medical Journal of Australia* 1:187–188.

Smallie, Paul. 1990a. *Introduction to Ratledge Files and Ratledge Manuscript*. Stockton, Calif.: World Wide Books.

———— 1990b. *Encyclopedia Chiropractica*. Stockton, Calif.: World Wide Books.

———— and Harold W. Evans. 1980. *Chiropractic Encyclopedia*. Stockton, Calif. Published by the authors.

Smith-Cunnien, Susan L. 1990. *Organized Medicine and Chiropractic: The Role of the Deviantization of Chiropractic in the Development of U.S. Medicine 1908 to 1976*. Doctoral Dissertation, University of Minnesota.

Smith, Oakley G. 1932. *Naprapathy Genetics: Being a Study of the Origin and Development of Naprapathy*. Chicago: Published by the author.

Smith, Ralph Lee. 1969. *At Your Own Risk: The Case Against Chiropractic*. New York: Pocket Books.

"Soviet Medical School to Offer Chiropractic Degree." 1991. *DC* 9(17):21.

Spears, Leo L. 1925. *Spears Painless System*. Denver: Published by the author.

Spears Free Clinic and Hospital for Poor Children, Inc., v. The State Board of Health of Colorado et al. 1950. No. 16204. Slip opinion, Colorado Supreme Court, July 1.

"Special Communication: Permanent Injunction Order Against AMA." 1988. *JAMA* 259:81–82.

Speranski, A.D. 1935. *A Basis for the Theory of Medicine*. Translated by C.P. Dutt. New York: International Publishers.

Spitzer, W.O., et al. 1987. "Scientific Approach to the Assessment and Management of Activity-Related Spinal Disorders: A Monograph for Clinicians. Report of the Quebec Task Force on Spinal Disorders." *Spine* 12(7S)(Suppl.):1–24.

Stalvey, Richard M. 1957. "What's New in Chiropractic?" *New York State Journal of Medicine* 57:49–59.

Stanford Research Institute. 1960. *Chiropractic in California*. South Pasadena, Calif.: The Haynes Foundation.

Stano, Miron. 1990. "A Review of the Chiropractic Services Pilot Program Study." *ACAJ* 27(11):65–68.

Starr, Paul. 1982. *The Social Transformation of American Medicine*. New York: Basic Books.

State of New York vs. AMA et al. 1979. Complaint #79C1732 filed July 5 in the United States District Court for the Eastern District of New York.

Steinbach, Leo J. 1941. "The Sacroiliac Mechanism: Some Important New Facts Are Revealed." *Chiropractic Journal* 10:11.

———1957. *Spinal Balance and Spinal Hygiene*. Pittsburgh: Published by the author.

Stephenson, Ralph W. 1927. *Chiropractic Textbook*. Davenport, Ia.: PSC.

Sternberg, David. 1969. *Boys in Plight: A Case Study of Chiropractic Students Confronting a Medically Oriented Society*. Ph.D. Dissertation, Department of Sociology, New York University.

Still, Andrew Taylor. 1897. *Autobiography of Andrew Taylor Still*. Kirksville, Mo.: Published by the author.

———1899. *Philosophy of Osteopathy*. Kirksville, Mo.: Published by the author.

———1910. *Osteopathy: Research and Practice*. Kirksville, Mo.: Published by the author.

Stonequist, Everett V. 1937. *The Marginal Man: A Study in Personality and Culture Conflict*. New York: Scribner.

Stouffer, Samuel, et al. 1950. *Measurement and Prediction*. Princeton, N.J.: Princeton University Press.

Stout, Robert J. 1988. "The Ph.C. Degree: An affirmation of Chiropractic Philosophy." *Ch Hist* 8(1):11–13.

Stowell, Chester C. 1983. "Lincoln College and the 'Big Four': A Chiropractic Protest, 1926-1962." *Ch Hist* 3:74–78.

Suh, Chung-Ha. 1974. "The Fundamentals of Computer-Aided X-Ray Analysis of the Spine." *Journal of Biomechanics* 7:161–169.

———1975. "Biomechanical Aspects of Subluxation." *NINCDS* pp. 103–119.

———1980. "Computer-Aided Spinal Biomechanics." In Scott Haldeman (Ed.). *Modern Developments in the Principles and Practice of Chiropractic*. New York: Appleton-Century-Crofts.

Sullivan, Edward C. 1989. "Stroke Screening Article Spurs Debate." *CJ* 3(10):12.

Sulzer, Jefferson L. 1965. "Chiropractic Healing as Psychotherapy." *Psychotherapy: Research and Practice* 2:38–41.

Supply and Characteristics of Chiropractors. 1986. DHHS, USPHS, Health Resources and Services Administration, Bureau of Health Professions (based on data supplied by the ACA). August.

"Survey on Straight Chiropractic Completed." 1989. *DCE* 32(3):7.

Swanberg, Harold. 1915. *The Intervertebral Foramina in Man*. Chicago: Chicago Scientific Publishing Co.

Sweaney, John A. 1989. "Report on Chiropractic in Australia: Unification of Professional Associations." *DC* 7(23):16–17.

Sweet, Waterman. 1929 (1833). *An Essay on the Science of Bonesetting*. Providence, R.I.: Marshall and Hammond.

Taksel, Leon. 1989. "US Medical School Finances." *JAMA* 263:1020–1028.

Tamulaitis, Christine. 1988. "World Federation of Chiropractic to Represent Global Chiropractic Interests." *ICA Review* 44(6):50–51.

———1989. (Ed.). "A Study of Chiropractic Worldwide." *FACTS Bulletin*. Vol. 3. Washington, D.C. Also in *ICA Review* 45(6):29–52.

Tappan, Frances M. 1988. *Healing Massage Techniques: Holistic, Classic, and Emerging Methods*. Norwalk, Conn.: Appleton and Lange.

Taylor, Hilton H. 1981. "Is a Subluxation a Lesion with a Fixation Causing Joint Dysfunction?" *ACAJ* 15(3):S29–S30.

Terrett, Allen C.J. 1986. "The Genius of D.D. Palmer." *Journal of the Australian Chiropractors' Association* 16(4):150–158.

———1988. "Vascular Accidents from Cervical Spine Manipulation: Report on 107 Cases." *ACAJ* 25(4):63–72.

————and Howard Vernon. 1984. "Manipulation and Pain Tolerance: A Controlled Study of the Effect of Spinal Manipulation on Paraspinal Cutaneous Pain Tolerance Levels." *American Journal of Physical Medicine* 63:217–225.

"That Aching Back." 1980. *Time Magazine* July 14.

Thewlis, M.W. 1923. "Chiropractic Philosophy." *Rhode Island Medical Journal* 6(5):79.

Thomas, M. Carroll. 1988. "What Happens When Chiros Get Hospital Privileges." *Medical Economics* Jan. 4, pp. 58–66.

Thompson, E.A. 1919. *Text on Chiropractic Spinography.* Davenport, Ia.: PSC.

Thompson, Richard E., and William Trickel, Jr. 1989. *Credentialing the Chiropractor: Specific Mechanisms and Clarifications for the Chiropractor Applicant.* Wheaton, Ill.: SENSS Publications.

Thomson, Samuel. 1822. *Narrative of the Life and Medical Discoveries of Samuel Thomson Containing an Account of His System of Practice.* Boston: Published by the author.

Tobis, Jerome S., et al. 1981. "Spinal Manipulation for Low Back Pain." *JAMA* 245:1835–1838.

————and Fred Hoehler. 1986. *Musculoskeletal Manipulation: Evaluation of the Scientific Evidence.* Springfield, Ill.: Charles C Thomas.

Trever, William. 1972. *In the Public Interest.* Los Angeles: Scriptures Unlimited.

Tuchfarber, Alfred J. 1989. "April 1989 Ohio Poll: Ohio State Chiropractic Association." Cincinnati: Institute for Policy Research, University of Cincinnati.

Turner, Chittenden. 1931. *The Rise of Chiropractic.* Los Angeles: Powell Publishing Co.

"Utilization of Selected Medical Practitioners: United States, 1974." 1978. Vital and Health Statistics of the National Center for Health Statistics, No. 24. Public Health Service, U.S. Department of Health, Education, and Welfare.

Vear, Herbert J. 1991. *Chiropractic Standards of Practice and Quality of Care.* Gaithersburg, Md.: Aspen.

Vedder, Harry. 1916. *A Textbook on Chiropractic Physiology*. Davenport, Ia.: Published by the author.

———1919. *A Textbook on Chiropractic Gynecology*. Davenport, Ia.: Published by the author.

———1930. "What Can a Minority Do?" *Universal Chiropractors' Association News* 6(Aug.).

Verner, J. Robinson. 1941. *The Science and Logic of Chiropractic*. Englewood, N.J.: Published by the author.

Vernon, Howard T. 1991. "Chiropractic: A Model of Incorporating the Illness Behavior Model in the Management of Low Back Pain Patients." *JMPT* 14:379–389.

———et al. 1986. "Spinal Manipulation and Beta Endorphin: A Controlled Study of the Effect of a Spinal Manipulation on Plasma Beta-Endorphin Levels in Normal Males." *JMPT* 9:115–123.

Viereck, G.S. 1957. "An Interview with Freud." *Psychoanalysis and the Future*. Special Double Issue of *Psychoanalysis: Journal of Psychoanalytic Psychology* 4(4) and 5(1):1–11.

Villiers, Alan, and Gordon W. Gahan. 1971. "The Voyages and Historic Discoveries of Capt. Jas. Cook." *National Geographic* 140(3):297–349.

"Vision to Action: A History of ICA, the First 60 Years." 1986. *ICA Review* 42(2):33–64.

Von Kuster, Thomas J. 1980. *Chiropractic Health Care: A National Study of Cost of Education, Service Utilization, Number of Practicing Doctors of Chiropractic, and Other Key Policy Issues*. Report to the Health Resources Administration, U.S. Public Health Service. Washington, D.C.: Foundation for the Advancement of Chiropractic Tenets and Science, ICA.

Waddell, G. 1987. "A New Clinical Model for the Treatment of Low Back Pain." *Spine* 12:632–644.

Walden, David M. 1989. *Utah's Health Care Revolution: Pluralism and Professionalism Since World War II*. Masters Thesis in History, Brigham Young University.

Walton, Alfred. 1915. *Chiropractic: The Spine in Its Relation to Disease, Showing Traumatism as an Important Factor: An Explanation of Chiropractic in Contradistinction to Osteopathy and Other Methods of Treating Disease.* Indianapolis: Shields and Hopkins.

Wardwell, Walter I. 1951. *Social Strain and Social Adjustment in the Marginal Role of the Chiropractor.* Ph.D. dissertation in Sociology, Harvard University.

——— 1952. "A Marginal Professional Role: The Chiropractor." *Social Forces* 30:339–348.

——— 1954. "Chiropractic's Struggle for Legal Recognition in Massachusetts." *Journal of the Chiropractic Association of New York* 1:7.

——— 1955. "The Reduction of Strain in a Marginal Social Role." *American Journal of Sociology* 61:16–25.

——— 1961. "Public Regulation of Chiropractic." *Journal of the National Medical Association* 53:166–172.

——— 1963. 1972. 1979. "Limited and Marginal Practitioners." In Howard E. Freeman, Sol Levine, and Leo G. Reeder (Eds.). *Handbook of Medical Sociology.* Englewood Cliffs, N.J.: Prentice-Hall.

——— 1964. "Christian Science Healing." *Journal for the Scientific Study of Religion* 4:175–181.

——— 1968. "Chiropractic Among the Healing Professions." *ACAJ* 5(10):13–19.

——— 1973. "Christian Science and Spiritual Healing." In Richard H. Cox (Ed.). *Religious Systems and Psychotherapy.* Springfield, Ill.: Charles C Thomas.

——— 1975. "Discussion: The Impact of Spinal Manipulative Therapy on the Health Care System." *NINCDS* pp. 53–58.

——— 1976a. "Orthodox and Unorthodox Practitioners: Changing Relationships and the Future Status of Chiropractors." In R. Wallis and P. Morley (Eds.). *Marginal Medicine.* London: Peter Owen.

——— 1976b. Review of J.B. Cowie and J. Roebuck, *An Ethnography of a Chiropractic Clinic: Definitions of a Deviant Situation. American Journal of Sociology* 82:500–502.

———— 1978. "Social Factors in the Survival of Chiropractic: A Comparative View." *Sociological Symposium* 22(Spring):6–7.

———— 1980a. "The Triumph of Chiropractic—And Then What?" *Journal of Sociology and Social Welfare* 7:427–439.

———— 1980b. "The Present and Future Role of the Chiropractor." In Scott Haldeman (Ed.). *Modern Developments in the Principles and Practice of Chiropractic*. New York: Appleton-Century-Crofts.

———— 1982a. "The Cutting Edge of Chiropractic Recognition: Prosecution and Legislation in Massachusetts." *Ch Hist* 2:54–65.

———— 1982b. "Chiropractors: Challengers of Medical Domination." In Julius Roth (Ed.). *Research in the Sociology of Health Care*. Vol. 2. Greenwich, Conn.: JAI Press.

———— 1987. "Before the Palmers: Overview of Chiropractic's Antecedents." *Ch Hist* 7(2):27–33.

———— 1988. "Chiropractors: Evolution to Acceptance." In Norman Gevitz (Ed.). *Other Healers: Unorthodox Medicine in America*. Baltimore: Johns Hopkins University Press.

———— 1989. "The Connecticut Survey of Public Attitudes toward Chiropractic." *JMPT* 12:167–173.

———— 1991. "Chiropractic Literature: An Historical Review of Its Categories." *ACAJ* 28(4):39–42.

Warner, Charles W. 1930. *Quacks*. Jackson, Miss.: Published by the author.

Watkins, Claude O. 1944. *The Basic Principles of Chiropractic Government*. Sidney, Mont.: Published by the author.

Weber, H. 1983. "Lumbar Disc Herniation: A Controlled Prospective Study with Ten Years of Observation." *Spine* 8:131–140.

Weber, Max. 1947. *The Theory of Social and Economic Organization*. Translated by A.M. Henderson and Talcott Parsons. Glencoe, Ill.: Free Press.

Weiant, Clarence W. 1941. "Chiropractic: A Reply." *New York State Chiropractic Journal* 10:4.

———1945. *The Case for Chiropractic in the Literature of Medicine*. New York: New York State Chiropractic Society.

———1947. "Chiropractic Presents Its Case." *Reader's Digest* Feb.

———1981. "Chiropractic Philosophy: The Misnomer That Plagues the Profession." *Archives of the California Chiropractic Association* 5(1):15–22.

———and Sol Goldschmidt. 1958. *Medicine and Chiropractic*. New York: Published by the authors.

Welch, Lorraine. 1955. *The History of Medical Organization and Counter-organization in the United States*. Doctoral Dissertation in Education, New York University.

Westbrooks, Bobby. 1982. "The Troubled Legacy of Harvey Willard: The Black Experience in Chiropractic." *Ch Hist* 2:47–53.

Whitcher, Sheryle J., and Jeffrey D. Fisher. 1979. "Multidimensional Reaction to Interpersonal Touch." *Journal of Personality and Social Psychology* 37:87–96.

White, Arthur H., and Robert Anderson. 1991. *Conservative Care of Low Back Pain*. Baltimore: Williams & Wilkins.

White, Jane See. 1983. "Competition: The Surprising Swing to Non-Physicians." *Medical Economics* 60:May 30, pp. 55–63.

White, Marjorie, and James K. Skipper, Jr. 1971. "The Chiropractic Physician: A Study of Career Contingencies." *Journal of Health and Social Behavior* 12:300–306.

Whitehead, Alfred North. 1917. *The Organization of Thought, Educational and Scientific*. London: Williams and Norgate.

———1925. *Science and the Modern World*. New York: Macmillan.

Whorton, James C. 1982. *Crusaders for Fitness: The History of American Health Reformers*. Princeton, N.J.: Princeton University Press.

———1988. "Patient, Heal Thyself: Popular Health Reform Movements as Unorthodox Medicine." In Norman Gevitz (Ed.). *Other Healers: Unorthodox Medicine in America*. Baltimore: Johns Hopkins University Press.

Wiese, Glenda, and Alana Ferguson. 1988. "How Many Chiropractic Schools? An Analysis of Institutions That Offered the D.C. Degree." *Ch Hist* 8(1):27–36.

Wilbur, Ray Lyman. 1946. *Report on a Community Rehabilitation Service and Center.* New York: The Baruch Commission on Physical Medicine.

Wilcher, C.C. 1989a. "Chiropractically Induced Iatrogenic Disease." *DCE* 31(6):121–122.

———— 1989b. "National Chiropractic Standards." *DC* 7(18):40.

Wild, Patricia B. 1978. "Social Origins and Ideology of Chiropractors: An Empirical Study of the Socialization of the Chiropractic Student." *Sociological Symposium* 22:33–54.

Wiles, Michael. 1990. "Visceral Disorders Related to the Spine." In Meridel I. Gatterman (Ed.). *Chiropractic Management of Spine Related Disorders.* Baltimore: Williams & Wilkins.

"Wilhelm Reich—The Psychoanalyst as Revolutionary." 1971. *Time* Magazine April 18.

Wilk, Chester C.A. 1973. *Chiropractic Speaks Out: A Reply to Medical Propaganda, Bigotry, and Ignorance.* Park Ridge, Ill.: Wilk Publishing Company.

Wilk, C.A. et al. vs. AMA et al. 1976. Complaint #76C3777 filed Oct. 12 in the United States District Court for the Northern District of Illinois, Eastern Division.

———— 1987. Agreement with the American Hospital Association signed June 12, 1987.

Wilk, C.A. et al. vs. Illinois State Medical Society. 1985. Joint Motion to Dismiss filed March 4, 1985, in the United States District Court for the Northern District of Illinois, Eastern Division.

Williams, Sid E. 1981. "Chiropractic Philosophy—The Road Not Yet Taken." *Archives of the California Chiropractic Association* 5(1):27–35.

———— 1990a. "Crossing the River." *Today's Chiropractic* 19(6):8–9, 76–77.

————1990b. "Eulogy for Dr. I.N. Toftness." *Today's Chiropractic* 19(6):110–111.

————1991. *Chiropractic Science and Practice in the United States*. Arlington, Va.: ICA.

Willis, Evan. 1983. *Medical Dominance: The Division of Labor in Australian Health Care*. Sydney: Allen and Unwin.

————1991. "Chiropractic in Australia." *JMPT* 14:59–69.

Willis, Jerry R. 1989. "Robert Contee Bowie: The 1989 Recipient of the Lee-Homewood Chiropractic Heritage Award." *Ch Hist* 9:59–60.

Wolinsky, Howard. 1988. "Injunction in JAMA Called a 'Major Victory' for AMA." *Physicians' Weekly* 5:1.

Wolk, Steve. 1988. *An Analysis of Florida Workers' Compensation Medical Claims for Back-Related Injuries*. Washington, D.C.: FCER.

Yesalis, Charles E. III, et al. 1980. "Does Chiropractic Utilization Substitute for Less Available Medical Services?" *AJPH* 70:415–417.

Yokum, Terry R., and Lindsay J. Rowe. 1987. *Essentials of Skeletal Radiology*. Baltimore: Williams & Wilkins.

Zarbuck, Merwyn V. 1986. "A Profession for 'Bohemian Chiropractic'—Oakley Smith and the Evolution of Naprapathy." *Ch Hist* 6:77–82.

————1988. "Chiropractic Parallax." *IPSCA (Illinois Prairie State Chiropractic Association) Journal of Chiropractic* April, pp. 4–5, 15–16.

————and Mary Beth Hayes. 1990. "Following D.D. Palmer to the West Coast: The Pasadena Connection, 1902." *Ch Hist* 10(2):17–22.

ABBREVIATIONS

AANP   American Association of Naturopathic Physicians

ABCA   American Black Chiropractors Association

ACA   American Chiropractic Association (formerly NCA)

ACAJ   *ACA Journal of Chiropractic* (formerly *JNCA*)

AECC   Anglo-European College of Chiropractic

AHA   American Hospital Association

AJCM   *American Journal of Chiropractic Medicine*

AJPH   *American Journal of Public Health*

AMA   American Medical Association

AOA   American Osteopathic Association

AOHA   American Osteopathic Hospital Association

B.J.   Bartlett Joseph Palmer

CA   Chiropractic Assistant

CCC-KC   Cleveland Chiropractic College, Kansas City, Missouri

CCC-LA   Cleveland Chiropractic College, Los Angeles, California

CCE   Council for Chiropractic Education

Ch Hist	*Chiropractic History: The Archives and Journal of the Association for the History of Chiropractic*
CJ	*The Chiropractic Journal*
CMCC	Canadian Memorial Chiropractic College
DC	Doctor of Chiropractic
DC	*Dynamic Chiropractic*
DCE	*Digest of Chiropractic Economics*
D.D.	Daniel David Palmer
DDT	Doctor of Drugless Therapy
DHEW	U.S. Department of Health, Education, and Welfare
DHHS	U.S. Department of Health and Human Services
DN	Doctor of Naprapathy
DO	Doctor of Osteopathy
DPM	Doctor of Podiatric Medicine
DPT	Doctor of Physical Therapy
FACTS	Foundation for the Advancement of Chiropractic Tenets and Science
FCER	Foundation for Chiropractic Education and Research
FDA	U.S. Food and Drug Administration
FSCO	Federation of Straight Chiropractic Organizations
FTC	Federal Trade Commission
HIO	Hole-in-one (atlas/axis) technique
HMO	Health Maintenance Organization
ICA	International Chiropractors Association

IPA   Independent Practice Association

JAMA   *Journal of the American Medical Association*

JAOA   *Journal of the American Osteopathic Association*

JCAH   Joint Commission on Accreditation of Hospitals

JCR   *Journal of Chiropractic Research* (formerly PCC's *Research Forum;*
              in 1990 it became *Chiropractic: A Journal of Chiropractic
              Research and Clinical Investigation*)

JMPT   *Journal of Manipulative and Physiological Therapeutics*

JNCA   *Journal of the National Chiropractic Association*

LACC   Los Angeles College of Chiropractic, Whittier, California

MAM   Malicious animal magnetism

MUA   Manipulation under anesthesia

MUST   Manipulation under sedation therapy

NAAMM   North American Academy of Manipulative (later Musculoskeletal)
              Medicine

NACM   National Association of Chiropractic Medicine

NCA   National Chiropractic Association

NCC   National College of Chiropractic, Lombard, Illinois

NCM   Neurocalometer

ND   Doctor of Naturopathy

NEJM   *New England Journal of Medicine*

NINCDS   National Institute of Neurological and Communicative Disorders and
              Stroke; publisher of Murray Goldstein (Ed.). *The Research Status
              of Spinal Manipulative Therapy* (A Workshop Held at the National
              Institutes of Health, Feb. 2–4, 1975). Bethesda, Md.: DHEW
              Publ. No. (NIH)76-998

NWCC	Northwestern College of Chiropractic, Bloomington, Minnesota
NYCC	New York Chiropractic College, Seneca Falls, New York (formerly Old Brookfield, Long Island)
OD	Doctor of Optometry
OMT	Osteopathic manipulative therapy
PCC	Palmer College of Chiropractic (became Palmer Chiropractic University), Davenport, Iowa
PCC-W	Palmer College of Chiropractic—West, Sunnyvale, California
PCSC	Pennsylvania College of Straight Chiropractic, Philadelphia
PCU	Palmer Chiropractic University, Davenport, Iowa
PPO	Preferred Provider Organization
PSC	Palmer School of Chiropractic (became Palmer College of Chiropractic), Davenport, Iowa
PT	Physical therapist
SCASA	Straight Chiropractic Academic Standards Association
SCCC	Southern California College of Chiropractic (formerly Pasadena Chiropractic College), Pico Rivera, California
SCSC	Sherman College of Straight Chiropractic, Spartanburg, South Carolina
SMT	Spinal manipulative therapy
TCC	Texas Chiropractic College, Pasadena, Texas
UCA	Universal Chiropractors Association
USPHS	United States Public Health Service, DHHS
VSC	Vertebral subluxation complex
WSCC	Western States Chiropractic College, Portland, Oregon

Index

A

Abbott, Andrew, 41, 52
Abrams, Albert, 19, 87
Accreditation, 7, 11, 101, 102, 141, 170, 244, 261, 280
Acupuncture, acupressure, 38, 122, 132, 257, 258
Activator, 209
Adams, Alan A., 100
ADIO (Chiropractic College), 98, 101, 183
Adjustment, 2, 12, 19, 21, 30, 34, 38, 45, 57, 63, 65, 68, 83, 88, 89, 101, 120, 121, 132, 184, 192, 208, 252, 259, 277, 280
Advertising, 12, 70, 126, 249, 258, 270–273
AFL-CIO, 165, 167
Aitken, Steven T., 258
Alabama, 130
Alameda County, 8, 113
Alcott, William Andrus, 250
Allopaths, 26, 37, 44, 113, 140, 250, 279
Altman, Edward, 133
American Academy of Physical Medicine and Rehabilitation, 168, 169, 172
American Back Society, 194, 202, 244, 261
American Bar Association, 163
American Black Chiropractors Association (ABCA), 148
American Bureau of Chiropractic, 114
American Cancer Society, 40, 244
American Chiropractic Association (ACA), 66, 86, 99, 100, 143, 144, 149, 166, 168, 178, 184, 192, 206, 239, 242, 243, 245, 262–264, 269, 273, 276
American College of Radiology, 167–169, 171, 174
American College of Physicians, 168, 171
American College of Orthopedic Surgeons, 168, 169, 171, 174
American College of Surgeons, 168, 169, 171, 174
American Hospital Association (AHA), 11, 37, 167, 168, 170
American Legion, 229

American Medical Association (AMA), 5, 9, 11, 17, 26–28, 40, 43, 45, 46, 73, 74, 161, 178, 220, 237, 241, 244, 246, 253, 255, 266, 278–286
American Naprapathic Association, 87
American Osteopathic Association (AOA), 3, 36, 37, 72, 73, 106, 107, 112, 135, 168, 169, 172, 176–178
American Osteopathic Hospital Association (AOHA), 37
American School of Chiropractic, 37, 59, 66, 86, 256
American School of Naturopathy, 37, 256
American Public Health Association, 167, 244
American Veterinary Chiropractic Association, 181
Anatomy, 16, 68, 77, 116, 117, 132, 134
Ancillary profession, 43, 44, 263, 275, 278, 282
Anderson, Robert, 19, 21, 22, 194, 205, 261
Andrew Taylor Still College of Osteopathy, 24
Anglo-European Chiropractic College (AECC), 98, 146, 261
Antisepsis, 17, 250
Anti-trust suits, 11, 45, 168–175, 244, 263, 276, 282
Antonio, Peter, 129–130
Aquilina, Anthony D., 37
Aristotle, 19
Arizona, 29, 231
Arkansas, 110
Arrests, 8, 42, 45, 59, 60, 65, 72, 99, 100, 113, 115, 118–126, 285
Art (see Technique)
Assendelft, William J.J., 205
Associations, 99–102, 163
Audiologists, 44, 281
Auerbach, Gary, 264
Australia, 9, 35, 98, 99, 102, 110, 130, 146, 193, 222, 231, 261, 264, 273, 280, 286
Authority, 212, 214